Critical Care Pharmacotherapeutics

Thomas J. Johnson, PharmD, MBA, BCPS, FASHP
Critical Care Pharmacy Specialist
PGY2 Critical Care Pharmacy Residency Program Director
Director of Hospital Pharmacy
Avera McKennan Hospital and University Health Center
Sioux Falls, SD

Adjunct Professor of Pharmacy Practice
South Dakota State University College of Pharmacy
Brookings, SD

D1556893

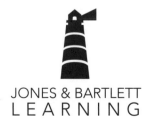

JONES & BARTLETT
LEARNING

World Headquarters
Jones & Bartlett Learning
5 Wall Street
Burlington, MA 01803
978-443-5000
info@jblearning.com
www.jblearning.com

Jones & Bartlett Learning books and products are available through most bookstores and online booksellers. To contact Jones & Bartlett Learning directly, call 800-832-0034, fax 978-443-8000, or visit our website, www.jblearning.com.

Substantial discounts on bulk quantities of Jones & Bartlett Learning publications are available to corporations, professional associations, and other qualified organizations. For details and specific discount information, contact the special sales department at Jones & Bartlett Learning via the above contact information or send an email to specialsales@jblearning.com.

Copyright © 2013 by Jones & Bartlett Learning, LLC, an Ascend Learning Company

All rights reserved. No part of the material protected by this copyright may be reproduced or utilized in any form, electronic or mechanical, including photocopying, recording, or by any information storage and retrieval system, without written permission from the copyright owner.

This publication is designed to provide accurate and authoritative information in regard to the Subject Matter covered. It is sold with the understanding that the publisher is not engaged in rendering legal, accounting, or other professional service. If legal advice or other expert assistance is required, the service of a competent professional person should be sought.

Production Credits
Publisher: David D. Cella
Acquisitions Editor: Katey Birtcher
Managing Editor: Maro Gartside
Editorial Assistant: Teresa Reilly
Editorial Assistant: Kayla Dos Santos
Production Manager: Tracey McCrea
Marketing Manager: Grace Richards
Manufacturing and Inventory Control Supervisor: Amy Bacus
Composition: Cenveo Publisher Services
Cover Design: Scott Moden
Rights and Permissions Manager: Katherine Crighton
Permissions and Photo Research Assistant: Amy Rathburn
Cover Image: © Bork/ShutterStock, Inc.
Printing and Binding: Malloy, Inc.
Cover Printing: Malloy, Inc.

Some images in this book feature models. These models do not necessarily endorse, represent, or participate in the activities represented in the images.

Critical Care Pharmacotherapeutics is an independent publication and has not been authorized, sponsored, or otherwise approved by the owners of the trademarks referenced in this product.

Library of Congress Cataloging-in-Publication Data
Critical care pharmacotherapeutics / [edited by] Thomas J. Johnson.
    p. ; cm.
Includes bibliographical references and index.
ISBN 978-1-4496-0478-3 (pbk.)
I. Johnson, Thomas J.
[DNLM: 1. Critical Care—methods. 2. Drug Therapy. WX 218]
615.5—dc23
                         2011034882

6048
Printed in the United States of America
16 15 14 13 12 10 9 8 7 6 5 4 3 2 1

Contents

Chapter 5   **Analgesia, Sedation, and Delirium Management** **73**
John Kappes

Chapter **13**   **Fundamentals of Antimicrobial Therapy
in the Critically Ill** **271**
Brad Laible

Chapter 16   **Neonatal and Pediatric Intensive Care Basics** **367**
Wendy Jensen-Bender

Preface

There are a lot of critical care textbooks—some are huge textbooks with every possible chapter—and there are smaller texts and dosing handbooks available as well. But in the more than a dozen years I have spent teaching critical care medicine to pharmacy students, I could never find quite the right one. They were either too complex, or included too many invasive procedures, or lacked a focus to pharmacotherapy, or didn't explain things in a way that a novice pharmacy student or resident would be able to understand. All of these issues would tend to either distract or bore pharmacy students and residents. I always found that even if the students started out with great energy tackling the readings and text chapters that I assigned, they usually couldn't keep that energy level up and would lose interest. Hence, this book was born.

The chapters are based off of the elective third professional year pharmacy course that I taught for many years titled, "Critical Care Pharmacotherapeutics." The course, and this book, is intended to lay a foundation for the practice of critical care pharmacy. Over the years, several of my past students have gone on to careers in critical care pharmacy and I am honored to have many of them as chapter authors in this text. The other chapter authors are all colleagues, former residents, nurses, and physicians with whom I have worked over the years to collaboratively teach the topics in critical care medicine and I am indebted to each of them for their time, expertise, and friendship.

This text is not intended to be an all-inclusive, definitive textbook on critical care pharmacy practice. Those books have already been written. Rather, it is intended to be a starting point. It could be a starting point for pharmacy students in a classroom setting or for the fourth year pharmacy student entering his or her first critical care experiential setting. This text should also be a great place to start with a PGY1 pharmacy resident entering a critical care experience. It could also serve as a guide to help PGY2 residents and new critical care practitioners become preceptors and facilitate topic discussions. The chapters are meant to begin the conversation between the student and the teacher or preceptor and help direct the learner toward the guideline statements and primary literature that make up the basis for daily practice and specific patient recommendations.

I hope that you will find this text to be a useful addition in helping teach critical care at an introductory level, and that perhaps this will be the seed that sparks more careers in this challenging and fascinating world of Critical Care Pharmacotherapeutics.

Contributor List

Billie Bartel, PharmD
Assistant Professor of Pharmacy Practice/Clinical Specialist in Critical Care
South Dakota State University College of Pharmacy
Avera McKennan Hospital and University Health Center
Sioux Falls, SD

Bradley Beck, PharmD
Clinical Specialist in Hematology/Oncology
Avera McKennan Hospital and University Health Center
Sioux Falls, SD

Joann Bennett, DO, FACOI
Avera McKennan Hospital and University Health Center
University of South Dakota Sanford School of Medicine
Sioux Falls, SD

James Clem, PharmD
Professor and Head—Department of Pharmacy Practice
South Dakota State University College of Pharmacy
Brookings, SD

Elizabeth Gau, PharmD
Clinical Specialist in Emergency Medicine/Critical Care
Avera McKennan Hospital and University Health Center
Sioux Falls, SD

Wendy Jensen-Bender, PharmD
Professor of Pharmacy Practice/Clinical Specialist in Pediatrics
South Dakota State University College of Pharmacy
Rapid City Regional Hospital
Rapid City, SD

John Kappes, PharmD
Assistant Professor of Pharmacy Practice/Clinical Specialist in Critical Care
South Dakota State University College of Pharmacy
Rapid City Regional Hospital
Rapid City, SD

David Kovaleski, MD, FASN
Avera McKennan Hospital and University Health Center
Sioux Falls, SD

Brad Laible, PharmD, BCPS
Associate Professor of Pharmacy Practice/Clinical Specialist in
   Infectious Disease
South Dakota State University College of Pharmacy
Avera McKennan Hospital and University Health Center
Sioux Falls, SD

Ron Neyens, PharmD, BCPS
Clinical Specialist in Neurocritical Care
Medical University of South Carolina
Charleston, SC

Becky Nichols, RN, MSN, CCNS, ANP-BC
Nurse Practitioner
Surgical Institute of South Dakota
Sioux Falls, SD

Erin Nystrom, PharmD, BCNSP
Clinical Specialist in Nutrition Support/Assistant Professor of Pharmacy
Mayo Clinic
Rochester, MN

Keith M. Olsen, PharmD, FCCM, FCCP
Professor and Chair—Department of Pharmacy Practice
University of Nebraska Medical Center College of Pharmacy
The Nebraska Medical Center
Omaha, NE

Gregory J. Peitz, PharmD, BCPS
Clinical Pharmacist in Critical Care/Adjunct Assistant Professor
The Nebraska Medical Center
University of Nebraska Medical Center College of Pharmacy
Omaha, NE

Garrett Schramm, PharmD, BCPS
Clinical Specialist in Critical Care/Residency Program Director
Mayo Clinic
Rochester, MN

Reviewers

Rebecca L. Attridge, PharmD, MSc, BCPS
University of the Incarnate Word, Feik School of Pharmacy
University of Texas Health Science Center San Antonio, Division of
Pulmonary Diseases and Critical Care
San Antonio, TX

James Bigelow, PhD
Department of Biomedical and Pharmaceutical Science
College of Pharmacy
Idaho State University
Pocatello, ID

Edward Eiland, PharmD, MBA, BCPS AQ Infectious Disease
Huntsville Hospital
Huntsville, AL

Brian L. Erstad, PharmD, FCCM, FCCP, FASHP
Professor, Program Director
University of Arizona College of Pharmacy
Tuscon, AZ

Farivar Jahansouz, PharmD
Critical Care Pharmacist
Health Sciences Associate Clinical Professor
Skaggs School of Pharmacy and Pharmaceutical Sciences
University of California, San Diego
La Jolla, CA

Myrna Y. Munar, PharmD
Associate Professor, Pharmacy Practice
Oregon State University/Oregon Health & Science University College of
Pharmacy
Portland, OR

Catherine M. Oliphant, PharmD
Associate Professor of Pharmacy Practice
College of Pharmacy
Idaho State University
Meridian, ID

Keith M. Olsen, PharmD, FCCM, FCCP
Professor and Chair
University of Nebraska Medical Center
Omaha, NE

Craig B. Whitman, PharmD, BCPS
Assistant Professor of Clinical Pharmacy
Philadelphia College of Pharmacy
University of the Sciences
Philadelphia, PA

About the Author

Thomas J. Johnson, PharmD, MBA, BCPS, FASHP has over 13 years of experience in pharmacy practice in the adult critical care setting, as well as in teaching pharmacy students and residents in the area of critical care medicine. Precepting student and resident experiences and developing didactic courses and lectures in the area of critical care have been the cornerstone of his career. He previously held the appointment of Professor of Pharmacy Practice at South Dakota State University (SDSU), but in 2011 transitioned to the position of Director of Hospital Pharmacy and now serves as an Adjunct Professor for SDSU. He continues to maintain an active critical care practice and serves as the residency program director for the critical care specialty residency, which he founded in 2008 at Avera McKennan Hospital and University Health Center. He is a Fellow of the American Society of Health-System Pharmacists and a Board Certified Pharmacotherapy Specialist.

Chapter 1

The Pharmacist's Role in Critical Care

Thomas Johnson

LEARNING OBJECTIVES

1. Define critical care pharmacy practice.
2. Describe the role pharmacists play in caring for the critically ill.
3. Describe a "typical day" for a critical care pharmacist.
4. Delineate and describe basic approaches to patient care.

INTRODUCTION

There are many terms used to describe the practice of pharmacy and the provision of patient care by a pharmacist. Terms like Medication Therapy Management (MTM), pharmaceutical care, direct patient care, and pharmacist care are all popular. They all have unique definitions, yet in day-to-day practice, they equate to similar activities, which generally include optimizing medication regimens; ensuring medication safety; monitoring for adverse medication events; and educating patients, families, and other clinicians about medication therapies. What exactly, then, is critical care pharmacy practice? Pharmacists that devote their time primarily or exclusively to the care of the sickest patients in a hospital are often referred to as critical care pharmacists; therefore, critical care pharmacy can be defined as a pharmacist working in an intensive care unit (ICU), providing patient care with a focus on ensuring the most effective use of medications through interactions with prescribers, nurses, patients, families, and others.

Critical care as a subspecialty of medicine is a relatively recent creation. Intensive care units began to develop in the early part of the 20th century, but really did not flourish until the 1950s with the advent of the modern mechanical ventilator.[1] At approximately the same time, clinical pharmacy pioneers began developing residency programs and clinical pharmacy services.[2] The development of increasingly complex medical issues, and therefore increasingly complex medication regimens, created a demand for pharmacist direct patient care services within ICUs and other patient care areas of the hospital. This expansion primarily began in the early 1970s and increased exponentially over the next 40 years.[3] Today, most critical care pharmacists complete a PGY1 residency, followed by a PGY2 critical care residency or fellowship, as a basis for entering practice. Many are board certified.

A significant amount of primary literature has been compiled over the past 30 years documenting the impact of the critical care pharmacist on patient care and patient outcomes. One of the most cited publications on the impact of an ICU pharmacist was published in 1999 in the *Journal of the American Medical Association* by Leape and colleagues.[4] In this study, the addition of a pharmacist to ICU patient care rounds led to a 66% reduction in preventable adverse drug events. Several other studies have also shown reductions in preventable adverse drug events, reduction of overall hospital costs, and improved patient outcomes when a critical care pharmacist was added to a patient care team.[5-9] Furthermore, as technology has advanced, so have pharmacist services in this setting. The addition of services such as remote monitoring of ICU patients has been shown to improve adherence to treatment guidelines and other outcomes.[10]

The increased prevalence of critical care pharmacy services over the years has been documented in several reports, surveys, and statements—two of which are described here.[11,12] In 1989, Dasta and colleagues published a survey of critical care pharmacy services and found that most ICU pharmacy services were associated with some type of satellite pharmacy, and the clinical services reported ranged from drug selection and monitoring to drug infusion rate calculations.[11] The most common response across the elements of the survey was "moderately involved." Compare this to data published in 2006, which indicated that 62.2% of survey respondents provided direct pharmacy services to the ICU, but satellite pharmacy services were not specifically mentioned.[12] Additional services that were more commonly provided by the ICU pharmacist in the 2006 survey included administrative functions, educational activities (including precepting students), and scholarly work. While these two surveys did not use the exact same scale, comparing the data side by side does indicate that the scope and function of an ICU pharmacist has advanced dramatically over the past 20 years.

ROLE AND FUNCTION OF AN ICU PHARMACIST

In the year 2000, the Society of Critical Care Medicine and the American College of Clinical Pharmacy published a joint statement that delineates the scope and practice of critical care pharmacists.[3] Services and practice were divided into fundamental, desirable, and optimal functions of a critical care pharmacist. This ambitious work has outlined an approach for the provision of critical care pharmacy services for a decade; Table 1–1 summarizes the recommendations from this statement.

The setup and function of the unit a pharmacist is assigned to cover will certainly impact their day-to-day activities and overall approach. Intensive care units are often divided by the types of patients that are treated. Common examples include Surgical (SICU), Medical (MICU), Neurology (which may include neurosurgical and general neurology), Trauma (which may be combined with surgical), Pediatric (PICU), Neonatology (NICU), Cardiac (CCU), Cardiovascular (CVICU), and Cardiothoracic Surgery (CTICU), just to name a few. More recently, remote electronic monitoring and provision of patient care has become another way for pharmacists and other healthcare professionals to interact with patients and bedside caregivers. In some hospitals, a mixed medical/surgical ICU model may be employed where all types of critically ill patients are cared for in one unit. Furthermore, particular units will have different types of physician services. A closed ICU is one in which only certain physicians (often those board-certified in critical care) have admitting privileges. Other units are open ICUs in which any physician with hospital admitting privileges and appropriate credentials can admit and care for patients. A third common model is a semi-closed unit, where any physician can admit patients, but some type of consultation of a critical care specialist physician is often mandatory. Each of the different types of units and physicians will affect the role and function of the pharmacist.

In each type of ICU, the pharmacist will need to understand the differences in patient management that exist between surgeons and medical physicians, and again among the different types of subspecialists. Differences in approach to anticoagulant or procoagulant use, fluid resuscitation,

Table 1–1 Critical Care Pharmacy Services[3]

Fundamental	Desirable	Optimal
• Pharmacist dedicated to ICU	• Participate in ICU rounds	• Assist physicians in patient discussions and decisions
• Prospective medication evaluation	• Review of previous medication therapy	• Provide formal accredited education
• Parenteral nutrition evaluation and monitoring	• Formal parenteral nutrition consultation service	• Teach Advanced Cardiac Life Support (ACLS)
• Adverse Drug Event (ADE) monitoring, avoidance, and reporting	• 24/7 response to resuscitation events	• Develop residencies or fellowships in critical care pharmacy
• Medical record documentation	• Didactic lectures in critical care pharmacy therapeutics	• Develop pharmacist and technician training programs
• Pharmacokinetic services	• Offer experiential rotations for students and residents	• Educate the public about the pharmacist's role in the ICU
• Provide drug information	• Coordinate development of drug therapy protocols	• Investigate impact of drug protocols used in ICU
• Drug therapy education	• Document clinical services that record clinical and financial impact	• Prospectively applies pharmacoeconomic principle to drug evaluation
• Ensure accreditation compliance	• Participate in design and conduct of research	• Secure funding for research
• Participate in quality assurance	• Contribute to the pharmacy and medical literature	• Report research findings at local and national meetings
	• Member of multidisciplinary committees	• Publish research findings in peer-reviewed journals

vasopressors, blood product usage, and sedation and analgesia are important to understand. Mixed medical/surgical units can be particularly challenging in trying to manage the different approaches to care and yet provide consistent pharmaceutical care that optimizes patient outcomes, no matter their underlying disease states.

Day in the Life of an ICU Pharmacist

It is often said that there is no such thing as a typical day for an ICU pharmacist, as the ICU setting and specific assigned responsibilities will affect both the day-to-day functions of the pharmacist as well as specific responsibilities and the overall function of the pharmacy department in that institution. However, a day in the life of an ICU pharmacist can be generally outlined as follows: The pharmacist begins their day reviewing the patient list and identifying new admissions to the unit and their initial diagnosis. Laboratory values and medication lists for the entire unit are often reviewed at this time. With the rapid advances in decision support software and mobile computing platforms, some or all of these functions may be automated. The pharmacist then prioritizes which patients need immediate attention based upon any requests for consultation or identification of potential problems with initial medication review, and these patients are prioritized and reviewed in more detail. If issues are identified that require immediate attention, the responsible physician would be contacted to address the issue. Other concerns that may not require immediate attention are noted so that recommendations can be made during rounds or via other means of communication. When formal rounds are conducted in the unit, the pharmacist attends rounds, addresses recommendations with the prescribing physician, and answers any medication related questions that may occur. During preparation time, within rounds, and during the remainder of the day, the pharmacist is often asked to clarify multiple medication issues, including intravenous compatibility; review home medication lists and medications for discharge from the ICU; provide formal consultation according to hospital policy for pharmacokinetics, nutrition, or other medication use; and answer questions for providers, nurses, and patients and their families. Many pharmacists also provide medication order entry or order verification services. All of these activities require documentation either directly in the medical record and/or in another database that helps with communication or to track productivity.

Depending on the pharmacist's defined responsibilities, time not spent on direct patient care could be spent attending committee meetings, developing and reviewing medication use protocols, providing educational sessions, conducting medication research, or precepting students and residents. As described by the American College of Clinical Pharmacy and Society of Critical Care Medicine recommendations and summarized in Table 1–1, there is not a shortage of goals to accomplish in critical care pharmacy.

APPROACHES TO PHARMACEUTICAL CARE

There are probably as many approaches to the care of individual patients as there are ICU pharmacists. Each clinician needs to adapt their methods and approach to their own personality, the type of unit, the common patients, and the other healthcare workers on the team. However, there are standardized approaches that at least provide a base for an individual approach to patient care.

One of the most common approaches is a head-to-toe assessment to review the patient's problem list and their medications. Working through the large number of disease states, medical problems, medications, and data for an ICU patient by reviewing and evaluating systems in this organized manner can help keep the pharmacy student or resident on track and focused to the primary patient care issues of the day. It also helps ensure that all issues are addressed appropriately. Further, a head-to-toe systems review is the common approach for the review of systems with history and physical examinations or clinical consultations.

FASTHUG-MAIDENS

There are so many elements to remember within the ICU that it is very easy to miss small details or to just plain forget to check on certain items. Mnemonics can be a very helpful addition to standard approaches such as the head-to-toe approach in a fast-paced and data-overloaded area like the ICU. While many mnemonics and checklists exist, one of the easiest is FASTHUG, and the derivation FASTHUG-MAIDENS.[13,14] The FASTHUG mnemonic ensures that the daily elements of **F**eeding, **A**nalgesia, **S**edation, **T**hromboembolic prophylaxis, **H**ypo/**H**yperactive delirium, **U**lcer prophylaxis, and **G**lucose control are addressed appropriately.[13] The MAIDENS term is related to medications and may particularly apply to pharmacists; the elements of **M**edication reconciliation, **A**nti-infectives, **I**ndication for medications, **D**ose, **E**lectrolytes and lab values, **N**o duplication/interactions/adverse events, and **S**top dates are all addressed within the MAIDENS mnemonic.[14] This can be a helpful checklist to be used independently of or as a supplement to a head-to-toe or other systematic approach to patient care. Most elements of FASTHUG-MAIDENS are discussed in detail throughout the text because they represent core practices for the ICU pharmacist, even if the mnemonic isn't used, but it also provides an opportunity to briefly present each element here.

Nutrition is a primary element of supportive, and sometimes therapeutic, intervention in critically ill patients. The initiation of early enteral nutrition and the use of adequate amounts of protein have been demonstrated to improve patient outcomes, and pharmacists can ensure that patients are receiving appropriate nutrition therapy by working with other members of the team, including nurses, dieticians, and physicians. As nutrition can be interrupted frequently in ICU patients, it is very important to evaluate this element on a daily basis. Nutrition therapy is discussed in detail in Chapter 12 of this text.

Analgesia and sedation are very important elements of patient care, as improved patient comfort has been shown to improve healing and overall patient progress, and are discussed in detail in Chapter 5. Appropriate analgesia and sedation practices have also been shown to reduce the incidence of delirium development. This becomes an even more important point as the development and duration of delirium has been shown to be independently associated with increased mortality.

Ensuring appropriate venous thromboembolic (VTE) prophylaxis is perhaps one of the most important interventions that the pharmacy team can make in critically ill patients. Risk of thromboembolism is increased in the critically ill, yet there are often significant risks for bleeding present as well. The benefit-to-risk evaluation for methods of VTE prophylaxis should occur at least daily to ensure that patients are receiving optimal prophylaxis regimens to minimize the complications associated with clotting and bleeding. As reimbursement increasingly depends upon meeting quality core measures like VTE prophylaxis, the pharmacist can play a key role in improving patient outcomes, as well as improving reimbursement rates for the hospital, by ensuring that appropriate prophylaxis is in place or contraindications are documented in the medical record. Specific approaches to VTE prophylaxis are addressed in Chapter 14.

Gastrointestinal (GI) stress-related bleeding is a common concern in the critically ill patient population, and several guidelines have been published regarding the indications and roles for acid suppression therapy.[15-18] While not a complete list, general indications for acid suppression include mechanical ventilation (particularly when a patient is ventilated for more than 48 hours), coagulopathy, past history of GI bleeding or disease, or need for medications known for adverse GI effects (such as corticosteroids). Common regimens include the histamine-2 (H-2) receptor antagonists, proton pump inhibitors, and occasionally sucralfate or antacids. Daily assessment should be performed for both the need to initiate and, once prescribed, the need to continue or discontinue acid suppression medications to avoid unnecessary use.

Glucose control has been shown to markedly reduce morbidity and mortality in the critically ill.[19,20] Events such as improved wound healing, decreased infections, and reduced mortality have all been reported. While controversy remains on the exact target for glucose control, current serum glucose targets for hospitalized patients are generally less than 180 to 200 mg/dL for all patients, depending upon the guidelines referenced.[19,20] Specific subsets of critically ill patients may have more aggressive targets. The overall management of hospitalized patients with hyperglycemia can be very challenging. Changes in diet, use of dextrose-containing intravenous (IV) solutions, previous medical history, medication use that can cause alterations in blood glucose, and even changes in blood flow and oxygen delivery can all lead to difficulties in managing glucose levels in the critically ill. The use of continuous IV insulin infusion to adequately manage glucose levels is common in the ICU, and many units utilize computer-based protocols for the titration of insulin dose. The pharmacist can actively contribute to improved patient management by assisting in the transition from one form of insulin to another and frequently assessing dose and route of delivery of insulin products. Chapter 12 includes a brief discussion on glucose control as it relates to nutrition therapy, and multiple guidelines and protocols have been published that are beyond the scope of this text to review.[21-24] Daily assessment (at a minimum) of blood glucose control is needed in the critically ill and pharmacists should play an active role ensuring that treatment targets are met.

Medication reconciliation is a difficult, yet necessary, part of the care of the critically ill. Many patients present to the ICU with minimal ability to communicate or remember the medications they take at home; even if they are able to convey their medication list, regimens can be complex and difficult for patients to fully understand. Furthermore, families and friends of the patients are often under stress because of an unplanned or urgent admission to the ICU, and so the pharmacist is uniquely positioned to help clarify and record the medications patients take prior to their ICU admission. Pharmacists can also help ensure that preadmission medications are resumed at the appropriate time, or identify potential adverse events or inappropriate therapy and correct those issues prior to ICU discharge. Medication reconciliation also needs to occur prior to the patient transferring out of the ICU and this process often includes stopping continuous IV infusions, removing sedatives or analgesics from the medication list, adjusting antimicrobial therapy, or stopping GI bleeding prophylaxis measures.

Many critical care patients are prescribed anti-infectives, and infectious diseases are causes both for ICU admission and common secondary complications. Daily review of the need for anti-infective medications is necessary to ensure that adequate coverage is provided while overuse is avoided. Chapter 13 provides a review of the approach to anti-infective selection and monitoring in the critically ill.

As discussed earlier, all critically ill patients are not the same, and individualized dosing regimens are necessary to ensure optimal therapy. While a comprehensive review of all possible scenarios that require dose adjustments is beyond the scope of this textbook, it is very important for the critical care pharmacist to evaluate dosing regimens on a daily basis and individualize for factors such as renal and hepatic function, indication for the medication, and intended outcome.

Electrolytes and fluid management are also a significant part of critical care practice. Essentially every ICU patient has intravenous fluid replacement in some form, and electrolytes are often altered for a variety of reasons. Chapters 7 and 12 provide more detail regarding electrolytes and fluid management.

Finally, all medications should be evaluated on a daily basis for indication, adverse events, therapeutic goals, and need for continuation. This is perhaps the pharmacist's most important role on the ICU team, as these details are often missed when a key focus to the details of medication therapy is not applied.

Critically ill patients tend to have many disease states, confounding factors, and data points as part of their medical record. The FASTHUG-MAIDENS approach covers the main elements of daily care for critically ill patients. The use of this or another, similar checklist protocol can help organize the pharmacist's approach to daily monitoring and ensure that key elements of patient care are not missed in the relatively fast-paced and often confusing environment of the ICU.

SUMMARY

Critical care pharmacists may use a variety of tools to organize their day and keep track of patient information. Some may use paper monitoring forms, others may use electronic information systems with dashboard displays that help sort and organize information for easier evaluation, and some will use a combination of paper and electronic monitoring tools. Mobile computing solutions are becoming an increasingly important part of patient care. As technology rapidly becomes the primary means of documentation, software programs will allow for greater efficiencies with the monitoring process and allow the ICU pharmacist to more rapidly identify opportunities to positively affect patient medication use and ultimately improve patient outcomes.

It is very important for each critical care pharmacist to develop their own strategies according to their setting and ICU structure to effectively monitor and treat patients and complete all other necessary tasks. Pharmacy students and residents will find that there are many successful approaches and each one is developed to efficiently manage the setting and the assigned workload. It is very important for students and residents to observe the different settings and practice types they encounter and learn to identify and adopt the approaches that will likely work best for them as they proceed in their careers.

KEY POINTS

- Critical care pharmacy is a diverse and rapidly changing area of practice.
- Pharmacists that practice in the critical care area have a significant impact on patient care and should work to design and improve medication use systems as well as educate a variety of people on the best use of medications in the critically ill.
- The exact day-to-day duties of a critical care pharmacist will vary depending upon the type of ICU they are assigned, as well as the defined scope of practice.
- Critical care pharmacists must develop systems and approaches to their job that best fit their environment.

SELECTED SUGGESTED READINGS

- Erstad BL. A primer on critical care pharmacy services. *Ann Pharmacother.* 2008;42:1871–1881.
- Rudis MI, Brandl KM. Position paper on critical care pharmacy services. Society of Critical Care Medicine and American College of Clinical Pharmacy Task Force on Critical Care Pharmacy Services. *Crit Care Med.* 2000;28:3746–3750.
- Moghissi ES, Korytkowski MT, DiNardo M, et al. American Association of Clinical Endocrinologists and American Diabetes Association consensus statement on inpatient glycemic control. *Endocr Pract.* 2009;15:1–17.
- Dager W, Bolesta S, Brophy G, et al. An Opinion Paper Outlining Recommendations for Training, Credentialing, and Documenting and Justifying Critical Care Pharmacy Services. *Pharmacotherapy.* 2011;31(8):829.

REFERENCES

1. History of Critical Care. Society of Critical Care Medicine. (Accessed July 20, 2011, at http://www.sccm.org/AboutSCCM/History_of_Critical_Care/Pages/default.aspx)

2. Erstad BL. A primer on critical care pharmacy services. *Ann Pharmacother.* 2008;42:1871–1881.
3. Rudis MI, Brandl KM. Position paper on critical care pharmacy services. Society of Critical Care Medicine and American College of Clinical Pharmacy Task Force on Critical Care Pharmacy Services. *Crit Care Med.* 2000;28:3746–3750.
4. Leape LL, Cullen DJ, Clapp MD, et al. Pharmacist participation on physician rounds and adverse drug events in the intensive care unit. *JAMA.* 1999;282:267–270.
5. Montazeri M, Cook DJ. Impact of a clinical pharmacist in a multidisciplinary intensive care unit. *Crit Care Med.* 1994;22:1044–1048.
6. Kane SL, Weber RJ, Dasta JF. The impact of critical care pharmacists on enhancing patient outcomes. *Intensive Care Med.* 2003;29:691–698.
7. MacLaren R, Bond CA, Martin SJ, Fike D. Clinical and economic outcomes of involving pharmacists in the direct care of critically ill patients with infections. *Crit Care Med.* 2008;36:3184–3189.
8. MacLaren R, Bond CA. Effects of pharmacist participation in intensive care units on clinical and economic outcomes of critically ill patients with thromboembolic or infarction-related events. *Pharmacotherapy.* 2009;29:761–768.
9. Kopp BJ, Mrsan M, Erstad BL, Duby JJ. Cost implications of and potential adverse events prevented by interventions of a critical care pharmacist. *Am J Health-Syst Pharm.* 2007;64:2483–2487.
10. Forni A, Skehan N, Hartman CA, et al. Evaluation of the impact of a tele-ICU pharmacist on the management of sedation in critically ill mechanically ventilated patients. *Ann Pharmacother.* 2010;44:432–438.
11. Dasta JF, Segal R, Cunningham A. National survey of critical-care pharmaceutical services. *Am J Hosp Pharm.* 1989;46:2308–2312.
12. Maclaren R, Devlin JW, Martin SJ, Dasta JF, Rudis MI, Bond CA. Critical care pharmacy services in United States hospitals. *Ann Pharmacother.* 2006;40:612–618.
13. Vincent JL. Give your patient a fast hug (at least) once a day. *Crit Care Med.* 2005;33:1225–1229.
14. Mabasa VH MD, Weatherby EM, Chan A. A Practical Method of Providing Pharmaceutical Care in the Intensive Care Unit: FASTHUG-MAIDENS. *CJHP.* 2010;63:1.
15. American Society of Health-System Pharmacists. ASHP therapeutic guidelines on stress ulcer prophylaxis. *Am J Health-Syst Pharm.* 1999; 56:347–379.
16. Welage LS. Overview of pharmacologic agents for acid suppression in critically ill patients. *Am J Health-Syst Pharm.* 2005;62(Suppl 2):S4–S10.
17. Martindale RG. Contemporary strategies for the prevention of stress-related mucosal bleeding. *Am J Health-Syst Pharm.* 2005;62(Suppl 2):S11–S17.
18. Ojiako K, Shingala H, Schorr C, Gerber DG. Famotidine versus pantoprazole for preventing bleeding in the upper gastrointestinal tract of critically ill patients receiving mechanical ventilation. *AM J Crit Care.* 2008;17:142–147.
19. Moghissi ES, Korytkowski MT, DiNardo M, et al. American Association of Clinical Endocrinologists and American Diabetes Association consensus statement on inpatient glycemic control. *Endocr Pract.* 2009;15:1–17.

20. Qaseem A, Humphrey LL, Chou R, Snow V, Shekelle P. Use of intensive insulin therapy for the management of glycemic control in hospitalized patients: A clinical practice guideline from the American College of Physicians. *Ann Int Med.* 2011;154:260–267.

21. Krinsley JS. Effect of an intensive glucose management protocol on the mortality of critically ill adult patients. *Mayo Clin Proc.* 2004;79(8):992–1000.

22. Goldberg PA, Bozzo JE, Thomas PG, et al. Glucometrics: Assessing the quality of inpatient glucose management. *Diabetes Technology & Therapeutics.* 2006;8(5):560–569.

23. Goldberg PA, Siegel MD, Sherwin RS, et al. Implementation of a safe and effective insulin infusion protocol in a medical intensive care unit. *Diabetes Care.* 2004;27:461–467.

24. Smith AB, Udekwu PO, Biswas S, et al. Implementation of a nurse-driven intensive insulin infusion protocol in a surgical intensive care unit. *Am J Health-Syst Pharm.* 2007; 64:1529–1540.

Chapter 2

Acute Illness Scoring Systems

Thomas Johnson

1. Describe the need for objective measures of severity of illness.
2. Describe the APACHE scoring system, including components and function.
3. Describe the usefulness of various illness scoring systems.
4. Determine the optimal use of scoring systems as applied to medication management.

INTRODUCTION

All patients admitted to the ICU are not the same. This seems obvious, and it probably should, but in reality, terms such as critically ill or seriously ill may produce significantly different pictures in someone's mind, depending on the interpretation and perspective of the reader. There is also a perception that a patient admitted to an intensive care unit must be equally as sick as the patient in the next room or in any ICU, for that matter. The perception may be that if the patient is admitted to a specific ward or unit that is dedicated to caring for the "critically ill," then they must be very ill. However, patients are admitted to ICUs for all kinds of primary diagnoses and they come with their own set of underlying conditions. Clearly, a patient population cannot be defined by the floor or unit to which they are admitted. Acuity of illness must be defined by some type of objective measure, and objective measurement of the level of acuity of illness is perhaps most important in the areas of research involving hospitalized patients, prediction of mortality and morbidity, and quality assurance data, especially when that data is comparing unit to unit or hospital to hospital. Therefore, scoring systems have been developed to provide objectivity to the process.

An accurate description of acuity of illness is particularly important in research trials. Without these definitions, there can be little applicability to practice because clinicians would not be able to accurately determine if the patients they commonly treat are similar to the patients included in research trials. Further, researchers and clinicians would not be certain that the comparison groups are equal or that the severity of disease did not affect the overall outcome of the study. Therefore, an understanding of the common scoring systems used in the ICU is very important for any clinician that needs to interpret and utilize literature related to the critically ill or for analysis of quality assurance/quality improvement initiatives.

From a patient and family perspective, receiving information about the probability of survival or of a positive or negative outcome is extremely important. Again, admission to a specific unit does not label a patient as survivable or not. Without objective scoring criteria, clinicians are left to their best guess on whether they think that a patient will survive or not, or if there is a significant risk of lasting sequelae. Clear information based upon objective measures can be very helpful to many families and patients faced with very difficult decisions about continuance or cessation of care. Scoring systems cannot make these decisions, and they should not be used to determine the ultimate disposition of the patient, but they are part of the overall decision process and can be helpful to ensure a fully informed decision regarding care.

Hospitals also find the information determined by scoring systems to be very helpful. Hospitals can use scoring system data to compare their patient outcomes to the outcomes of peer institutions, or to regional and national benchmarks for care. Because an institution has little to no control over the acuity of the patients admitted to their ICU, it is important to accurately understand how their patient population compares to other units within the same or outside institutions, as well as with national benchmarks. This is becoming increasingly important as the public reporting of patient outcomes becomes more and more commonplace.

As a very simple example, let's look at the reporting of two institutions for ICU mortality. Institution A reports an actual mortality rate of 45% in their ICU, and Institution B reports an actual mortality rate of 20%. Without the benefit of some sort of acuity score, the logical conclusion would be that

Institution B provides superior outcomes for their patients. However, if an acuity scoring system is utilized, and it is determined that the predicted mortality rate for Institution A should be 58%, and the predicted mortality rate for Institution B should be 14%, then it would be concluded that Institution A is actually delivering better outcomes than Institution B even though it would not appear that way on first look.

The scoring systems described in this chapter should not be confused with monitoring tools that are used in day-to-day practice for managing patients. Examples of these monitoring tools include sedation scales, pain scales, nerve stimulators, ventilator weaning assessment tools, and other monitoring devices. Most of these scales and devices provide a very specific outcome or endpoint, while the scoring systems primarily provide for population descriptions.

SCORING SYSTEMS

Acute Physiology and Chronic Health Evaluation

The Acute Physiology and Chronic Health Evaluation (APACHE®–Cerner Corporation) scoring system is perhaps the most commonly used scoring system to assess severity of illness in critically ill patients.[1] The APACHE system was first developed during the late 1970s–early 1980s and is currently in the fourth revision of the system, although the APACHE II score remains in common use within practice.[2-4]

The current version of the APACHE (APACHE IV) scoring system provides the most accurate information regarding predicted mortality of a patient population.[1] However, there are many data points, and calculating the score "by hand" is very cumbersome and requires specific training and significant practice. By comparison, the APACHE II score is relatively easy to calculate for individual patients or by investigators that do not have access to the APACHE IV data system. The 1985 publication of the APACHE II system included a worksheet to calculate the score and is illustrated in Figure 2–1.[3] As with any scoring system, there is some intra- and inter-rater variation in calculating the score, which can limit the usefulness of the score if strict attention to methodology is lacking.[5]

To minimize variability in calculating the APACHE II score, clinicians should be trained on how to accurately calculate and use the score. The APACHE II score consists of three domains: the Acute Physiology Score (APS), the Age score, and the Chronic Health Score (CHS). The APS component is determined by identifying the worst values (high or low) recorded within the previous 24 hours and scoring them according to the worksheet. Values not available result in a score of zero for that element. One of the most difficult

THE APACHE II SEVERITY OF DISEASE CLASSIFICATION SYSTEM

PHYSIOLOGIC VARIABLE	HIGH ABNORMAL RANGE				0	LOW ABNORMAL RANGE			
	+4	+3	+2	+1	0	+1	+2	+3	+4
TEMPERATURE – rectal (°C)	$\geq 41°$	39°-40.9°		38.5°-38.9°	36°-38.4°	34°-35.9°	32°-33.9°	30°-31.9°	$\leq 29.8°$
MEAN ARTERIAL PRESSURE – mmHg	≥ 160	130-159	110-129		70-109		50-69		≤ 49
HEART RATE (ventricular response)	≥ 180	140-179	110-139		70-109		55-69	40-54	≤ 39
RESPIRATORY RATE – (non-ventilated or ventilated)	≥ 50	35-49		25-34	12-24	10-11	6-9		≤ 5
OXYGENATION: A-aDO$_2$ or PaO$_3$ (mmHg) a. FiO$_2 \geq 0.5$ record A-aDO$_2$	≥ 500	350-499	200-349		<200				
b. FiO$_2$ < 0.5 record only PaO$_2$					PO$_2$ >70	PO$_2$ 61-70		PO$_2$ 55-60	PO$_2$ < 55
ARTERIAL pH	≥ 7.7	7.6-7.69		7.5-7.59	7.33-7.49		7.25-7.32	7.15-7.24	<7.15
SERUM SODIUM (mMol/L)	≥ 180	160-179	155-159	150-154	130-149		120-129	111-119	≤ 110
SERUM POTASSIUM (mMol/L)	≥ 7	6-6.9		5.5-5.9	3.5-5.4	3-3.4	2.5-2.9		<2.5
SERUM CREATININE (mg/100 ml) (Double point score for acute renal failure)	≥ 3.5	2-3.4	1.5-1.9		0.6-1.4		< 0.6		
HEMATOCRIT (%)	≥ 60		50-50.9	46-49.9	30-45.9		20-29.9		<20
WHITE BLOOD COUNT (total/mm^3) (in 1,000s)	≥ 40		20-39.9	15-19.9	3-14.9		1-2.9		<1
GLASGOW COMA SCORE (GCS): Score = 15 minus actual GCS									
Serum HCO$_3$ (venous-mMol/L) [Not preferred, use if no ABGs]	≥ 52	41-51.9		32-40.9	22-31.9		18-21.9	15-17.9	<15

A Total ACUTE PHYSIOLOGY SCORE (APS): Sum of the 12 individual variable points

B AGE POINTS: Assign points to age as follows:

AGE(yrs)	Points
≤ 44	0
45-54	2
55-64	3
65-74	5
≥75	6

C CHRONIC HEALTH POINTS
If the patient has a history of severe organ system insufficiency or is immuno-compromised assign points as follows:
a. for nonoperative or emergency postoperative patients — 5 points
or
b. for elective postoperative patients — 2 points

DEFINITIONS
Organ insufficiency or immuno-compromised state must have been evident prior to this hospital admission and conform to the following criteria:

LIVER: Biopsy proven cirrhosis and documented portal hypertension; episodes of past upper GI bleeding attributed to portal hypertension; or prior episodes of hepatic failure/encephalopathy/coma.

CARDIOVASCULAR: New York Heart Association Class IV.

RESPIRATORY: Chronic restrictive, obstructive, or vascular disease resulting in severe exercise restriction, i.e., unable to climb stairs or perform household duties; or documented chronic hypoxia, hypercapnia, secondary polycythemia, severe pulmonary hypertension, (>40mmHg), or respirator dependency.

RENAL: Receiving chronic dialysis.

IMMUNO-COMPROMISED: The patient has received therapy that suppresses resistance to infection, e.g., immuno-suppression, chemotherapy, radiation, long term or recent high dose steroids, or has a disease that is sufficiently advanced to suppress resistance to infection, e.g., leukemia, lymphoma, AIDS.

APACHE II SCORE

Sum of A + B + C :

A APS points _____
B Age points _____
C Chronic Health points _____

Total APACHE II _____

Figure 2-1 APACHE II Scoring Worksheet

Source: Reproduced from Knaus WA, et al. *Crit Care Med.* 1985;13:818–829 with permission.

data elements to determine is the Glasgow Coma Score (GCS) in patients that are mechanically ventilated and sedated. The GCS is a scale that measures basic neurologic function based on verbal response, response to pain, and eye opening response, with total scores ranging from 3 to 15. To avoid false elevation of the APS, the pre-sedation GCS level should be recorded whenever possible, as medications can certainly have an effect on the level of response of the patient. The CHS is clearly defined when using the worksheet, but may not be very well defined on homemade calculators or shortened versions of the scoring tool. It is important to accurately identify the CHS and classify correctly. It should be noted that multiple chronic conditions are not additive for this score, as the patient can only receive a maximum of five points within the CHS. An Internet search of "APACHE II Calculator" will result in several websites that offer online tools to calculate the score, with good explanations of how to proceed. Further, online calculators will offer a calculated mortality rate, but the rates determined via the APACHE II system are not as accurate as the data that would be obtained with the APACHE IV.

Simplified Acute Physiology Score

The Simplified Acute Physiology Score (SAPS) was first developed in 1984[6] and revised in 1993 to the SAPS II.[7] The SAPS II score utilizes 15 variables (like APACHE, these should be the worst values within the previous 24 hours) to provide an estimated mortality rate. The accuracy of the mortality rate of the SAPS II score is questionable at this point, since the data used to determine the mortality rates is now almost 20 years old. However, SAPS II remains a relatively simple score to calculate and allows clinicians to compare severity of illness within two groups of patients for purposes of research or quality improvement.

Sequential Organ Failure Assessment Score

The Sequential Organ Failure Assessment (SOFA) score is a score based upon six organ systems, each of which receives a score (0 to 4) with the maximum total score being 24.[8,9] This score was originally referred to as the Sepsis-related Organ Failure Assessment, but as applications to other disease states became common, the term Sequential replaced Sepsis-related. The SOFA score is intended to be tracked on a daily basis within the ICU and the change of score from day to day can be used as an objective measure to track the improvement or worsening of an individual patient. Mortality rates have been correlated with both the peak SOFA score as well as the change in score from ICU admission.[9] This score is also useful in research trials where tracking progress of the patient day-to-day during their ICU stay is important to the study outcomes.

Multiple Organ Dysfunction Score

The Multiple Organ Dysfunction Score (MODS) is similar to the SOFA score. Each organ system is scored on a 0–4 scale with a maximum total score of 24.[10] The main difference between the MODS and SOFA scores is how the cardiovascular system is scored. The MODS approach uses a computation involving the heart rate and vascular pressures, while the SOFA score uses a somewhat simpler approach of recording blood pressure and if vasopressor support is necessary. The authors of the original 1995 publication describing the MODS are quite clear in describing this score as an outcomes measurement as opposed to a predictive instrument. However, a predictive component is available, with associated mortality rates based upon the score and the number of ICU days for the patient. The MODS and SOFA scores have been compared in clinical practice and found to be similar in predicting and measuring outcomes.[11]

Therapeutic Intervention Scoring System

The Therapeutic Intervention Scoring System (TISS) is an example of a scoring system that can be used to help determine staffing needs (particularly for nursing) by way of measuring specific nursing activities.[12] The TISS score, and especially the abbreviated version (TISS-28), has also been used to measure acuity, admission rates, and serve as a measure to describe comparability between two arms of a study population.

Injury Severity Score

The Injury Severity Score (ISS) is the primary score used to describe the initial injury in trauma patients, and has been in use for over 30 years.[13] Trauma programs use this number when submitting patients to the national trauma registry. Use of the ISS allows programs to compare outcomes data at the institution level to nationwide outcomes data. Online calculators are readily available, but it should be noted that individual patients should not be treated based upon the calculation of an ISS.[14]

Risk, Injury, Failure, Loss, End-stage Renal Disease Score

The Risk, Injury, Failure, Loss, End-stage renal disease (RIFLE) score is a system used to stratify acute kidney injury.[15] This is one example of a scoring system that can be used to describe either a patient population or individual patients. In describing a patient population for a research study, an investigator may use the RIFLE system to describe how many patients met each of the various criteria. However, the bedside clinician may use the RIFLE score to determine the degree of organ dysfunction for an individual patient. It is important to understand how a specific scoring tool is used in a particular context to understand the implications of the data that are presented.

The RIFLE score is defined by a specific set of criteria listed in Table 2–1. Note that serum creatinine changes and/or urine output are used to describe the risk, injury, and failure portions of the scale. This allows for a more timely identification of kidney dysfunction compared to kidney injury definitions that rely solely on laboratory values. It should also be noted that changes in glomerular filtration rate (GFR) are included in the RIFLE criteria, although they have been left off of Table 2–1 for simplicity because rapid and consistent monitoring of measured GFR is typically not available in most ICUs. Prior to the development of the RIFLE system, acute kidney injury was not consistently defined. Many studies have been completed examining the ability to predict outcome and stratify patients with acute kidney injury according to the RIFLE criteria.[16-18]

The RIFLE criteria can be a very important tool for the critical care pharmacist to remember and understand. Many medications used in the critically ill patient have the potential to induce damage to the kidney. Further, many medications used in the critically ill are eliminated via the kidneys,

Table 2–1 RIFLE Criteria for Acute Kidney Injury[15]

	Serum Creatinine (SCr) changes	Urine output
Risk	150% increase in SCr from baseline	Less than 0.5 ml/kg/hr for at least 6 hours
Injury	200% increase in SCr from baseline	Less than 0.5 ml/kg/hr for at least 12 hours
Failure	300% increase in SCr from baseline	Less than 0.3 ml/kg/hr for at least 24 hours
	or a SCr of ≥ 4 mg/dL	or anuria for 12 hours
Loss	Complete loss of kidney function for at least 4 weeks	
End-stage renal disease	Complete loss of kidney function for greater than 3 months	

and these should be adjusted or replaced with alternative agents (if available) for changes in renal function. Appropriate monitoring of urine output and serum creatinine levels, using the RIFLE criteria as a guide, are important parts of the overall patient care plan.

While the RIFLE criteria can be helpful in determining degree of kidney injury or failure, it does not directly help with medication dose adjustments. Typically the Cockroft–Gault equation will be used for most medication dose adjustments. However, this equation was not developed with critically ill patients with multiple changing variables in mind.[16] While several other equations have been developed over the years to try to account for patients with increased body weight, changing urine output, or hypermetabolic conditions, the Cockroft–Gault equation remains in use for most clinicians in day-to-day practice.[17] There are many opinions as to the best equation to use, or the best assumptions to make with any of the creatinine clearance or GFR estimators. Ultimately, this is left to the bedside clinician's best judgment based upon their understanding of the individual patient, the medication regimens, and desired outcomes for the patient. A thorough review and understanding of kidney function estimation tools and their application to medication therapy is a key component of providing successful medication management services for critically ill patients.

SUMMARY

There is a large alphabet soup of common measurement systems utilized to evaluate and study critically ill patient populations. Pharmacists should have a basic understanding of the common scoring systems to be able to interpret the critical care literature and apply population data for quality improvement initiatives. Population scoring systems should not be confused with individual monitoring tools related to individual patient outcomes. This chapter only covers some of the main scoring systems that are commonly used, and a critical care practitioner will need to devote significant time to understanding all the nuances and appropriate use of each system.

KEY POINTS

- Scoring systems are commonly used in individual patients and in research studies to accurately describe both the patient and population being studied.
- The critical care pharmacist should have a working understanding of the various scores and scales available to assist in their

understanding of the literature and day-to-day patient assessment and monitoring.

- Scoring systems and scales can have a significant impact on patient care, and the importance of understanding the appropriate use of each scale cannot be underestimated.

SELECTED SUGGESTED READINGS

- Vincent JL, Ferreira F, Moreno R. Scoring systems for assessing organ dysfunction and survival. *Crit Care Clin.* 2000;16:353–366.
- Richardson MM. Precision versus approximation: The trade off in assessing kidney function and drug dosing. *Pharmacotherapy.* 2010;30(8):758–761.

REFERENCES

1. CareAware™ APACHE® Outcomes. Cerner Corporation. (Accessed July 20, 2011, at https://store.cerner.com/items/5)
2. Knaus WA, Zimmerman JE, Wagner DP, Draper EA, Lawrence DE. APACHE-acute physiology and chronic health evaluation: a physiologically based classification system. *Crit Care Med.* 1981;9:591–597.
3. Knaus WA, Draper EA, Wagner DP, Zimmerman JE. APACHE II: a severity of disease classification system. *Crit Care Med.* 1985;13:818–829.
4. Knaus WA, Wagner DP, Draper EA, et al. The APACHE III prognostic system. Risk prediction of hospital mortality for critically ill hospitalized adults. *Chest.* 1991;100:1619–1636.
5. Kho ME, McDonald E, Stratford PW, Cook DJ. Interrater reliability of APACHE II scores for medical-surgical intensive care patients: a prospective blinded study. *Am J Crit Care.* 2007;16:378–383.
6. Le Gall JR, Loirat P, Alperovitch A, et al. A simplified acute physiology score for ICU patients. *Crit Care Med.* 1984;12:975–977.
7. Le Gall JR, Lemeshow S, Saulnier F. A new Simplified Acute Physiology Score (SAPS II) based on a European/North American multicenter study. *JAMA.* 1993;270:2957–2963.
8. Vincent JL, Moreno R, Takala J, et al. The SOFA (Sepsis-related Organ Failure Assessment) score to describe organ dysfunction/failure. On behalf of the Working Group on Sepsis-Related Problems of the European Society of Intensive Care Medicine. *Intensive Care Med.* 1996;22:707–710.
9. Vincent JL, Ferreira F, Moreno R. Scoring systems for assessing organ dysfunction and survival. *Crit Care Clin.* 2000;16:353–366.
10. Marshall JC, Cook DJ, Christou NV, Bernard GR, Sprung CL, Sibbald WJ. Multiple organ dysfunction score: a reliable descriptor of a complex clinical outcome. *Crit Care Med.* 1995;23:1638–1652.
11. Peres Bota D, Melot C, Lopes Ferreira F, Nguyen Ba V, Vincent JL. The Multiple Organ Dysfunction Score (MODS) versus the Sequential Organ

Failure Assessment (SOFA) score in outcome prediction. *Intensive Care Med.* 2002;28:1619–1624.

12. Miranda DR, de Rijk A, Schaufeli W. Simplified Therapeutic Intervention Scoring System: the TISS-28 items—results from a multicenter study. *Crit Care Med.* 1996;24:64–73.

13. Baker SP, O'Neill B, Haddon W, Jr., Long WB. The injury severity score: a method for describing patients with multiple injuries and evaluating emergency care. *J Trauma.* 1974;14:187–196.

14. Brohi K. Injury Severity Score. (Accessed July 20, 2011, at http://www.trauma .org/index.php/main/article/383/)

15. Bellomo R, Ronco C, Kellum JA, Mehta RL, Palevsky P. Acute renal failure—definition, outcome measures, animal models, fluid therapy and information technology needs: the Second International Consensus Conference of the Acute Dialysis Quality Initiative (ADQI) Group. *Crit Care.* 2004;8:R204–212.

16. Cockroft DW, Gault MH. Prediction of creatinine clearance from serum creatinine. *Nephron.* 1976;16:31–41.

17. Bagshaw SM, George C, Dinu I, Bellomo R. A multi-centre evaluation of the RIFLE criteria for early acute kidney injury in critically ill patients. *Nephrol Dial Transplant.* 2008;23:1203–1210.

18. Joannidis M, Metnitz B, Bauer P, Schusterschitz N, Moreno R, Druml W, Metnitz PG. Acute kidney injury in critically ill patients classified by AKIN versus RIFLE using the SAPS 3 database. *Intensive Care Med.* 2009;35:1692–1702.

19. Ostermann M, Chang RWS. Acute kidney injury in the intensive care unit according to RIFLE. *Crit Care Med.* 2007; 35:1837–1843.

20. Richardson MM. Precision versus approximation: The trade off in assessing kidney function and drug dosing. *Pharmacotherapy.* 2010;30(8):758–761.

Chapter 3

Tubes and Lines, Invasive Monitoring, and Hemodynamics

Becky Nichols

LEARNING OBJECTIVES

1. Describe various intravascular (IV) devices, including indications, complications, and special considerations.
2. Explore indications and uses of other invasive tubes and lines commonly found in the intensive care unit (ICU) setting, including urinary catheters, rectal tubes, chest tubes, and intracranial bolts.
3. Describe intra-abdominal pressure (IAP) measurement and recognition of intra-abdominal hypertension (IAH) and treatment.
4. Summarize basic concepts in intra-aortic balloon pump (IABP) counter-pulsation therapy for the treatment of low cardiac output (CO) states.
5. Explain basic concepts in hemodynamics and oxygen profile evaluation.

INTRODUCTION

Patients admitted to the intensive care unit (ICU) present a complex dynamic of chronic co-morbidities complicated by acute illness and injury. There are many tools and devices used for monitoring and treatment of critically ill patients and they grow in intricacy and number as patient acuity climbs. This chapter will describe and illustrate a variety of equipment used to measure and maintain hemodynamic stability and oxygenation.

In addition, some of the various lines and tubes commonly used in critically ill patients will also be described. Although this chapter is not intended to provide extensive detail on every type of monitoring and treatment apparatus found in the ICU, it will afford the reader a basic understanding of and familiarity with what is commonly observed in critical care practice.

INTRAVASCULAR DEVICES

One of the most commonly observed interventions in the ICU is the placement of intravascular (IV) access devices. An intravascular device can be placed intravenously (also denoted as IV) or intra-arterially. Most commonly, "IV" will indicate intravenous placement, but it should be noted that other vascular placement is possible. Intravenous access devices are used to deliver fluids and medications, and some can be used for monitoring as well as for blood draws. When evaluating which type of access to insert, consideration is given to infusions being administered, therapies to be provided, duration of therapy, patient anatomy, cost, and expertise required for placement. Table 3–1 provides a list of types of intravenous devices, along with a brief description, dwell time, and indications of each.[1-3]

Table 3–1 Intravenous Access Devices[1-3]

Device	Description	Dwell Time	Indications and Special Considerations
Peripheral cannula	1. Access to peripheral circulation 2. 1" to 2" in length	72 to 96 hours	1. Short-term venous access (typically fewer than 5 days) 2. Infusion of non-irritating solutions
Midline	1. Peripherally inserted catheter that terminates in the upper arm 2. Approximately 20 cm in length 3. 1 to 2 lumens	About one month	1. Moderate-term venous access 2. Infusion of irritating solutions 3. Frequent phlebotomy
Peripherally Inserted Central Catheter (PICC) (Figure 3-1)	1. Peripherally inserted catheter that terminates in the superior vena cava (SVC) 2. Approximately 40–50 cm in length 3. 1 to 3 lumens	Months	1. Long-term venous access 2. Infusion of irritating solutions 3. Frequent phlebotomy

Table 3–1 Intravenous Access Devices[1-3] (*continued*)

Device	Description	Dwell Time	Indications and Special Considerations
Central Venous Catheter (Figure 3–2)	1. Non-tunneled catheter inserted into the subclavian, jugular, or femoral vein 2. Access to central circulation 3. Catheters placed in the upper chest or neck are typically 20 cm in length, while those placed in the groin site are 30 cm 4. 2 to 4 lumens	Weeks	1. Moderate-term venous access 2. Infusion of irritating solutions 3. Frequent phlebotomy 4. Central venous pressure and SVO_2 monitoring
Introducer (i.e., Trauma Catheter)	1. Non-tunneled catheter inserted into the subclavian, jugular, or femoral vein 2. Access to central circulation 3. Large bore (6 to 8.5 Fr) single lumen	Weeks	1. Short-term venous access 2. Infusion of irritating solutions 3. Frequent phlebotomy 4. High-rate, high-volume infusion
Dialysis Catheter (i.e., Quintin)	1. Non-tunneled catheter inserted into the subclavian, jugular, or femoral vein 2. Access to central circulation 3. Curved or straight with 2 ports used for dialysis and optional side port for medication delivery	Weeks	1. Short-term venous access 2. Dialysis or phoresis therapy 3. Bridge to fistula or tunneled catheter placement
Tunneled Catheters (i.e., Hickman or Groshong)	1. Tunneled under the skin into the subclavian vein 2. May have a cuff near the exit site to decrease risk of infection 3. Multiple ports	Months	1. Long-term access 2. Infusion of irritating solutions 3. Dialysis or phoresis 4. Frequent phlebotomy
Implanted ports	1. Port placed in surgically created pocket 2. Catheter off port is tunneled into subclavian vein 3. Access to central circulation 4. Requires special needle to access port	Months to years	1. Long-term access 2. Infusion of irritating solutions 3. Frequent phlebotomy

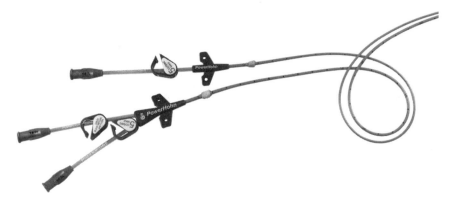

Figure 3–1 Central Venous Catheter

Source: © C. R. Bard, Inc.

Although a common procedure, IV placement is not without potential complications. Minor complications such as bleeding and bruising may be easily controlled with direct pressure and time. More concerning adverse effects, such as phlebitis, infiltration, and extravasation, require concentrated interventions, while less common complications such as infections, air emboli, and pneumothorax can be life-threatening.[4,5] Air emboli occur when air is introduced directly into the intravascular space. The incidence of air emboli can be related to a number of different pathologies, ranging from invasive procedures to indwelling catheters. Although small air emboli may not result in severe consequence and be "reabsorbed" by the lungs, a single large or continuous infusion of air can gain access into the systemic arterial circulation. In the presence of a patent foramen ovale, air emboli have the ability to infiltrate the coronary or cerebral circulation. Clinical symptoms vary from none all the way to respiratory distress, confusion, seizures, tachycardia, hypotension, and death. The immediate treatment of suspected venous air emboli is positioning

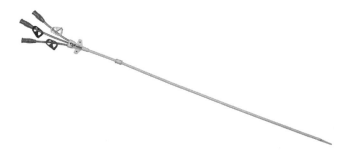

Figure 3–2 Triple Lumen Central Line

Source: © C. R. Bard, Inc.

of the patient into the left-lateral decubitus position and placing the bed into Trendelenburg while administering 100% oxygen. Additional measures to remove the emboli, such as aspiration from a central venous catheter positioned near the right atrium, may be attempted, hyperbaric oxygen therapy may be considered, and anticonvulsants for seizures may be ordered.[6]

Phlebitis, or inflammation of a vein, causes redness and swelling along the line of the vein, throbbing and burning at the IV site, and possibly low-grade fever. Extended dwell time, localized infections, clots, irritating solutions, and even the catheter material itself can cause phlebitis.[1] Phlebitis treatment consists of removal of the access device, antibiotics if needed for associated infections, and anticoagulants if blood clots are present.[7-11]

Infiltration, another potential complication of IV therapy, is "inadvertent administration of a nonvesicant solution into surrounding tissue that may or may not cause damage."[1,5] Although the solution itself may not cause tissue damage, excessive fluid build-up into a confined space may cause a compartment-like syndrome leading to decreased perfusion and ultimately tissue ischemia and necrosis. Symptoms are characterized by cool, blanched skin, leaking from the insertion site, and pain. Infiltration treatment consists of removal of the access device, encouraging the use of the extremity to promote reabsorption of fluid, and warm packs for comfort.[1,9]

Extravasation is the "inadvertent administration of a vesicant solution or medication into surrounding tissues that can cause tissue damage and destruction."[1,4,5] Treatment of extravasation requires knowledge of the medication or solution that was administered and the antidote required to attempt to counteract damaging effects. Patients who experience extravasation will describe significant pain at the IV site, the skin may appear inflamed and swollen, and ulceration may develop hours to days after the event.[1] Antidotes are typically given subcutaneously into the tissue surrounding the affected area and through the catheter before it is removed. Early consultation with a certified wound ostomy continence (WOC) registered nurse (RN) may be helpful in developing a treatment regimen to prevent further tissue damage.[2] Some of the more common drugs involved in extravasation in the ICU and their antidotes are presented in Table 3–2.[1,2,4,5,7]

Central venous catheters, other non-tunneled catheters, and tunneled catheters may be associated with insertion-related adverse events such as pneumo- and hemothorax and cardiac dysrhythmias, as well as removal-related events such as air emboli. Early recognition and emergency intervention are necessary to prevent patient demise should any of these severe complications arise.[5,8-10]

Pulmonary artery (PA) and intra-arterial catheters are also considered intravascular devices. Their indications, complications, and considerations will be presented later in this chapter.

Table 3–2 Extravasation Antidotes[1,2,4–5,7]

Drug	Antidote
Aminophylline, calcium, contrast media, dextrose (>10% concentration), nafcillin, potassium, total parenteral nutrition	Hyaluronidase 15 units/mL Provided as 0.2 mL subcutaneously around site
Dobutamine, dopamine, epinephrine, norepinephrine	Phentolamine 5 to 10 mg diluted in 10–15 mL of normal saline Administered at 0.2 ml subcutaneously around site as soon as possible, but within 12 hours of event

MISCELLANEOUS LINES AND TUBES

Urinary Catheters

Probably the second most common device inserted into an ICU patient is the urinary catheter (often called a Foley catheter). The urinary catheter is useful in monitoring a patient's fluid volume status and renal function.[3] Typically inserted by an RN using sterile technique, the catheter is guided through the urethra and into the bladder. Once in place, a balloon near the tip of the catheter is inflated with sterile normal saline to secure its position.[3,9,10]

Typically considered a routine procedure, urinary catheters are not without risk. Urethral trauma and perforation during insertion, urinary outflow obstruction due to kinked catheters leading to bladder distention and possible hydronephrosis, bladder spasms causing patient discomfort and urine leakage, and urinary tract infections are all potential adverse effects of urinary catheter placement.[12,13] Quality initiatives for ICU patients often include re-evaluating the need for urinary catheters at least daily.

Rectal Tubes

Rectal tubes may be considered for patients with excessive stooling who are immobile and at risk for tissue breakdown. Additionally, these tubes are helpful in the administration of medications via enemas, as they provide a direct route to the colon. They can be clamped to assist in retention and then released after a prescribed amount of time. Generally, these tubes do not cause any discomfort for the patient; however, if the tube is incorrectly placed or kinks off inadvertently, leakage, extrinsic bowel obstruction, and discomfort may occur. A balloon on the end of the rectal tube helps secure its position. Overinflation of the balloon or prolonged insertion may lead to mucosal ulceration and lower gastrointestinal bleeding.[14]

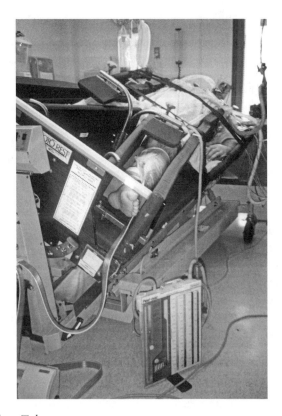

Figure 3-3 Chest Tube

Source: © B. Slaven, MD/Custom Medical Stock Photo.

Chest Tubes

Chest tubes (Figure 3-3) may be inserted into the pleural space for a variety of reasons. Re-expansion of the lung in pneumothorax, removal of blood in hemothorax, drainage of fluid in pleural effusion, and post-operatively in thoracotomy or cardiac bypass are some of the more common indications for chest tube placement in ICU patients.[15] Chest tubes may be placed by physicians or surgeons and the size of the tube is dependent upon patient size. After cleansing the area and providing a local anesthetic, a small incision is made in the mid-axillary line between the 4th and 5th intercostal space. The chest tube with a trocar in it is inserted into the pleural cavity, the trocar is removed, and the chest tube is connected to a suction unit via an extension tube. Typically, chest tubes are maintained on low wall suction for several days, followed by water seal to ensure patient stability before removal of the tube.[16] A water seal acts as a one-way valve: When the patient exhales, the air travels through the extension tube into the suction device and bubbles out through the water, and when the patient inhales, the water prevents air from traveling back up the tube and into the pleural space. Figure 3–3 illustrates this system. Complications of chest tubes include bleeding; injury to the lung, heart, or arteries; infection; air leaks; and tension pneumothorax development.[4]

PRESSURE MONITORING

Neurologic Monitoring Devices

The brain is a highly metabolic organ that requires consistent oxygen delivery. Damage caused by lack of oxygen to the central nervous system is measured in minutes. Rapid intervention and aggressive treatment are required to provide patients with the optimal chance of survival. Fortunately, there are several methods of monitoring and improving perfusion and oxygenation to the cells of the brain to ensure the very best possible outcome for patients with brain injury. Brain injury can occur from a multitude of causes ranging from trauma to tumors, blood clots to bleeds; the most common neurologic injuries are described in Chapter 15. Although the mechanisms may differ, prescribed interventions are intended to optimize perfusion and oxygenation of brain tissue, reverse ischemia, and minimize the area of cellular death.[17] While it is possible to utilize clinical exam in some patients to evaluate neurological status and identify deterioration, unresponsive patients prove to be more challenging.

Normally, a pressure of 5 to 15 mmHg is maintained within the rigid box of the skull through displacement of one of three space-occupying entities: cerebral spinal fluid (CSF), blood, or brain tissue.[17] This ability of the brain to compensate for an increase in one compartment through reduction in another is described by the Monroe–Kelly Doctrine. One can assume that the shifting of CSF would be the best compartment for reduction as opposed to reduced blood flow, which places brain cells at risk of ischemia. Additionally, shifting of brain tissue may lead to altered perfusion and ultimately herniation with irreversible brain damage and death.

Monitoring of intracranial pressure (ICP) to allow for expedient treatment of increased pressure can be achieved through the placement of a fiberoptic monitor through a bolt into one of three spaces in the brain (i.e., ventricular, epidural, or subarachnoid).[15,17,18] The ICP bolt gives an indication of perfusion. The equation to determine cerebral perfusion pressure (CPP) is mean arterial pressure (MAP) minus ICP.[18] Normal CPP is greater than 70 mmHg, and treatment targets of CPP are usually about 60 mmHg.[19] Unfortunately, ICP tells us nothing about the oxygenation of brain tissue, but several methods are available for monitoring brain tissue oxygen levels. Management of intracranial pressure is discussed in detail in Chapter 15, with methods of monitoring ICP discussed further here.

Because blood from the brain drains through the internal jugular veins, it is possible to measure the partial pressure of oxygen within them. Called SjO_2, it can be used to evaluate for brain tissue hypoxia.[19,20] This can be performed continuously with an oximetric central catheter placed in the jugular vein or intermittently via blood draw. Normal SjO_2 ranges from 60% to 70%.[19] Unfortunately, this method does not provide information about the oxygenation of tissue near the area of injury; rather, it provides a global representation of whole brain oxygenation.[19] An alternative method of measuring brain oxygenation is through the use of an intraparenchymal sensor placed in conjunction with an ICP bolt near the area of injury. Normal brain tissue oxygen levels are greater than 30 mmHg, with treatment goals typically aimed at maintaining a level of 20 to 25 mmHg.[20]

Intra- and extraventricular drains may be placed to reduce the amount of circulating CSF, thus decreasing ICP.[18,21,22] It is possible to have drains placed with ICP bolts or obtain manual ICP readings from standard drains. The main risks of these devices include infection, CSF leakage, brain tissue injury, and bleeding.[18,21,22] In cases of infection, antibiotics may be directly administered into the brain by a neurosurgeon in patients who have any of these devices in place.

Intra-Abdominal Pressure (IAP)

When pressure inside the abdominal compartment exceeds normal levels, intra-abdominal organ tissues become compromised because the increased pressure impedes normal blood flow. Clinical manifestations of intra-abdominal hypertension (IAH) include: respiratory failure (mechanically ventilated patients will have increasing peak airway pressures and decreasing tidal volumes), oliguria or anuria, hypotension, and tachycardia. Laboratory values such as blood urea nitrogen (BUN), creatinine, lactic acid, and arterial blood gases (ABGs) may be helpful to evaluate the extent of organ dysfunction and metabolic disturbance. Without intervention, the patient may go on to develop abdominal compartment syndrome (ACS) with irreversible organ failure and, ultimately, death.[23,24] Early recognition and treatment is essential with IAH to prevent ACS development.

Patients who have had direct injury to the abdominal cavity, such as with trauma, intra-abdominal procedures, or large volume resuscitation, have increased risk for IAH.[23,24] Normal IAP is <10 mmHg, with results of 10 to 20 mmHg classified as mild IAH, 20 to 40 mmHg as moderate, and >40 mmHg as severe.[23,24]

Methods are available to provide objective evaluation of IAP monitoring. Direct IAP via the use of invasive line placement directly into the peritoneal space is not practical for patients; however, good correlations have been demonstrated using commercial transducers (such as the AbVisor®) specifically designed to attach to the bladder catheter. The bladder pressures provide a reasonable indication if IAH is present, and readings are typically monitored for trends with correlation to clinical symptoms to aid in the determination of appropriate interventions.[23,24]

INTRA-AORTIC BALLOON PUMP (IABP)

Conditions that commonly contribute to decreased cardiac output (CO) include myocardial infarction (MI), left ventricular failure, cardiogenic shock, and septic shock with depressed myocardial function. Although medications can provide some benefit, mechanical intervention through the use of an IABP may be required to ensure adequate perfusion and oxygen delivery (Figure 3–4). Additionally, the IABP can be placed to improve oxygen delivery and reduce oxygen demand in the coronary arteries in unstable angina.[25]

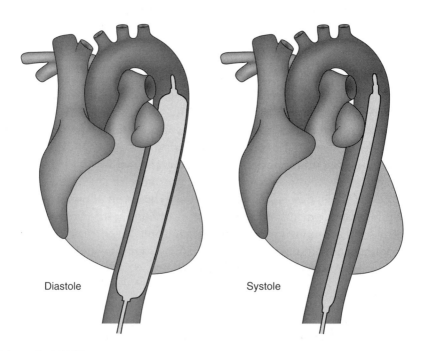

Diastole   Systole

Figure 3–4 IABP

To insert, a cardiologist threads a catheter encased in a long tubular balloon into the femoral artery and situates it in the descending aorta just distal to the left subclavian artery. This ensures that the balloon does not occlude the carotid arteries as they branch off the aorta or the renal arteries in the descending aorta.[15,18]

Timing for balloon inflation can be obtained several different ways. The first is via telemetry. The pump recognizes the R wave on the electrocardiograph (ECG) and the balloon is set to begin inflation in the middle of the T wave and deflate just prior to the end of the QRS complex.[26] Complications with timing using ECG can occur with tachycardias, cardiac dysrhythmias, and poor ECG quality.[27] Another method of timing can be performed using the arterial waveform. Deflation of the balloon occurs just prior to the arterial upstroke (ventricular contraction or systole) and inflation occurs on the diacritic notch (relaxation or diastole).[26] However, a poor arterial waveform will cause problems in IABP timing using this method.[27] The third and final method for timing is through intrinsic pump programming, which is used when there is loss of the arterial waveform or ECG tracing, such as with cardiac arrest.[26] The timing of balloon deflation just before systole provides for reduced afterload, while inflation at the beginning of diastole augments circulation by providing an extra "push" within the aorta to drive blood into the periphery.

Typically, the IABP is set for one to one (identified as "1:1") augmentation.[18,26] This means that for every heartbeat, the balloon will inflate and deflate. Over time, as cardiac function improves, the pump will be weaned to a 1:2 (augmenting every other beat) or 1:3 (augmenting every third beat) and so on, until the balloon can be removed.[18,26] Trending of both augmented and non-augmented blood pressure is performed along with monitoring of the augmented waveform to evaluate effectiveness, weanability, and timing.[18]

Some complications of IABP include balloon rupture, bleeding or infection at the insertion site, limb ischemia, thrombosis formation, and catheter migration.[18,27,28] The insertion site should be monitored for hematoma development and signs of infection, just as pedal pulses, neurologic status, and urine output should be watched closely to assess for complications of balloon migration.[18] The augmented waveform is assessed for early and late balloon inflation and deflation. Early inflation and late deflation have the potential to increase cardiac workload and oxygen demand; less harmful are late inflation and early deflation, which prevent adequate coronary artery perfusion and oxygenation.[25,26,28,29] Typically, an IABP will be in place for 1 to 5 days, although in patients who are awaiting cardiac transplant, the dwell time could be much longer.

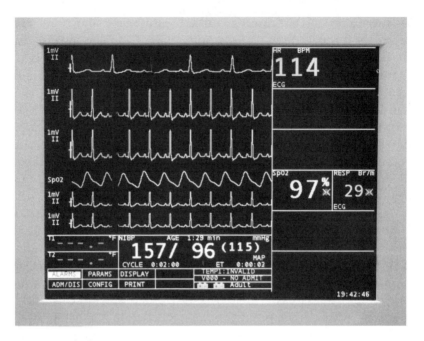

Figure 3–5 Bedside Monitor

Source: © Lorelyn Medina/ShutterStock, Inc.

Devices that measure hemodynamics are visualized om a bedside monitor similar to the one shown in Figure 3–5.

HEMODYNAMIC MONITORING

For a gasoline engine to run properly, the correct mixture of gasoline and oxygen must be present when the spark plugs fire to move the cylinders and put the car into motion. The same is true of our cells. Think of blood flow as being like gasoline: even though it may adequately flow into the capillaries and subsequently perfuse tissue, without the right amount of oxygen, this "gas" is useless. Alternatively, even though there may be enough oxygen entering into the lungs, without blood flow to pick up and carry it to the cells, the outcome is the same. Eventually, the cells will become ischemic and die and the human "engine" will stop. Not only do cars need the correct mixture, it is important to have enough fuel to meet the demands that we place on our vehicles. If one is planning on a cross-country drive, it will become necessary to refuel at some point along the way or risk being stranded. The more demanded of the automobile, the more supply it needs; it is about balance. This is also true of the human body—supply must equal demand.

Devices for Measuring Hemodynamics

The Arterial Line

There are several different devices that can be used to monitor fluid balance and hemodynamics.[15,18,30,31] One of the most common in the ICU setting is the arterial line. A cannula, much like one used for IV therapy, is threaded into an artery (most commonly the radial artery) and attached to a transducer connected to a bedside monitor. This system allows for real-time monitoring of blood pressure and can be used for blood draws for patients requiring frequent laboratory monitoring.[15,18,30,31] Arterial lines are not used to administer medication.

The arterial waveform is created when the left ventricle contracts. As blood leaves the ventricle, travels through the aorta, and finally enters into the arteries, the elastic properties of the blood vessels maintain the hemodynamic energy of that contraction. The arterial line visually transforms that energy into a waveform that can be observed on the bedside monitor. Not only does the waveform show ventricular contraction, but it also shows the closing of the aortic valve. The upstroke on the left side of the waveform follows the QRS complex on the ECG.[15,18,30,31] This represents ventricular contraction. The downward slope after the peak of the waveform represents the cessation of contraction (systole) followed by a small bump, called the diacritic notch. The closing of the aortic valve creates the notch and indicates the beginning of diastole. The waveform then proceeds to have a smooth downward flow, called "run off." To have a proper waveform, the transducer must be in line with the right atrium of the patient and regularly "zeroed" to atmospheric pressure. Transducers that are below the right atrium will read erroneously high, while the opposite is true of those above the right atrium; there are numerous additional reasons why an arterial line may read inaccurately, which is beyond the scope of this text. Pharmacists and other clinicians need to understand that these nuances exist to help with management of blood pressure and hemodynamics and to remember that equipment needs to be adjusted properly to obtain accurate readings. Complications of arterial lines include bleeding, infection, thrombosis, air emboli, hematomas, and foreign body emboli from cannula disruption.[15,18,30,31]

Pulmonary Artery Pressure Monitoring

The arterial line is not always adequate in providing all of the necessary information to evaluate and treat critically ill patients. When providers need to know more about fluid volume status, cardiac function, and whole body perfusion, they turn to the pulmonary artery (PA) catheter (Figure 3–6).

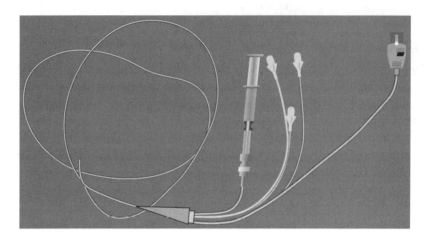

Figure 3–6 PA Catheter

Considered the "gold standard" for hemodynamic monitoring, the PA catheter provides information on all of the parameters that make up cardiac output (CO): preload, afterload, contractility, and heart rate.[15,18,30,31] With this information, the provider can initiate combinations of fluid and medications to optimize CO and ultimately perfusion.

The PA catheter is typically inserted into the patient at the bedside or during procedures such as cardiac catheterization or coronary bypass. The catheter is threaded through a large vein (typically the jugular or subclavian, though the femoral may also be used) into the heart via the right atrium, continuing on through the right ventricle and into the pulmonary artery. A balloon on the tip of the catheter is inflated during insertion to aid in "floating" the catheter into place while protecting the walls of the heart from perforation. The catheter is attached to a transducer system, allowing the PA waveform and data to appear on the bedside monitor just like the arterial waveform. The location of the catheter tip is determined by observing changes in the waveform as the catheter passes from one area of the heart to the next. Once in place, a "wedge" waveform appears as the balloon slides into a small arteriole in the pulmonary artery, blocking off forward blood flow. After the balloon is deflated, the PA waveform appears. Similar to an arterial line waveform, the PA waveform has a smooth upstroke, correlating with the right ventricle contraction, followed by a short downward slope, diacritic notch (pulmonary valve closure), and runoff.[15,18,30,31]

Complications of PA Catheters The PA catheter comes with several risks. Hemo- or pneumothorax, cardiac dysrhythmias, valvular damage, and perforation of the heart are all possible complications that may occur during

PA catheter insertion. Infection, dysrhythmias, pulmonary artery rupture, thrombosis, and air emboli may occur while the catheter is in place or during removal.[15,18,30,31]

PA Catheter Hemodynamics   When observing the dynamics being evaluated by the PA catheter, it is important to understand the following components of cardiac output: preload, afterload, and contractility (which make up stroke volume (SV)) and heart rate (HR). Expressed as an equation, CO = HR × SV, where SV is the difference between end-diastolic volume (preload) and end-systolic volume (afterload). Finally, ejection fraction (EF) is SV expressed as a percentage.[15,18,30,31]

However, before discussing these concepts in detail, remember that the heart is divided into left and right sections. Both sides of the heart have blood volume entering and both have ventricles that contract to push blood out past a valve and into a system (either pulmonary or systemic). The right atrium receives blood from the body, and that volume then enters into the right ventricle to finally pass through the pulmonary artery into the low-pressure system of the pulmonary vasculature. The left atrium receives blood from the pulmonary vein, ejects that volume into the left ventricle which contracts to push blood through the aortic valve into the higher-pressure system of systemic circulation.[30,31]

Preload is defined as the "load imposed on the ventricular muscle before the onset of contraction."[30,31] In other words, it is the pressure of blood at maximum fill, just before the ventricle contracts to eject that volume out. Preload on the right side of the heart may be called by a variety of names, such as right atrial pressure (RAP) or central venous pressure (CVP). The preload on the left side of the heart also has several names, including pulmonary artery occlusive pressure (PAOP), pulmonary capillary wedge pressure (PCWP), and pulmonary artery wedge pressure (PAWP).[15,18,30,31] For the purpose of this book, CVP and PAWP will be used to describe right and left preload. Typically, preload is used to evaluate fluid volume status; however, in cases of mitral or aortic valvular disease, as well as obstructive or cardiovascular shock, preload may appear elevated without changes in volume. In contrast, cardiac dysrhythmias may decrease preload without being an accurate reflection of volume status.[30,31]

Afterload is defined as "the opposing force that determines the force of muscle contraction needed to initiate muscle shortening" or the pressure that the ventricle must overcome to eject its volume of blood.[30,31] On the right side of the heart, this pressure is called pulmonary vascular resistance (PVR) and on the left, systemic vascular resistance (SVR). Typically, afterload is elevated in situations where vasoconstriction is occurring, such as hypothermia, hypovolemia, vasopressor use, and hypoxia. Decreases in afterload can be seen when vasodilation is present, such as anaphylactic shock, sepsis, and vasodilator medication administration.[30,31] Contractility is the ability of cardiac muscle fibers to shorten. Alterations in contractility can occur deliberately through the use of medications. A decrease in contractility can occur in conjunction with myocardial injury, fluid volume overload or hypovolemia, and electrolyte imbalance, while increased contractility may be seen with hyperthyroidism or decreased afterload. Although contractility cannot be measured with a traditional PA catheter, there are special oximetric PA catheters that have the ability to measure Stroke Work Index (SWI), which is the amount of work performed by the ventricle per contraction at constant end diastolic volume and provides information about myocardial contractility.[30,31]

Starling's Law states that the greater the amount of stretch on the ventricle, or end-diastolic volume, the greater the force of the contraction. However, this law is only true to a certain extent; too much preload and contraction may actually become suboptimal. The heart attempts to compensate for this through manipulation of heart rate and afterload. A decrease in preload stimulates a rise in afterload in an attempt to promote improved venous return. To overcome the rise in afterload, the left ventricular muscle fibers increase in size. Additionally, as preload decreases and CO drops, the heart rate will increase in compensation, ultimately increasing cardiac workload.[30,31] Uninterrupted, this vicious cycle leads to left ventricular hypertrophy and heart failure.

It is essential that fluid volume status be optimized to promote adequate CO while minimizing any increase in cardiac workload. The PA catheter is one way to evaluate and determine the effects of interventions to support CO, however, there are other, less invasive methods available that measure many of the variables also monitored by the PA catheter.

Pulse Pressure Variation and Less Invasive Hemodynamic Monitoring

When a mechanically ventilated patient is delivered a breath, positive pressure in the lungs slightly decreases the amount of venous return to the heart, which in turn decreases CO and, ultimately, blood pressure. The arterial waveform registers this decrease with a slightly dampened arterial waveform. From one beat to the next, the variation that occurs is called stroke volume variation (SVV) and it is measured as a percentage. In euvolemia, the normal variation from beat to beat is less than 13%, whereas in hypovolemia, the variation becomes more pronounced and is often greater than 13 to 15%.[30-33] In essence, the higher the SVV, the more likely the patient will respond with improved CO from the administration of volume. Special transducers and monitors have the capability to monitor SVV using the arterial line. Additionally, some of these devices may also

Table 3–3 Hemodynamic Measurements[15,18,30,31]

Hemodynamic Measure	Component Being Evaluated	Normal Range
Central Venous Pressure (CVP)	Right Heart Preload	4–10 mmHg
Pulmonary Artery Wedge Pressure (PAWP)	Left Heart Preload	8–12 mmHg
Pulmonary Vascular Resistance (PVR)	Right Heart Afterload	150–250 dynes/sec/cm^{-5}
Systemic Vascular Resistance (SVR)	Left Heart Afterload	900–1400 dynes/sec/cm^{-5}
CO	Volume of blood, in liters, pumped out of the heart in one minute	5–8 L/minute
Cardiac Index (CI)	CO based on BSA	2.5–4.2 L/minute
SV	Amount of blood pumped out of the left ventricle in one beat	60–80 mL/beat
SVV	Volume variation from one heart beat to the next	<13%
EF	SV expressed as a percentage	60–80%

measure CO and EF. Since the arterial line is far more commonly placed in the ICU and has fewer complications compared to a PA catheter, using these monitoring devices may provide less risk for the patient to obtain similar information.

Electrical impedance may also be used to measure blood flow within the chest cavity. The blood flow rates can then analyzed via equations to determine variables such as preload, afterload, and contractility.

Normal Hemodynamic Values

Table 3-3 provides the expected values for each hemodynamic measurement.[15,18,30,31] It is important to remember that these "normal" ranges were first determined in relatively young, healthy males and the typical ICU patient is anything but "normal." Additionally, some values, such as CO, are indexed, or based upon the body surface area (BSA), to individualize the results to the patient.

Oxygenation Profile

Optimization of perfusion through the use of an arterial line, PA catheter, or less invasive methods does not guarantee adequate oxygen delivery to the tissues. The overall goal is to ensure that oxygen delivery meets demand. There are several ways to monitor that this balance is being maintained, but understanding of the following terms is required. The most important determinant of oxygen delivery (DO_2) to the body is cardiac output.[30,31] At the tissue level, the cells require a certain amount of oxygen to maintain aerobic metabolism. The oxygen demand (VO_2) of the cells remains relatively constant in a resting state and the percentage of oxygen that is removed from the hemoglobin is called extraction ratio (O_2ER).[30,31] In summary, if VO_2 goes up, O_2ER will rise regardless of the amount of DO_2.

The amount of oxygen "left over" upon return to the heart is referred to as mixed venous oxygen (SvO_2), which is the balance of whole body tissue oxygenation. In a balanced state, SvO_2 plus O_2ER should be close to 100%. Fick's equation includes those components that determine SvO_2 in that $SvO_2 = SaO_2$ (arterial oxygen) $- VO_2/13.9$ (constant) $\times CO \times$ hemoglobin.[30,31]

Several additional factors affect DO_2. Hemoglobin, arterial oxygenation, fraction of inspired oxygen (FiO_2), body temperature, and acid–base balance all affect SvO_2.[15,18,30,31] In alkalosis, hemoglobin's affinity for oxygen increases, and in acidosis, hemoglobin's affinity for oxygen decreases. Low levels of hemoglobin also result in less oxygen being transported. Decreased FiO_2 does not allow the lungs to inhale enough oxygen to meet the body's needs. There is higher affinity for hemoglobin to oxygen in hypothermia and a lower affinity in hyperthermia.[31]

Oxygen balance can also be evaluated through the use of laboratory analysis of lactic acid.[30,31] Too much demand or not enough delivery of oxygen and the tissues revert to anaerobic metabolism and lactic acid production occurs. Although it is possible to obtain laboratory specimens to measure arterial blood gases (ABGs), SvO_2, and lactic acid, these only provide a snapshot of the patient's current status and ongoing evaluation is often necessary. Alternatively, oximetric PA and central line catheters attached to special monitors have the ability to observe and trend, in real time, the oxygen profile. The oxygen profile normal ranges are provided in Table 3–4.[30,31]

Compensation

The body is a wondrous machine. Back-up and compensatory mechanisms exist to preserve normal function for as long as possible and the same is true for perfusion and oxygenation. Because CO is composed of preload, afterload, contractility and heart rate, any alteration in one part of the equation

Table 3-4 Oxygen Profile Normal Ranges[30,31]

Oxygen Profile Component	Normal Range
DO_2 (oxygen delivery)	950–1150 mL/min
VO_2 (oxygen demand)	200–250 mL/min
O_2ER (oxygen extraction ratio)	22–30%
SvO_2 (mixed venous oxygen)	60–80%

leads to compensation by another component. For example, in severe sepsis, as massive vasodilation (decreased afterload) occurs, there is initially a rise in CO as cardiac workload decreases; however, over time, capillary leak, in addition to vasodilation, leads to decreased preload and ultimately a drop in CO. If no intervention is provided, perfusion and oxygen delivery decrease, anaerobic metabolism begins and lactic acid rises. SvO_2 drops due to the rise in O_2ER to meet the oxygen requirements of the tissues.

Using the basics of hemodynamics and the oxygen profile and applying that knowledge to individual patients in the ICU setting will promote a deeper understanding of disease pathology and the intended effects of the interventions being implemented.

HEMODYNAMIC CASE SCENARIO

Presented below is an example case, which integrates several of the topics described in this chapter, outlines the patient's parameters, and describes the steps taken to treat the patient.

GB is a 79-year-old, Caucasian male who presented to the emergency department (ED) with acute onset of left-sided chest pain, which radiated down his left arm and up his left neck. His blood pressure was 95/53 and his heart rate was 45 beats per minute. He looked pale and diaphoretic, and felt dizzy. Work-up in the ED included a 12 lead electrocardiogram (ECG), chest X-ray, and cardiac enzymes. It was determined that GB was suffering an acute myocardial infarction (AMI) and that he needed to be taken to the cardiac catheterization lab for intervention.

Although no direct measurement was available in the ED, based upon GB's clinical appearance, it is possible to determine the effects of AMI on his CO and the compensation that occurred. Bradycardia as a result of cardiac damage decreased CO. The body attempted to compensate through vasoconstriction and increased heart rate; unfortunately, in a heart that is already stressed, the rise in afterload and resulting work further damage cardiac muscle as the oxygen demand overshadows supply. As in this example, a damaged heart may not have the ability to increase heart rate. Vasoconstriction leads to pale appearance, as well as cool skin, while decreased CO lessens perfusion and oxygen delivery. In the case of GB, decreased perfusion to the brain caused dizziness, blood shunting away from the intestinal organs caused nausea, and, finally, decreased peripheral perfusion added to the cool, clammy skin.

Immediately after stent placement, GB suffered ventricular fibrillation (VF) cardiac arrest. In VF, there is complete loss of CO, as the left ventricle is no longer contracting. Immediate resuscitation included electrical defibrillation, which unfortunately converted the rhythm to asystole in this patient. In asystole, as in VF, there is no left ventricular contraction, thus no CO. Artificial means of providing CO must be implemented; these include chest compressions or compressions with an automated device. With appropriate intervention, GB regained a perfusing rhythm identified as normal sinus rhythm with frequent premature ventricular complexes (PVCs). His blood pressure was 85/56 and he remained unresponsive. An oximetric PA catheter was inserted to assist with optimization and monitoring of hemodynamics and oxygenation. Initial values were as follows: CO 3.0 L/minute, CI 1.8 L/minute, SVR 1935 dynes/sec/cm^{-5}, PVR 245 dynes/sec/cm^{-5}, and CVP 1 mmHg. Oxygen profile indicated a DO_2 of 800 mL/minute, VO_2 225 mL/min, O_2ER 45%, and SvO_2 55%. It was assumed that improvement of CO would improve DO_2 as the hemoglobin, temperature, and ABGs were within normal limits. To augment DO_2 until CO could be improved, the FiO_2 was increased to 100% per mechanical ventilation. This increased the SvO_2 to 65%. Normal saline was bolused until CVP was greater than 10 mmHg; however, the patient's blood pressure remained low and he continued to require high-dose vasopressor administration. It was determined that GB would benefit from IABP placement. The augmented blood pressure rose to 115/63, CO increased to 6.2 L/min, CI 3.0 L/min, SVR 950 dynes/sec/cm^{-5}, PVR 250 dynes/sec/cm^{-5}, and CVP 12 mmHg.

In the ICU, over the course of several days, GB continued to improve and was weaned off of the IABP, but he continued to be minimally responsive and remained intubated. On hospital day 5, the patient experienced a fever of 101 degrees F, his blood pressure decreased to 98/57, and the cardiac rhythm became uncontrolled atrial fibrillation with a ventricular rate of 135 beats per minute. The CO increased to 10 L/min, CI 5.8 L/min, SVR 665 dynes/sec/cm^{-5}, PVR 150 dynes/sec/cm^{-5}, CVP 3 mmHg, and SvO_2 decreased to 40%. A lactic acid concentration was obtained and was elevated at 7.9 mmol/L. It was determined that the patient was septic from a urinary tract infection related to bladder catheter placement. Multiple normal saline boluses were required to get the CVP greater than 12 mmHg, the catheter was removed, and antibiotics initiated. Acetaminophen was given to reduce the fever, which also decreased VO_2, and within 2 hours, the SvO_2 increased to 70%. Although the CVP was within range, the blood pressure and SVR remained low. Norepinephrine was initiated, and the SVR increased to 1200 dynes/sec/cm^{-5}, CO decreased to normal limits, and blood pressure improved. Within 24 hours, the patient was weaned off norepinephrine and was extubated the next day.

This patient utilized several of the invasive monitoring and supportive therapy tools available for critically ill patients. While this is just an example, it is easy to see how many variables can be involved in the care of these patients.

SUMMARY

A basic understanding of intravenous, intra-arterial, and invasive monitoring and support equipment is essential for any practitioner in the ICU. Applying this knowledge to pharmacotherapy and optimizing patient outcomes is a significant component of the day-to-day care of critically ill patients.

KEY POINTS

- Intravascular access is an important part of critical care management.
- There are multiple tubes and catheters that are used to treat and monitor critically ill patients.
- A fundamental knowledge of invasive and noninvasive hemodynamic monitoring is important to understanding pharmacology in treatment of the critically ill.
- Monitoring of oxygenation provides management goals for critically ill patients and is a primary therapeutic goal for supporting therapies, including medications.

SELECTED SUGGESTED READINGS

- Gould CV, Umscheid CA, Agarwal RA, et al. Guideline for the prevention of catheter-associated urinary tract infections 2009. *Infect Control Hosp Epidemiol.* 2010;31:319–326.
- Perkins LA, Barker JA. Intraabdominal Hypertension and Abdominal Compartment Syndrome. American College of Chest Physcians,

PCCSU. www.chestnet.org/accp/pccsu/intraabdominal-hypertension-
and-abdominal-compartment-syndrome?page=0,3. Published
November 1, 2010; Accessed July 25, 2011.

REFERENCES

1. Infusion Nurses Society. *Infusion Nursing Standards of Practice. 2nd ed.* Infusion Nurses Society; 2006.
2. Zuccarini M, ed. *Plumer's Principles & Practice of Intravenous Therapy. 8th ed.* Philadelphia: Lippincott Williams & Wilkens; 2001.
3. Nettina SM. *Manual of Nursing Practice. 9th ed.* Philadelphia: Lippincott, Williams & Wilkens; 2010.
4. Polowich M, White J, Kelleher L, eds. *Chemotherapy and Biotherapy Guidelines and Recommendations for Practice. 2nd ed.* Pittsburgh: Oncology Nursing Society; 2005.
5. McGee DC, Gould MK. Preventing complications of central venous catheterizations. *N Engl J Med.* 2003;304:1123-1133.
6. Goldman L, Ausiello D, eds. *Cecil Medicine. 23rd ed.* Philadelphia: Saunders Elsevier; 2008.
7. Gahart B, Nazareno A. *Intravenous medications. 12th ed.* St Louis: Mosby; 2004.
8. Camp-Sorrell D, Cope D, eds. *Access Device Guidelines: Recommendations for Nursing Practice. 2nd ed.* Pittsburgh, PA: Oncology Nursing Press; 2004.
9. Perry AG, Potter PA. *Clinical Nursing Skills and Techniques.* St. Louis: Mosby; 1998:790-99.
10. Smith Temple J, Johnson J. *Nurse's Guild to Clinical Procedures. 4th ed.* Philadelphia: Lippencott, Williams & Wilkens; 2002: 275-279.
11. Center for Disease Control. Guidelines for prevention of intravascular catheter-related infections. *Morbidity & Mortality Weekly Report.* 2002;501.
12. Cravens DD, Zweig S. Urinary catheter management. *Am Fam Physician.* 2000;61:369-376.
13. Gould CV, Umscheid CA, Agarwal RA, et al. Guideline for the prevention of catheter-associated urinary tract infections 2009. *Infect Control Hosp Epidemiol.* 2010;31:319-326.
14. Beitz JM. Fecal incontinence in acutely and critically ill patients: Options in management. *Ostomy Wound Manage.* 2006;52:56-58, 60, 62-66.
15. Lynn-McHale D, Carlson K, eds. *AACN Procedure Manual for Critical Care. 4th ed.* Philadelphia: WB Saunders; 2001: 99-140.
16. Dural R, Hogue H, Davies T. Managing a chest tube and drainage system. *AORN.* 2010;275-283. (Accessed November 7, 2010, at www.aornjournal.org/article/PIIS0001209209009284/fulltext).
17. Bratton SL, Chestnut RM, Ghajar J, et al. Indications for intracranial pressure monitoring. *J Neurotrauma,* 2007;24(Suppl 1):37-44.
18. Lynn-McHale D, Weigand D, Carlson K, eds. *AACN Procedure Manual for Critical Care. 5th ed.* St. Louis: WB Saunders; 2005.

19. Deem S. Management of acute brain injury and associated respiratory issues. *Respir Care.* 2006;51:357–367.

20. Hession D. Management of traumatic brain injury: Nursing practice guidelines for cerebral perfusion and brain tissue oxygenation ($PbtO_2$) systems. *Pediatr Nurs.* 2008: 34(6). (Accessed November 7, 2010, at www.medscape.com/viewarticle/704918).

21. Ehtisham A, Taylor S, Bayless L, Klein MW, Janzen JM. Placement of external ventricular drains and intracranial pressure monitors. *Neurocrit Care.* 2009;10:241–247.

22. Pope W. External ventriculostomy: A practical application for the acute care nurse. *J Neurosci Nurs.* 1998;30:185.

23. Perkins LA, Barker JA. Intraabdominal Hypertension and Abdominal Compartment Syndrome. American College of Chest Physcians, PCCSU. www.chestnet.org/accp/pccsu/intraabdominal-hypertension-and-abdominal-comprtment-syndrome?page=0,3. Published November 1, 2010. (Accessed July 25, 2011).

24. Mulbrain M, Cheatham M, Kirkpatrick A, et al. Results from the international conference of experts on intra-abdominal hypertension and abdominal compartment syndrome. *Intens Care Med.* 2006;32:1722–1732.

25. Davidson J, Baumgariner F, Omari B, Milliken J. Intra-aortic balloon pump: Indications and complications. *J Natl Med Assoc.* 1998;90:137–140.

26. IABP timing and linear pocket reference guide. *Maquet Getinge Group* 2009.

27. Surbu H, Busch T, Aleksic I. Ischemic complications with intraaortic balloon counterpulsation: Incidence and management. *Cardiovac surg.* 2000;8:66–71.

28. Arceo A, Urban P, Dorsaz PA, et al. In-hospital complications of percutaneous intraaortic balloon counterpulsation. *Angiology.* 2003;54:577–585.

29. Pantalos GM, Koenig SC, Gillars KJ, Dowling R, Gray LA. Characterization of intraaortic balloon pump (IABP) timing errors using an adult cardiovascular simulator. *ASAIO Journal Abstracts.* 2001;47:143.

30. Marino PL. *The ICU Book. 3rd ed.* Philadelphia: Lippencott, Williams & Wilkens; 2006.

31. American Association of Critical Care Nurses. *Core Curriculum for Critical Care. 6th ed.* St. Louis: WB Saunders; 2005.

32. Gan T, Soppitt A, Maroof M, et al. Goal-directed intraoperative fluid administration reduces length of hospital stay after major surgery. *Anesthesiology.* 2002;97:820–826.

33. Michard F. Changes in arterial pressure during mechanical ventilation. *Anesthesiology.* 2005;103:419–428.

Chapter 4

Mechanical Ventilation

Thomas Johnson and Joann Bennett

LEARNING OBJECTIVES

1. Describe the indications for mechanical ventilation.
2. Understand the fundamental physics behind mechanical ventilation.
3. Develop a basic understanding of the function of positive pressure mechanical ventilation.
4. Describe the basic settings of mechanical ventilation and the impact on development of patient care plans.
5. Determine appropriate approaches to medication delivery related to the mechanical ventilator.

INTRODUCTION

Mechanical ventilation is a basic therapeutic and supportive intervention used in the critically ill patient. While pharmacists do not spend significant time working directly with the mechanical ventilator, a basic understanding of the settings used in and the function of mechanical ventilation is very helpful in the development of patient care plans. For example, sedation and analgesia regimens must take into account current ventilator settings, and nutrition regimens can impact or be impacted by mechanical ventilation. Complications, or avoiding complications, related to mechanical ventilation can be a significant component of developing patient care plans.

Understanding mechanical ventilation will also allow the pharmacist to better interpret medical literature and participate in interdisciplinary rounds. This chapter will cover the basics of mechanical ventilation with a focus on the impact on medication use.

History of Mechanical Ventilation

The history of mechanical ventilation dates at least as far back to a 1555 description of a tracheotomy and ventilation procedure, and initial work can be traced back at least one thousand years earlier.[1,2] However, the first workable negative pressure ventilator, the iron lung, was developed and produced by Drinker and Shaw in the late 1920s.[2,3] Positive pressure ventilation came of age during the polio epidemics of the 1950s with the large scale production of portable positive pressure mechanical ventilators.[1-4] Over the next 50 years, various modes and techniques of positive pressure ventilation have been attempted, revised, refined, abandoned, and revived. Current ventilators are capable of perhaps hundreds of combinations of settings and airflow patterns, but the fundamental principle of mechanical ventilation remains the same: moving air in and out of a patient's lungs.

Indications for Mechanical Ventilation

Mechanical ventilation is indicated in the patient requiring support to maintain oxygenation or eliminate carbon dioxide.[1,5-7] Mechanical ventilation may also be initiated for airway protection in an unresponsive or incoherent patient. A summary of the generally accepted indications and objectives for mechanical ventilation is listed in Table 4-1.

Table 4-1 Indications for and Objectives of Mechanical Ventilation[5-7]

Indications:	Reduce or change the work of breathing
Acute Respiratory Failure/Apnea	Reverse hypoxemia
Coma/Inability to protect airway	Reverse acute respiratory acidosis
Acute exacerbation of COPD	Relieve respiratory distress
Ventilatory dysfunction secondary to neuromuscular disorders	Prevent or correct atelectasis
Objectives:	Reverse or minimize ventilatory muscle fatigue
Alveolar ventilation	Permit sedation or neuromuscular blockade
Arterial oxygenation	Decrease systemic or myocardial oxygen consumption
Increase lung volume	Stabilize the chest wall

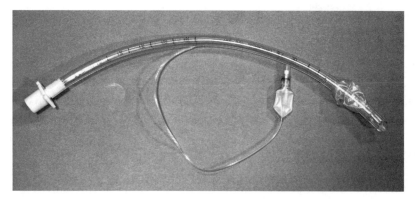

Figure 4-1 Endotracheal Tube

Source: © Jones & Bartlett Learning, courtesy of Maryland Institute for Emergency Medical Services Systems.

Physics of Mechanical Ventilation

Positive pressure invasive mechanical ventilation necessitates insertion of an endotracheal tube (ETT) illustrated in Figure 4-1. Ventilation without ETT insertion has been achieved with the advent of noninvasive ventilation techniques, and less critically ill patients may be managed without intubation. However, in this discussion, we will focus on the intubated patient on mechanical ventilation.

The ETT is smaller than the patient's natural airway, and as a result, airflow patterns change. These changes lead to increased airway resistance and increased work of breathing. The resistance in the tube can be illustrated by the equation $R = 8\eta\ell/\pi r^4$ (where η = viscosity, ℓ = length of tube, and r = internal radius of the tube), which is derived from Poiseuille's Law.[1,8,9] When the tube is lengthened or narrowed, resistance increases. Over time, new ventilator techniques have evolved to reduce the work of breathing associated with intubation and mechanical ventilation.

POSITIVE PRESSURE VENTILATION TERMINOLOGY

Airway Pressures

Positive pressure volume ventilation delivers tidal volume to the patient's lungs under pressure. Ventilated patients often have pulmonary pathology such as areas of damaged lung tissue, obstructed airways, and other structural abnormalities. It is important to remember that air behaves as a fluid, and therefore follows the path of least resistance as it enters the lungs. Therefore, it becomes necessary to understand and monitor several ventilation parameters.

Peak inspiratory pressure (PIP or P_{peak}) is the maximal airway pressure during the respiratory cycle.[5] PIP generally measures the pressures in the major airways. Significant or acute changes in PIP may indicate complications such as mucus plugging or bronchospasm, and elevated PIP necessitates clinical evaluation to identify the cause. Specific intervention or ventilator adjustment may be needed to decrease airway pressures in order to avoid the complications caused by prolonged airway pressure elevation.

Plateau pressure (P_{plat}) provides a measure of airway pressures at end inspiration, which reflects the pressure in the alveoli. P_{plat} is a major determinant of volutrauma and other ventilator complications (see Complications section). P_{plat} should be kept at or below 30 to 35 cm H_2O pressure.[10-16] In recent years, much attention has been directed toward avoiding ventilation with high pressure.

Volumes

Tidal volume (Vt) is defined as the volume of air breathed in and out during a respiratory cycle. Minute ventilation (MV—also abbreviated as Ve) is derived by multiplying respiratory rate by Vt. Minute ventilation is the primary respiratory determinant of blood CO_2 levels. Increasing MV will tend to decrease blood CO_2 by increasing CO_2 elimination. Decreasing MV will increase blood CO_2 by decreasing CO_2 elimination. The normal respiratory tract has several non-perfused areas referred to as physiologic dead space (V_{DS}),[17] which is the sum of anatomic (trachea, bronchus) and alveolar components that do not participate in CO_2 elimination. Adequate ventilation requires air ventilation and blood perfusion (sometimes denoted as V/Q) to be matched. Dead space to Tidal Volume ratio (V_{DS}/Vt) defines the ability of the lung to carry CO_2 from the pulmonary artery to the alveolus. Pathologic processes affect this ratio, as do ventilator settings. A good example of abnormal dead space is pulmonary embolism. In this situation, there is alveolar ventilation without blood perfusion, which leads to an increased V_{DS}/Vt ratio, resulting in abnormal oxygenation as well as ventilation.

Oxygen

The fraction of inspired oxygen (FiO_2) is the percentage of oxygen present in the air that is inhaled by the patient; for reference, room air has an FiO_2 of 0.21 (21%). An FiO_2 greater than 60% is associated with increased oxygen free radical production and potential cellular harm (oxygen toxicity).[1,10,18] Patients with poor respiratory function, including patients with severe acute respiratory distress syndrome (ARDS), often require FiO_2 values greater than 60% to maintain appropriate blood oxygen levels, and high FiO_2 levels should not be avoided at the expense of tissue oxygenation. The use of positive end expiratory pressure (PEEP) or other advanced ventilator recruitment techniques are directed toward reduction of FiO_2 to safe levels (i.e., <60%).[10,12,13,15]

Alveolar recruitment techniques allow alveoli that are not participating in ventilation to re-open and add to the functioning surface area for ventilation and oxygenation.[19-23] Recruitment is achieved by maximizing alveolar capillary function. Titration of PEEP is a form of alveolar recruitment that acts by adjusting the amount of pressure remaining within the lungs at the end of expiration. Using recruitment techniques encourages a higher number of alveoli to be opened or stay open. Prone positioning is also utilized in patients with ARDS to improve oxygenation via potential improvement in ventilation–perfusion match.[22,24-26]

VENTILATOR MODES AND SETTINGS

There are many ventilator settings and combinations of settings that are used in the management of critically ill patients. For simplicity, each setting will be discussed as a separate entity, but there are certainly instances where two or more settings will be used simultaneously. Table 4–2 summarizes the ventilator modes discussed in this section.

Controlled Mechanical Ventilation

In controlled mechanical ventilation (CMV), the ventilator does all of the work of breathing.[27,28] CMV restricts ventilation to only the set rate and volume prescribed. The patient cannot breath spontaneously in this mode, which typically leads to the need to deeply sedate and frequently paralyze the patient, as it is not a comfortable mode of ventilation. Strict CMV is not commonly employed, as most ventilators currently used in practice utilize settings that allow the patient to breath spontaneously and are often more comfortable for the patient.

Assist/Control

In current practice, CMV and the Assist/Control (A/C) mode of ventilation are essentially synonymous. In A/C, the patient receives a set rate and volume, but the patient may initiate spontaneous breaths as well.[28] All breaths delivered to the patient (spontaneous or ventilator initiated) provide the

Table 4–2 Summary of Ventilator Modes/Settings[23-27, 31-42]

Mode	Summary	Role	Sedation/Paralytics
CMV Controlled Mechanical Ventilation	Full support Set rate and volume	Complete ventilation	Often required
A/C Assist/Control	Full support Set rate and volume Patient may initiate breaths	Complete ventilation	Often required Minimal paralytics if vent adjusted
SIMV Synchronized Intermittent Mandatory Ventilation	Partial support Set rate and volume Patient breaths not fully supported	Weaning Post-operative	Sedation OK No paralytics
APRV Airway Pressure Release Ventilation	Full support P_{high} pressure maintained P_{low} pressure is the release pressure	Improve oxygenation in specific patients	Mode often reduces need for sedation and paralysis

Mode	Description	Use	Sedation
High-Frequency	Full support. Rapid, shallow breaths delivered to expanded lung	Improve oxygenation in acute respiratory distress syndrome patient	Deep sedation and paralysis commonly required
PS Pressure **S**upport	Minimal support. Pressure delivered to assist breath at beginning of inspiration	Weaning and combination with other modes	Light sedation. No paralytics
PEEP **P**ositive **E**nd **E**xpiratory **P**ressure	Pressure applied to exhalation phase to improve oxygenation	Increase oxygenation. Lung recruitment	N/A
CPAP **C**ontinuous **P**ositive **A**irway **P**ressure	Minimal support. PEEP without a set tidal volume	Weaning	Minimal sedation. No paralytics
ATC **A**utomatic **T**ube **C**ompensation	Pressure applied to overcome increased airway resistance	Weaning. Alternative to T-piece trial	Minimal sedation. No paralytics

full set tidal volume. Therefore, if the ventilator set rate is 12 breaths per minute (bpm), the patient is guaranteed 12 full breaths, but if their spontaneous rate is 20 bpm, they will receive 20 full breaths. The use of low tidal volumes and titrating PEEP with A/C mode is a standard approach to ventilation in the ARDS patient.

Intermittent Mandatory Ventilation

Sometimes referred to as synchronized intermittent mechanical ventilation (SIMV), intermittent mandatory ventilation (IMV) is a mode of ventilation where the ventilator is set to deliver a specific number of full breaths each minute (rate) with a set Vt. In addition, the patient may initiate and take spontaneous breaths that they generate without ventilator assistance.[28] Pressure support (PS), which may be added to each IMV breath, is, in essence, added support at the initiation of the spontaneous breath, which is the most difficult part of inhalation in terms of energy expenditure. This decreases the work of breathing and increases the tidal volume that can be spontaneously generated by the patient.

Illustration of Synchronized Intermittent Mechanical Ventilation

Because SIMV can be a difficult mode to visualize, a patient example is provided. A patient set to the ventilator mode of SIMV, rate of 12, Vt of 600, PS 10 means that the patient will receive 12 full breaths of a Vt of 600 ml each minute, and these breaths will be synchronized with the patient's own breathing rate. If the patient breathes 20 times per minute, 12 breaths will be fully supported and 8 breaths will be supported by 10 cm H_2O pressure support only. The number of set breaths can then be weaned down over time (typically by intervals of two) so that the patient slowly takes over the additional work of breathing.

Intermittent mandatory ventilation was originally thought of as a weaning mode of ventilation.[7,29] However, newer weaning techniques have now begun to replace the use of this ventilator approach.[29,30] The work of breathing is higher in modes that do not completely support the patient's respiratory needs, and so the use of IMV in the weaning process was based on the concept that "conditioning" the respiratory muscles would facilitate extubation. However, new approaches to ventilator management suggest that the use of SIMV in this way actually leads to muscle fatigue and may delay extubation.[29] Many intensive care physicians favor resting the patient on A/C and performing daily or twice daily spontaneous breathing trials (SBT) to assess weanability.[30,31]

Pressure vs. Volume Control

In modes such as A/C, volume ventilation provides a volume (Vt) without regard to the airway pressure required to deliver that volume. Pressure control ventilation delivers a tidal volume via a set pressure, which generates a tidal breath. The advantage of pressure control ventilation is that it generates less alveolar injury by decreasing the amount of alveolar stretching during inflation in an already fragile lung (such as in ARDS). Figures 4–2a and 4–2b illustrates the contrasting air-flow patterns of pressure versus volume delivery.[27] Many of the ventilator settings discussed in this chapter, but specifically CMV and A/C, can be delivered with either a pressure control setting or a volume control setting.

Airway Pressure Release Ventilation

Airway pressure release ventilation (APRV) is defined as continuous positive airway pressure (CPAP) with intermittent releases of pressure that produce gas exchange.[32,33] Instead of setting a specific Vt, the ventilator is set to maintain a P_{high} pressure and then release to a P_{low} pressure at regular intervals; the Vt is obtained by the change in pressure. The P_{high} pressure is

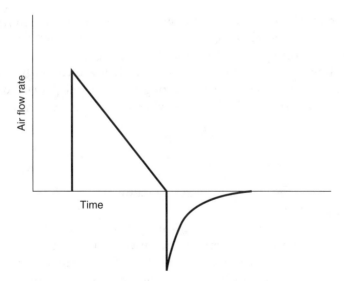

Figure 4–2a Pressure control with a decelerating air flow rate. A constant pressure is maintained in the ventilator circuit and a resulting Vt is delivered.

Data from: Chatburn RL, Branson RD. Classification of mechanical ventilation. In: MacIntyre NR and Branson RD, eds. *Mechanical Ventilation*. Philadelphia: WB Saunders Company; 2001:2–50.

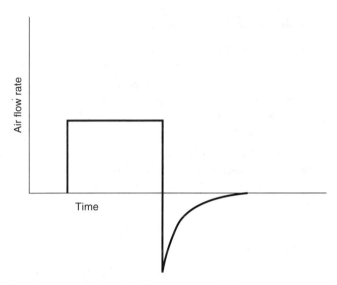

Figure 4–2b Volume control mode with a constant air flow rate, represented by the square waveform seen here. Constant air flow continues until the set Vt is delivered.

Data from: Chatburn RL, Branson RD. Classification of mechanical ventilation. In: MacIntyre NR and Branson RD, eds. *Mechanical Ventilation*. Philadelphia: WB Saunders Company; 2001:2–50.

maintained for the majority of time, and therefore maintains lung expansion and encourages alveolar recruitment. Generally, patients should be allowed to breathe spontaneously on top of the P_{high} pressure.[33] Paralytic use and deep sedation are needed significantly less often with APRV (as compared to some other ventilator settings) to allow the patient to accept this type of ventilation. Figure 4–3 provides a visual representation of airway pressure during APRV.

High-Frequency Ventilation

High-frequency ventilation is most commonly used in the neonatal and pediatric patient population.[34] The underlying concept is somewhat similar to that of APRV in that the lungs are expanded and then small, rapid breaths (~300 bpm) are delivered to the patient.[35] This high rate of breath delivery maintains open alveoli, yet still allows for oxygen delivery and the elimination of carbon dioxide. Unlike APRV, deep sedation and paralytics are usually required for the patient to tolerate this setting. Current indications in adults are rather limited, and further data and trials demonstrating improved outcomes with high-frequency ventilation are needed to support widespread use in adults.[34–37]

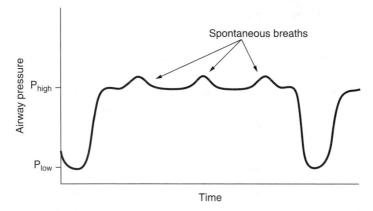

Figure 4–3 Airway Pressure Release Ventilation (APRV). This representative waveform shows the set P_{high} and P_{low} pressure levels as well as the spontaneous breaths generated by the patient.

Data from: Habashi NM. Other approaches to open-lung ventilation: Airway pressure release ventilation. *Crit Care Med* 2005;33(Suppl.):S228–S240. DOI: 10.1097/01.CCM.0000155920.11893.37.

Pressure Support

Pressure support (PS) may be used alone or in combination with other ventilation settings.[28] In this setting, the ventilator is set to deliver a specific pressure (e.g., 10 cm H_2O) at the initiation of a spontaneous breath to assist with overcoming initial airway resistance. Pressure support is generally considered a weaning mode of ventilation,[29,30] and as a lone setting has no set ventilatory rate. As the level of PS is decreased, the patient must assume more of the work of breathing.

Positive End Expiratory Pressure

Positive end expiratory pressure (PEEP) is positive pressure maintained in the airways during the exhalation phase of the respiratory cycle. It is used in conjunction with other modes of ventilation to improve oxygenation and prevent lung collapse. As described earlier, increasing levels of PEEP is a lung recruitment strategy and allows alveoli to remain open longer;[19-23] by remaining open, more lung surface area is available for oxygen exchange. The ARDSnet protocol for ventilation in patients with ARDS utilized a low tidal volume combined with progressively higher levels of PEEP and oxygen to maintain oxygenation.[12] This low tidal volume strategy reduces the sheering injury caused by high pressures that is felt to lead to worsened lung injury.[38]

58 | **Chapter 4:** Mechanical Ventilation

Continuous Positive Airway Pressure

Both inspiratory pressure (PS) and end expiratory pressure (PEEP) can be delivered alone or in conjunction with other ventilator modes. When PEEP is delivered without a set Vt, it is referred to as continuous positive airway pressure (CPAP). CPAP is also considered a weaning mode of ventilation, as patients often are placed on this setting to determine if they have a reasonable chance of progressing to extubation.

Automatic Tube Compensation

Automatic tube compensation (ATC) is available on newer ventilators. Similar to the PS setting, ATC delivers set pressure to the distal end of the artificial airway. In ATC, the pressure is calculated specifically to compensate for the increased resistance caused by the ETT, therefore simulating breathing without the tube in place.

Ventilator Parameters

While subjective criteria such as level of alertness and strength of cough are certainly used to determine if a patient may be ready for extubation, objective measures are also available. The rapid shallow breathing index (RSBI) is one example. The RSBI is calculated by dividing the respiratory rate by the Vt (in liters); an RSBI less than 100 is a reasonable indication that the patient is ready for extubation. Another example is the negative inspiratory force (NIF), which is a measure of the patient's ability to generate a breath. Pharmacists will often hear these terms, as well as others, and should at least have a working knowledge of the application of these measures.

Ventilator Settings Summary

An example of how ventilator settings may be ordered or otherwise reported would include the following elements: setting, rate, volume, FiO_2 (e.g., CMV, rate - 12, Vt - 700 mls, O_2 - 60%). Beyond the specific ventilator settings, it is important for the new practitioner with minimal experience working with and around ventilators to remember some simple concepts. First of all, ventilators are means to support the movement of air in and out of a patient's lungs. This is accomplished by delivering and allowing for exhalation of a Vt, which must be done at a set rate. Secondly, ventilators are capable of being set to do all of the work of breathing, or essentially none of the work of breathing, so it is important to understand how much a patient is participating in their own air exchange. Finally, remembering and understanding terms like recruitment, PEEP, low-volume ventilation, weaning, and breathing trials will be helpful during the care decision discussions that occur in ventilated, critically ill patients.

VENTILATOR COMPLICATIONS

Three of the most common complications associated with ventilatory support include volutrauma, hypotension, and ventilator-associated pneumonia (VAP).[39] Volutrauma is the result of overdistension of the alveoli unit in the lung, leading to overstretching of the alveoli and compression of the capillary bed, which then results in a ventilation/perfusion (V/Q) mismatch and increased shear force on adjacent collapsed alveoli.[4] Appropriate ventilator techniques can prevent this by maintaining low plateau pressures.

Initiation of positive pressure ventilation or titration of PEEP can affect the pleural (intrathoracic) pressure and result in systemic hypotension due to reduced venous return.[7] Hypotension secondary to mechanical ventilation can typically be addressed by fluid administration and ventilator adjustment, although occasionally vasopressors may be needed. However, hypotension in the critically ill patient is often multi-factorial, and mechanical ventilation may be only one element of a patient's hypotension.

Ventilator-associated pneumonia is a major complication of ventilation. The development of VAP is associated with increased morbidity and mortality as well as leading to longer ventilatory support time. Ventilator-associated pneumonia is nosocomial bacterial pneumonia that occurs in patients receiving mechanical ventilation for more than 48 hours after intubation.[40,41] Definitive diagnosis can be difficult as there are multiple comorbidities often present in ventilated patients.[42] Invasive treatment strategies including bronchoscopy procedures and appropriate initial antibiotics have been shown to decrease mortality and shorten treatment courses.[43] Appropriate initial antibiotic selection based upon suspected pathogens and local resistance patterns is extremely important to minimize mortality and complications associated with VAP.[44,45] Prediction of these pathogens may be based on time of pneumonia onset, as well as many other factors.[46,47] The clinician must carefully consider all of these factors in ventilated patients to ensure appropriate treatment of VAP.

The financial implications of VAP in the United States are significant, and so multiple strategies have been developed to prevent VAP. Shortening ventilation times is an obvious method for preventing VAP.[40,41] Body position also has been described in the prevention of VAP; a semirecumbent position, as compared to supine body position, decreased both clinically-suspected and microbiologically-confirmed VAP in one study.[48] Subsequent studies have not reproduced these results, but the trial designs were different.[49,50] Semirecumbency is an easy, noninvasive intervention, so elevation of the head of the bed to 30 to 45 degrees is generally recommended for the prevention of VAP and aspiration.[40,41,51]

Continuous subglottic suctioning utilizes a special endotracheal tube with a suction port in the dorsal area just above the ETT cuff. Continuous aspiration of subglottic secretions has been shown to decrease the rate of VAP.[52] While these special ET tubes are more expensive than standard tubes, there is some evidence that the reduction of VAP results in overall cost savings.[53] New types of ventilator strategies, oral cares, silver-coated tubes, and other interventions are being developed continuously, and many institutions utilize checklists of procedures and patient care techniques commonly referred to as "ventilator bundles" to help minimize or eliminate VAP as a complication.

NON-INVASIVE VENTILATION STRATEGIES

Bi-Level Positive Airway Pressure and Continuous Positive Airway Pressure

Non-invasive positive pressure ventilation (NPPV) strategies are becoming more common for several reasons. One reason is that more patients are using non-invasive ventilation at home to treat sleep disordered breathing (i.e., sleep apnea and related conditions). Further, because of the adverse events and discomfort associated with invasive mechanical ventilation, the use of non-invasive ventilation or ventilatory support continues to be investigated and trialed.

The two most common modes of non-invasive ventilation are continuous positive airway pressure (CPAP) and bi-level positive airway pressure (BiPAP). Both of these forms of non-invasive mechanical ventilation do not require an ET tube, but instead use a tight-fitting mask that covers either the nose or both the nose and mouth. This allows for higher pressures to be applied to the upper and lower airways, resulting in relief of upper airway obstruction and an increase in Vt and PEEP, which ultimately results in improvements in ventilation and oxygenation. The patient needs to be reasonably alert and not have any significant risk of aspiration in order to be a candidate for this type of ventilatory support.

Depending on the mode used, different pressures can be applied. The pressures are adjusted by a physician or respiratory therapist in order to decrease patient work of breathing, improve patient comfort, and improve variables such as ventilation and oxygenation. Non-invasive positive pressure ventilation can be used as a treatment for sleep disordered breathing, as an attempt to prevent intubation (especially in patients with chronic lung disease or congestive heart failure), and as a supportive therapy to prevent re-intubation in patients previously intubated and mechanically ventilated.

MECHANICAL VENTILATION IMPACT ON PHARMACOTHERAPY

Sedation and Analgesia

In the past, the initiation of mechanical ventilation most often meant that deep sedation and muscle paralysis were required for the patient to accept ventilation, which often resulted in prolonged ventilator times. Appropriate and comfortable ventilator adjustment is an important component of controlling anxiety and agitation in the ventilated patient. There are multiple studies indicating that daily wake-up and use of short-term sedatives lead to decreased ventilator times.[54-58] Less sedated patients are able to undergo more aggressive physical therapy and mobilization.[59] Despite attention to ventilation and patient comfort with the mode of ventilation, patient anxiety and agitation may still exist and require treatment.[60]

Ventilator strategies vary in the way they affect patient/ventilator synchrony, and therefore comfort. The overall goals of sedation and medication choice are dependent on many factors. When the patient is receiving ventilation through a full support mode such as CMV or A/C, the ventilator is completely supporting ventilation, thus allowing for deeper sedation without fear of respiratory depression. Patients on these modes may require and will tolerate paralysis, continuous sedative infusions, and continuous analgesics without adverse effects on the ventilation. It is important to note that mechanical ventilation by itself is not an indication for sedation; the indications for sedation are anxiety or agitation not relieved by non-pharmacologic methods.[59,60] As described in detail in Chapter 5, inappropriate use of sedatives and analgesics increases the risk of delirium, prolongs ventilation times, and further places the patient at risk for ventilator-associated complications.[61-63]

Modes of ventilation such as IMV, PS, or CPAP require different treatment strategies for anxiety, agitation, and delirium as deep sedation will suppress patient respiratory drive, and these modes require the patient to initiate their own breaths. Continuous benzodiazepines, propofol, and narcotic analgesics may be needed for patients on these weaning modes, but caution must be used to minimize the potential for respiratory depression. Dexmedetomidine (DEX), a central alpha-2 agonist, is a potential alternative as there is no respiratory depression associated with this agent.[64] DEX has been successfully used in small studies and case reports to facilitate weaning from mechanical ventilation after long-term sedation with other agents,[65-69] and may be particularly useful in patients suffering from physical withdrawal symptoms of recreational drugs such as alcohol or narcotics[70] or medications used for prolonged sedation and analgesia.[67-68] Additional studies have suggested a lower rate of delirium in certain populations treated with DEX.[71-75] Drug cost, especially at higher doses, is a disadvantage of DEX, and so additional larger scale studies are needed to more clearly define the role of this agent in mechanically ventilated patients to identify cost-effective strategies for use. It should be noted that any patient on non-invasive ventilation should only receive sedation medications under the specific guidance of a physician, as alterations in wakefulness can lead to disastrous results in patients with a confined mask over their mouth and nose.

Neuromuscular Blockade

Neuromuscular blockade is appropriate only in patients who are difficult to ventilate due to poor lung compliance, high airway pressures, or the inability to maintain a comfortable respiratory cycle with sedation and analgesia alone. Only after initiation of adequate sedative medications should neuromuscular blockers (NMBs) be used, as they have no sedative or analgesic properties. Common NMBs used for acceptance of ventilation include pancuronium, vecuronium, atracurium, and cisatracurium, and are discussed in detail in Chapter 5.[76] A peripheral nerve stimulator should be used to ensure patients achieve therapeutic goals with the minimum amount of medication, as excessive paralytic doses can lead to prolonged muscle weakness, prolonged ventilator times, and possible hemodynamic compromise. NMBs must be stopped prior to changing ventilator settings to a mode that does not provide full support as patients will not be able to breathe spontaneously.

Nutrition

Nutrition provision to the mechanically ventilated patient will be impacted by multiple factors. Ventilator settings or medications used to facilitate mechanical ventilation may alter nutrition measurements via indirect calorimetry or affect total caloric requirements. Mechanical ventilation and lung function may also affect the delivery or type of nutrition provided.

Indirect calorimetry (IC) directly measures oxygen consumed and carbon dioxide produced during the respiratory cycle to derive the patient's resting energy expenditure (REE) via the modified Weir equation.[77-79] The results are very helpful in designing patient-specific nutrition regimens, especially in patients with multiple co-morbidities or extremes of body habitus, although unfortunately many institutions do not have this technology readily available. General requirements to perform an accurate IC are FiO_2 <60%, consistent ventilator settings, a ventilator circuit that ensures direct gas measurement, a patient at rest or baseline level of arousal, and appropriate equipment and personnel. While mechanical ventilation is not required to perform this procedure, the intubated patient typically ensures a closed ventilatory circuit to minimize gas leaks that adversely affect test results. To maximize accuracy of IC, the test should not be performed within two hours of ventilator setting changes.[80]

There is minimal data directly correlating energy expenditure to specific ventilator modes, though increasing levels of sedation and chemical paralysis have both been shown to reduce energy expenditure in ventilated patients.[81,82] While this may indicate a relationship between energy expenditure and the work of breathing, further studies are needed to determine a direct correlation between ventilator modes and nutrition requirements of the patient. Increased minute ventilation has been linked to increased energy expenditure and has been included in some energy estimation equations,[83,84] though it is unclear if the increase in minute ventilation is the cause or the result of an increased metabolic rate.

Other factors that may affect nutrition delivery in the mechanically ventilated patient include concerns about aspiration, prone positioning, and weaning from mechanical ventilation. Gastric residual volume (GRV) is often used to assess tolerance of gastric tube feedings; however, the risk of aspiration does not correlate to measured GRV.[85] Clinicians are now generally using more liberalized limits for GRV in critically ill patients.[86] Prone positioning of mechanically ventilated patients presents challenges for providing enteral feeding, and published data is somewhat conflicting on the safety and effectiveness of enteral feeding in proned patients.[87,88] Interventions such as prokinetics, transpyloric feeding tube placement, and placing the patient in a semi-recumbent position may aid in tolerance of enteral feeds. Enteral feedings are also often held for weaning and discontinuation of ventilation. One study in a pediatric population has shown the safety of continuing transpyloric feedings during the weaning and extubation process, with equivalent adverse events in the group that continued nutrition versus the group that held nutrition.[89] Additional studies in adults will need to be completed to compel clinicians to alter the common practice of holding enteral feeds during the weaning and extubation process.

PRACTICAL CONSIDERATIONS

Nebulizers vs. Inhalers

Several medications may be delivered by aerosol administration, most commonly beta-2 agonists and anticholinergic medications, and guidelines for selection of appropriate delivery devices have been published.[90] Either metered dose inhalers (MDI) or nebulizers may be used in mechanically ventilated patients.[91,92] A spacer device should be used with MDIs and the inhaler should be actuated precisely with initiation of inspiration, with the dose for bronchodilators and anticholinergics roughly doubled from doses used in non-ventilated patients. Institution-specific equipment will influence the decision regarding routine use of nebulizers or MDIs for beta-2 agonist administration.[91] Techniques for the delivery of medication via a dry powder inhaler (DPI) have been described, but further studies are needed to determine optimal technique to achieve adequate drug deposition in the lungs with DPIs.[93]

Inhaled Antibiotics

There has been increasing interest over the last few years in the use of aerosolized antibiotics in mechanically ventilated patients.[94,95] With increases in multi-drug resistant organisms, the use of higher doses and more toxic medications is becoming more commonplace. To try to minimize systemic exposure and also to try to get high concentrations of antibiotic directly to the site of infection, inhaled antimicrobials have been employed. The most common medications used are the aminoglycosides, and positive effects have primarily been seen in clearing upper airway cultures and decreasing secretions in tracheobronchitis.

Some level of technical expertise is required to ensure adequate drug delivery to the target tissues, be it for antibiotics or other medications. The specifics of these techniques can be found in other reviews on the topic.[91-93,96]

NOVEL PHARMACOLOGIC INTERVENTIONS

Heliox

If we recall the physics of air flow in mechanical ventilation ($R = 8\eta\ell/\pi r^4$), resistance is determined by pressure and laminar flow, and laminar flow is affected by both the density and viscosity of the gas.[9] Since a helium/oxygen mixture has a lower density and higher viscosity than a standard nitrogen/oxygen mixture, flow is improved and resistance is reduced. Heliox in mechanically ventilated patients has been shown to decrease peak inspiratory airway pressures.[97,98] Large, randomized, controlled trials have not yet been completed, so the indications for heliox remain relatively limited to some severe asthma patients.[98,99]

Surfactant

Surfactant replacement has been used for many years in neonates to correct surfactant deficiencies in premature lungs. Adult patients with ARDS-associated respiratory failure exhibit alterations in both production and function of the different subtypes of surfactant.[100,101] Trials involving the recombinant form of surfactant protein C over the last several years have shown promise in animal models[102-104] and in subgroups of human trials,[105,106] but confirmatory trials are still needed to address the patient selection and usefulness of surfactant in adult patients with respiratory failure requiring intubation.[107]

SUMMARY

The pharmacist that works with mechanically ventilated patients should have a fundamental knowledge of mechanical ventilation to provide optimal pharmaceutical care. Many medication regimens impact or are impacted by the modes or types of mechanical ventilation. Ventilation and pharmacologic therapies continue to evolve quickly for critically ill patients, and new treatment strategies may be on the horizon.

KEY POINTS

- Mechanical ventilation is a key component of critical care practice.
- The various mechanical ventilation settings can affect the approach to sedation and analgesia, as well as how certain medications are delivered to the patient.
- Weaning or liberation from the mechanical ventilator is important to shorten length of ICU stay and minimize complications.
- Non-invasive ventilation is becoming a larger part of critical care management.

SELECTED SUGGESTED READINGS

- Cawley MJ. Mechanical ventilation: a tutorial for pharmacists. *Pharmacotherapy.* 2007;27:250–266.
- Gattinoni L, Caironi P, Cressoni M, et al. Lung recruitment in patients with the acute respiratory distress syndrome. *N Engl J Med.* 2006;354:1775–1786.

- AARC Clinical Practice Guideline: Metabolic measurement using indirect calorimetry during mechanical ventilation – 2004 revision & update. *Respir Care.* 2004;49(9):1073–1079.
- Dhand R. Aerosol delivery during mechanical ventilation: from basic techniques to new devices. *J Aerosol Med Pulm Drug Deliv.* 2008;21:45–60.

REFERENCES

1. Marino PL, Sutin KM. *The ICU book. 3rd ed.* Philadelphia: Lippincott Williams & Wilkins; 2007.
2. Cawley MJ. Mechanical ventilation: a tutorial for pharmacists. *Pharmacotherapy.* 2007;27:250–266.
3. Barbarash RA, Smith LA, Godwin JE, Sahn SA. Mechanical ventilation. *Ann Pharmacother.* 1990;24:959–970.
4. Gluck E, Sarrigianidis A, Dellinger RP. Mechanical Ventilation. In: Parrillo JE and Dellinger RP, eds. *Critical care medicine: Principles of diagnosis and management in the adult. 2nd ed.* St. Louis: Mosby, Inc.; 2002:137–161.
5. Tobin MJ. Advances in mechanical ventilation. *N Engl J Med.* 2001;344(26): 1986–1996.
6. Pierson DJ. Indications for mechanical ventilation in adults with acute respiratory failure. *Resp Care.* 2002;47(3):249–265.
7. Slutsky AS. ACCP Consensus Conference: mechanical ventilation. *Chest.* 1993;104:1833–1859.
8. Nave CR. Poiseuille's Law. (Accessed July 18, 2011 at http://hyperphysics.phy-astr.gsu.edu/hbase/ppois.html).
9. Hess DR, Fink JB, Venkataraman ST, Kim IK, Myers TR, Tano BD. The history and physics of Heliox. *Respir Care.* 2006;51(6):608–612.
10. Brower RG, Rubenfeld GD. Lung-protective ventilation strategies in acute lung injury. *Crit Care Med.* 2003;31(Suppl.):S312–S316.
11. Cordingley JJ, Keogh BF. The pulmonary physician in critical care – 8: ventilatory management of ALI/ARDS. *Thorax.* 2002;57:729–734.
12. The Acute Respiratory Distress Syndrome Network. Ventilation with lower tidal volumes as compared with traditional tidal volumes for acute lung injury and the acute respiratory distress syndrome. *N Engl J Med.* 2000;342:1301–1308.
13. McIntyre RC, Pulido EJ, Bensard DD, Shames BD, Abraham E. Thirty years of clinical trials in acute respiratory distress syndrome. *Crit Care Med.* 2000;28:3314–3331.
14. Ware LB, Matthay MA. The acute respiratory distress syndrome. *N Engl J Med.* 2000;342(18):1334–1349.
15. Villar J, Kacmarek RM, Perez-Mendez L, Aguirre-Jaime A. A high positive end-expiratory pressure, low tidal volume ventilatory strategy improves outcome in persistent acute respiratory distress syndrome: a randomized, controlled trial. *Crit Care Med.* 2006;34:1311–1318.
16. Slutsky AS, Ranieri VM. Mechanical Ventilation: Lessons from the ARDSNet trial. *Respir Res.* 2000;1:73–77.

17. Peruzzi WT, Shapiro BA. Arterial blood gases. In: Parrillo JE and Dellinger RP, eds. *Critical care medicine: Principles of diagnosis and management in the adult.* *2nd ed.* St. Louis: Mosby, Inc.; 2002:202–223.

18. Gammon RB, Strickland JH, Kennedy JI, Young KR. Mechanical ventilation: a review for the internist. *Am J Med.* 1995;99:553–562.

19. Gattinoni L, Caironi P, Cressoni M, et al. Lung recruitment in patients with the acute respiratory distress syndrome. *N Engl J Med.* 2006;354:1775–1786.

20. Richard JC, Maggiore SM, Jonson B, Mancebo J, LeMaire F, Brochard L. Influence of tidal volume on alveolar recruitment: respective role of PEEP and a recruitment maneuver. *Am J Respir Crit Care Med.* 2001;163: 1609–1613.

21. Richard JC, Brochard L, Vandelet P, et al. Respective effects of end-expiratory and end-inspiratory pressures on alveolar recruitment in acute lung injury. *Crit Care Med.* 2003;31:89–92.

22. Lim CM, Jung H, Koh Y, et al. Effect of alveolar recruitment maneuver in early acute respiratory distress syndrome according to antiderecruitment strategy, etiological category of diffuse lung injury, and body position of the patient. *Crit Care Med.* 2003;31:411–418.

23. Mols G, Priebe HJ, Guttmann J. Alveolar recruitment in acute lung injury. *Br J Anaesth.* 2006;96(2):156–166.

24. Galiatsou E, Kostanti E, Svarna E, et al. Prone position augments recruitment and prevents alveolar overinflation in acute lung injury. *Am J Respir Crit Care Med.* 2006;174:187–197.

25. Alsaghir AH, Martin CM. Effect of prone positioning in patients with acute respiratory distress syndrome: a meta-analysis. *Crit Care Med.* 2008;36: 603–609.

26. Fan E, Mehta S. High-frequency oscillatory ventilation and adjunctive therapies: inhaled nitric oxide and prone positioning. *Crit Care Med.* 2005;33(Suppl.):S182–S187.

27. Chatburn RL, Branson RD. Classification of mechanical ventilation. In: MacIntyre NR and Branson RD, eds. *Mechanical Ventilation.* Philadelphia: WB Saunders Company; 2001:2–50.

28. Branson RD, Campbell RS. Modes of ventilator operation. In: MacIntyre NR and Branson RD, eds. *Mechanical Ventilation.* Philadelphia: WB Saunders Company; 2001:51–84.

29. Hess D. Ventilator modes used in weaning. *Chest.* 2001;120:474S–476S.

30. MacIntyre NR, Cook DJ, Ely EW, et al. Evidence-based guidelines for weaning and discontinuing ventilatory support: a collective task force facilitated by the American College of Chest Physicians; the American Association for Respiratory Care; and the American College of Critical Care Medicine. *Chest.* 2001;120:375S–395S.

31. Girard TD, Kress JP, Fuchs BD, et al. Efficacy and safety of a paired sedation and ventilator weaning protocol for mechanically ventilated patients in intensive care (Awakening and Breathing Controlled trial): a randomised controlled trial. *Lancet.* 2008;371:126–134.

32. McCunn M, Habashi NM. Airway pressure release ventilation in the acute respiratory distress syndrome following traumatic injury. *Int Anesthesiol Clin.* 2002 Summer;40(3):89–102.

33. Habashi NM. Other approaches to open-lung ventilation: airway pressure release ventilation. *Crit Care Med.* 2005;33(Suppl.):S228–S240.

34. Derdak S. High-frequency oscillatory ventilation for acute respiratory distress syndrome in adult patients. *Crit Care Med.* 2003;31(Suppl.):S317–S323.

35. Salim A, Martin M. High-frequency percussive ventilation. *Crit Care Med.* 2005;33(Suppl.):S241–S245.

36. Chan KPW, Stewart TE. Clinical use of high-frequency oscillatory ventilation in adult patients with acute respiratory distress syndrome. *Crit Care Med.* 2005;33(Suppl.):S170–S174.

37. Imai Y, Slutsky AS. High-frequency oscillatory ventilation and ventilator-induced lung injury. *Crit Care Med.* 2005;33(Suppl.):S219–S314.

38. Piantoadosi CA, Schwartz DA. The acute respiratory distress syndrome. *Ann Intern Med.* 2004;141:460–470.

39. Chatila WM, Criner GJ. Complications of long-term mechanical ventilation. *Resp Care Clin.* 2002;8:631–647.

40. Kollef MH. The prevention of ventilator-associated pneumonia. *N Engl J Med.* 1999;340:627–633.

41. Kollef MH. Prevention of hospital-associated pneumonia and ventilator-associated pneumonia. *Crit Care Med.* 2004;32:1396–1405.

42. Wunderink RG. Clinical criteria in the diagnosis of ventilator-associated pneumonia. *Chest.* 2000;117:191S–194S.

43. Fagon JY, Chastre J, Wolff M, et al. Invasive and noninvasive strategies for management of suspected ventilator-associated pneumonia. *Ann Intern Med.* 2000;132:621–630.

44. Fowler RA, Flavin KE, Barr J, Weinacker AB, Parsonnet J, Gould MK. Variability in antibiotic prescribing patterns and outcomes in patients with clinically suspected ventilator-associated pneumonia. *Chest* 2003;123:835–844.

45. Kuti EL, Patel AA, Coleman CI. Impact of inappropriate antibiotic therapy on mortality in patients with ventilator-associated pneumonia and blood stream infection: a meta-analysis. *J Crit Care.* 2008;23:91–100.

46. Singh N, Falestiny MN, Rogers P, et al. Pulmonary infiltrates in the surgical ICU: prospective assessment of predictors of etiology and mortality. *Chest.* 1998;114:1129–1136.

47. Ibrahim EH, Ward S, Sherman G, Kollef MH. A comparative analysis of patients with early-onset vs late-onset nosocomial pneumonia in the ICU setting. *Chest.* 2000;117:1434–1442.

48. Drakulovic MB, Torres A, Bauer TT, Nicolas JM, Nogue S, Ferrer M. Supine body position as a risk factor for nosocomial pneumonia in mechanically ventilated patients: a randomized trial. *Lancet.* 1999;354:1851–1858.

49. van Nieuwenhoven CA, Vandenbroucke-Grauls C, van Tiel FH, et al. Feasibility and effects of the semirecumbent position to prevent ventilator-associated pneumonia: a randomized study. *Crit Care Med.* 2006;34:396–402.

50. Girou E, Buu-Hoi A, Stephan F, et al. Airway colonization in long-term mechanically ventilated patients. *Intensive Care Med.* 2004;30:225–233. Epub 29 Nov 2003.

51. Scolapio JS. Methods for decreasing risk of aspiration pneumonia in critically ill patients. *JPEN.* 2002;26:S58–S61.

52. Lacherade JC, De Jonghe B, Guezennec P, et al. Intermittent subglottic secretion drainage and ventilator-associated pneumonia: a multicenter trial. *Am J Respir Crit Care Med.* 2010;182:910–917.

53. Shorr AF, O'Malley PG. Continuous subglottic suctioning for the prevention of ventilator-associated pneumonia. *Chest.* 2001;119:228–235.

54. Schweickert WD, Gehlbach BK, Pohlman AS, Hall JB, Kress JP. Daily interruption of sedative infusions and complications of critical illness in mechanically ventilated patients. *Crit Care Med.* 2004;32:1272–1276.

55. Carson SS, Kress JP, Rodgers JE, et al. A randomized trial of intermittent lorazepam versus propofol with daily interruption in mechanically ventilated patients. *Crit Care Med.* 2006;34:1326–1332.

56. Wittbrodt ET. Daily interruption of continuous sedation. *Pharmacotherapy.* 2005;25(5):3S–7S.

57. Muellejans B, Matthey T, Schlopp J, Schill M. Sedation in the intensive care unit with remifentanil/propofol versus midazolam/fentanyl: a randomised open-label, pharmacoeconomic trial. *Crit Care.* 2006;10:R91.

58. Richman PS, Baram D, Varela M, Glass PS. Sedation during mechanical ventilation: a trial of benzodiazepine and opiate in combination. *Crit Care Med.* 2006;34:1395–1401.

59. Kress JP, Hall JB. Sedation in the mechanically ventilated patient. *Crit Care Med.* 2006;34:2541–2546.

60. Society of Critical Care Medicine and American Society of Health-System Pharmacists: Clinical Practice Guidelines for the Sustained Use of Sedatives and Analgesics in the Critically Ill Adult. *Am J Health-Syst Pharm.* 2002;59:150–178.

61. Arroliga A, Frutos-Vivar F, Hall J, Esteban A, Apezteguia C, Soto L, Anzueto A. Use of sedatives and neuromuscular blockers in a cohort of patients receiving mechanical ventilation. *Chest.* 2005;128:496–506.

62. Pandharipande P, Shintani A, Peterson J, et al. Lorazepam is an independent risk factor for transitioning to delirium in intensive care unit patients. *Anesthesiology.* 2006;104:21–26.

63. Riker RR, Fraser GL. Adverse events associated with sedatives, analgesics, and other drugs that provide patient comfort in the intensive care unit. *Pharmacotherapy.* 2005;25(5):8S–18S.

64. Venn RM, Newman PJ, Grounds RM. A phase II study to evaluate the efficacy of dexmedetomidine for sedation in the medical intensive care unit. *Intensive Care Med.* 2003;29:201–207.

65. Multz AS. Prolonged dexmedetomidine infusion as an adjunct in treating sedation-induced withdrawal. *Anesth Analg.* 2003;96:1064–1065.

66. Tobias JD. Dexmedetomidine to treat withdrawal following prolonged opioid administration to infants and children. *Anesthesiology.* 2005;103:A1369 [abstract].

67. Siobal MS, Kallet RH, Kivett VA, Tang JF. Use of dexmedetomidine to facilitate extubation in surgical intensive-care-unit patients who failed previous weaning attempts following prolonged mechanical ventilation: a pilot study. *Respir Care.* 2006;51(5):492–496.

68. Kent CD, Kaufman BS, Lowy J. Dexmedetomidine facilitates the withdrawal of ventilatory support in palliative care. *Anesthesiology.* 2005;103:439–441.

69. Marcel R, Weido J, Hebeler RF, Ramsay MA. Early extubation in cardiovascular surgery facilitated by dexmedetomidine. *Anesthesiology.* 2004;101:A392 [abstract].

70. Rovasalo A, Tohmo H, Aantaa R, Kettunen E, Palojoki R. Dexmedetomidine as an adjuvant in the treatment of alcohol withdrawal delirium: a case report. *Gen Hospl Psych.* 2006;28:362–363.

71. Shehabi Y, Ruettimann U, Adamson H, Innes R, Ickeringill M. Dexmedetomidine infusion for more than 24 hours in critically ill patients: sedative and cardiovascular effects. *Intensive Care Med.* 2004;30:2188–2196.

72. Guinter JR, Kristeller JL. Prolonged infusions of dexmedetomidine in critically ill patients. *Am J Health Syst Pharm.* 2010;67:1246–1253.

73. Riker RR, Shehabi Y, Bokesch PM, et al. Dexmedetomidine vs midazolam for sedation of critically ill patients: a randomized trial. *JAMA.* 2009;301:489–499.

74. Pandharipande PP, Pun BT, Herr DL, et al. Effect of sedation with dexmedetomidine vs lorazepam on acute brain dysfunction in mechanically ventilated patients: the MENDS randomized controlled trial. *JAMA.* 2007;298:2644–2653.

75. Darrouj J, Puri N, Prince E, Lomonaco A, Spevetz A, Gerber DR. Dexmedetomidine infusion as adjunctive therapy to benzodiazepines for acute alcohol withdrawal. *Ann Pharmacother.* 2008;42:1703–1705.

76. Society of Critical Care Medicine and American Society of Health-System Pharmacists. Clinical practice guidelines for sustained neuromuscular blockade in the adult critically ill patient. *Am J Health Syst Pharm.* 2002;59:179–195.

77. McClave SA, McClain CJ, Snider HL. Should indirect calorimetry be used as part of nutritional assessment? *J Clin Gantroenterol.* 2001;33(1):14–19.

78. AARC Clinical Practice Guideline: Metabolic measurement using indirect calorimetry during mechanical ventilation – 2004 revision & update. *Respir Care.* 2004;49(9):1073–1079.

79. Smyrnios NA, Curley FJ, Shaker KG. Accuracy of 30-minute indirect calorimetry studies in predicting 24-hour energy expenditure in mechanically ventilated, critically ill patients. *JPEN.* 1997;21:168–174.

80. Brandi LS, Bertolini R, Santini L, Cavani S. Effects of ventilator resetting on indirect calorimetry measurement in the critically ill surgical patient. *Crit Care Med.* 1999;27:531–539.

81. Barton RG, Craft WB, Mone MC, Saffle JR. Chemical paralysis reduces energy expenditure in patients with burns and severe respiratory failure treated with mechanical ventilation. *J Burn Care Rehabil.* 1997;18:461–468.

82. Terao Y, Miura K, Saito M, Sekino M, Fukusaki M, Sumikawa K. Quantitative analysis of the relationship between sedation and resting energy expenditure in postoperative patients. *Crit Care Med.* 2003;31:830–833.

83. Frankenfield DC, Coleman A, Alam S, Cooney RN. Analysis of estimation methods for resting metabolic rate in critically ill adults. *JPEN*. 2009;33:27–36.
84. Frankenfield D, Smith S, Cooney RN. Validation of 2 approaches to predicting resting metabolic rate in critically ill patients. *JPEN*. 2004;28:259–264.
85. McClave SA, Lukan JK, Stefater JA, et al. Poor validity of residual volumes as a marker for risk of aspiration in critically ill patients. *Crit Care Med*. 2005;33:324–330.
86. Montejo JC, Minambres E, Bordeje L, et al. Gastric residual volume during enteral nutrition in ICU patients: the REGANE study. *Intensive Care Med*. 2010;36:1386–1393.
87. Reignier J, Thenoz-Jost N, Fiancette M, et al. Early enteral nutrition in mechanically ventilated patients in the prone position. *Crit Care Med*. 2004;32:94–99.
88. van der Voort PH, Zandstra DF. Enteral feeding in the critically ill: comparison between the supine and prone positions: a prospective crossover study in mechanically ventilated patients. *Crit Care*. 2001;5:216–220.
89. Lyons KA, Brilli RJ, Wieman RA, Jacobs BR. Continuation of transpyloric feeding during weaning of mechanical ventilation and tracheal extubation in children: a randomized controlled trial. *JPEN*. 2002;26:209–213.
90. Dolovich MB, Ahrens RC, Hess DR, et al. Device selection and outcomes of aerosol therapy: evidence-based guidelines: American College of Chest Physicians/American College of Asthma, Allergy, and Immunology. *Chest*. 2005;127:335–371.
91. Duarte AG. Inhaled bronchodilator administration during mechanical ventilation. *Respir Care*. 2004;49(6):623–634.
92. Dhand R. Basic techniques for aerosol delivery during mechanical ventilation. *Respir Care*. 2004;49(6):611–622.
93. Dhand R. Inhalation therapy with metered-dose inhalers and dry powder inhalers in mechanically ventilated patients. *Respir Care*. 2005;50(10): 1331–1344.
94. Palmer LB. Aerosolized antibiotics in critically acutely ill ventilated patients. *Curr Opin Crit Care*. 2009;15:413–418.
95. Palmer LB, Smaldone GC, Chen JJ, et al. Aerosolized antibiotics and ventilator-associated tracheobronchitis in the intensive care unit. *Crit Care Med*. 2008;36:2008–2013.
96. Dhand R. Aerosol delivery during mechanical ventilation: from basic techniques to new devices. *J Aerosol Med Pulm Drug Deliv*. 2008;21:45–60.
97. Pizov R, Oppenheim A, Eidelman LA, Weiss YG, Sprung CL, Cotev S. Helium versus oxygen for tracheal gas insufflation during mechanical ventilation. *Crit Care Med*. 1998;26:290–295.
98. Venkataraman ST. Heliox during mechanical ventilation. *Respir Care*. 2006;51(6):632–639.
99. Brenner B, Corbridge T, Kazzi A. Intubation and mechanical ventilation of the asthmatic patient in respiratory failure. *Proc Am Thorac Soc*. 2009;6:371–379.
100. Poynter SE, LeVine AM. Surfactant biology and clinical application. *Crit Care Clin*. 2003;19(3):459–472.

101. Eisner MD, Parsons P, Matthay MA, Ware L, Greene K. Plasma surfactant protein levels and clinical outcomes in patients with acute lung injury. *Thorax.* 2003;58:983–988.

102. Elsasser S, Schächinger H, Strobel W. Adjunctive drug treatment in severe hypoxic respiratory failure. *Drugs.* 1999;58(3):429–446.

103. Häfner D, Germann PG, Hauschke D. Comparison of rSP-C surfactant with natural and synthetic surfactants after late treatment in a rat model of the acute respiratory distress syndrome. *British J Pharm.* 1998;124:1083–1090.

104. Mikawa K, Nishina K, Takao Y, Obara H. Intratracheal application of recombinant surfactant protein-C surfactant to rabbits attenuates acute lung injury induced by intratracheal acidified infant formula. *Anesth Analg.* 2004;98:1273–1279.

105. Spragg RG, Lewis JF, Wurst W, Häfner D, Baughman RP, Wewers MD, Marsh JJ. Treatment of acute respiratory distress syndrome with recombinant surfactant protein C surfactant. *Am J Respir Crit Care Med.* 2003;167:1562–1566.

106. Spragg RG, Lewis JF, Walmrath HD, et al. Effect of recombinant surfactant protein C-based surfactant on the acute respiratory distress syndrome. *N Eng J Med.* 2004;351:884–892.

107. Spragg RG, Taut FJH, Lewis JF, et al. Recombinant surfactant protein C based surfactant for patients with severe direct lung injury. *Am J Respir Crit Care Med.* 2011;183(8):1055–1061.

Chapter 5

Analgesia, Sedation, and Delirium Management

John Kappes

LEARNING OBJECTIVES

1. Describe the indications for analgesia and sedation.
2. Understand the physiologic responses to pain and stress that commonly occur in the critically ill.
3. Describe the effective use of scales to assess and manage pain, sedation, and delirium in the intensive care unit.
4. Determine appropriate analgesia regimens for critically ill patients.
5. Utilize multiple patient factors to develop and monitor the need for sedation regimens in the critically ill.
6. Develop medication regimens for the treatment of delirious, critically ill patients.
7. Delineate the appropriate use and monitoring of neuromuscular blockade in patients in the intensive care unit.

INTRODUCTION

Increased heart rate, alertness, sweating, and rate and depth of respiration are all signs and symptoms of a well-conditioned athlete running an endurance race. These signs are not unlike the symptoms observed in the critical care patient population, such as tachycardia, diaphoresis, and tachypnea, which arise via activation of the sympathetic nervous system in order to increase cardiac output and maintain vital organ perfusion. Release of endorphins provides pain relief, and increased metabolic functions are initiated to aid in healing.[1,2] Therefore, the physiologic stress response of a distance runner and a critically ill patient are remarkably similar, but unlike the well-conditioned athlete, critically ill patients may not stop "running" for days and are not always capable of enduring this continuous stress response.

In the setting of acute illness and continuous stimulation, this physiologic response can cause deleterious effects. These effects may include: hypertension, myocardial ischemia, hyperglycemia, nitrogen wasting, and many others.[1] Couple these effects with extreme exhaustion, sleep deprivation, confusion, numerous sources of pain, fear, lights, alarms, memory loss, mechanical devices, and surgery—just to name a few—and little effort is required to understand the feelings of anxiety a patient may have.[3] The persistence and perpetuation of these stimuli often lead to further feelings of anxiety, which may give way to agitation and eventually delirium.

Pain, anxiety, agitation, and delirium seem inevitable in the setting of the intensive care unit (ICU), but these symptoms may be alleviated with adequate analgesia and sedation. The indication for analgesia is pain and discomfort, whereas the indication for sedation is not well defined but is generally considered appropriate for unrelieved anxiety and/or agitation.[4] Sedation may also be utilized to decrease oxygen consumption, which may be elevated in acute lung injury or shock.[5] While mechanical ventilation and anxiety/agitation frequently coexist, mechanical ventilation alone is not an indication for sedation. In fact, it is not uncommon for a patient to have less anxiety or agitation once intubated because air hunger is alleviated.

Despite proper use of analgesia and sedation, the incidence of delirium in the ICU is reported to be as high as 80%. Signs and symptoms of delirium include acute changes in mental status, erratic and disorganized thinking, distorted level of awareness, and possibly agitation. Routine assessment and treatment of delirium is recommended in guidelines on analgesia and sedation.[4]

Occasionally, treatment regimens require patients to be completely passive, and this can be accomplished with neuromuscular blocking agents. Most often the indication for neuromuscular blockade is to facilitate mechanical ventilation or allow tolerance of different modes of mechanical ventilation.[6] Chemical paralysis may also be used to control shivering when inducing hypothermia status post-cardiac arrest or neurologic injury.[7]

This chapter will focus on the pharmacotherapy of medications used for analgesia, sedation, treatment of delirium, and neuromuscular blockade.

PAIN AND SEDATION SCALES

Pain

In order to properly utilize sedative and analgesic agents, quick, reliable, and valid assessment scales are fundamental. Development of pain scales for an unresponsive or nonverbal patient that meet these criteria is difficult. There are several pain scales available, including visual analog scales (VAS), verbal rating scales (VRS), numeric rating scales (NRS), objective pain rating scales, pictorial rating scales, pain questionnaires, and others. In a trial comparing several of these scales in burn patients, Gordon and colleagues[8] found the pictorial faces pain rating scale to be the most preferred, while the visual analog scale was the least preferred. Failure to identify what contributed to this preference limits the results of this trial, yet other reports have suggested the numeric scale to have the least variance and therefore was concluded to be the best tool utilized.[2]

Each of these scales has advantages and disadvantages, but each can be impractical in the unresponsive/nonverbal patient. Patient self-reporting is the most reliable and valid indicator of pain and is optimal when the patient can respond. Surrogates (i.e., friends and family) may help in determining pain when the patient is unable to respond; it has been estimated that surrogates accurately identified the presence or absence of pain in 73.5% of patients, but only described the level of pain correctly 53% of the time.[9] Other scales have been utilized for nonverbal patients with some success, including the observer-reported face scales and a behavioral pain scale. Both of these scales were validated and found to have at least some correlation with a self-reporting scale.[10,11]

Ultimately, healthcare practitioners must rely on indicators or behaviors that may reflect pain in nonverbal patients. Indicators of pain can be divided into physiologic and behavioral indicators (Table 5–1).[12] It is important to note that physiologic measures have been found to be the least sensitive indicators of pain because resolution of these measures may be seen before the patient experiences pain relief.[12,13]

Beyond identification of pain and degree or level of pain, healthcare practitioners also need to evaluate the type, duration, intensity, and site of pain. Further defining the type of pain into somatic, visceral, or neuropathic may help to identify the source of tissue damage and the cause of pain.[2] Determining acute versus chronic status, as well as duration, of pain will aid in the selection of short or long-acting agents, scheduling of each agent, and need for a continuous infusion. Intensity of pain may assist in dosage of the medication, while site of pain and medication properties may help in selection of the most appropriate agent. Clearly, the more details obtained about the pain sensation

Table 5-1 Pain Indicators in a Nonverbal Patient[12]

Behavior Indicators	Physiologic Indicators
Restlessness	Increase or decrease in heart rate by 15% or more from baseline
Sighing	Increase or decrease in blood pressure by 15% or more from baseline
Gasping	Increase stroke volume
Bracing	Increased or decreased respiratory rate
Grimacing	Dilated pupils
Frowning	Pallor
Wincing	Perspiration
Muscle tension	Nausea
Clenching of teeth	Vomiting
Wrinkling of forehead	Flushing
Tearing	
Decreased, hesitant, or cautious movements	
Withdrawal reflexes	
Thrashing	
Assuming special positions or postures	
Rocking or rhythmic movements	
Kicking	
Massaging or rubbing areas of body	

will aid the practitioner in selecting the most appropriate treatment, as well as increasing the possibility of alleviating the cause of pain.

While considerable debate and time have been consumed on proper assessment of pain, the most important fact remains that any assessment is better than no assessment. Many believe pain should be considered the fifth vital sign.[14]

Sedation

While the indication for sedation is not as well-defined as that of analgesics, the need to monitor levels of sedation is equally as important. This importance was demonstrated in a trial that found significantly less pain and sedation in the intervention group, which used a sedation scale, compared to a control group (pain 42% vs. 63%, p < 0.02; agitation 12% vs. 29%, p < 0.02).[15] An observation of significantly reduced mechanical ventilation times was also found (65 vs. 120 hours, P < 0.01). In another trial, proper use of a sedation scale and a sedation protocol not only found a reduction of mechanical ventilation times, but also a decrease in length of stay.[16]

Numerous scales have been developed to increase the consistency of assessment and to aid in the titration of sedative agents. Interrater reliability is a key characteristic in the validity of each scale. Examples of sedation scales include: Riker Sedation-Agitation Scale (SAS), Motor Activity Assessment Scale (MAAS), Ramsay Scale, Richmond Agitation Sedation Scale (RASS), Vancouver Interaction and Calmness Scale (VICS), and others, which are described in Table 5–2.[18-21] No consensus has been established as to the best scale to utilize;[4,17] therefore, an institution should select one standard, validated scale in order to maximize effective use.

The goal or target sedation level is ideally determined before initiation and revaluated on a routine basis. Selection of the target level will vary depending on the patient's condition and/or disease states. Sedation goals can also be selected based on the mode of mechanical ventilation and a patient's compliance or synchrony with ventilation. Current guidelines support maintaining the lightest sedation possible in order to maintain patient comfort and a typical pattern of sleep and wakefulness.[4] Development of protocols that allow for fluctuation and titration in sedation agents to obtain goal sedation levels is recommended in national guidelines.

ANALGESIA

Pain

Tissue damage produces a neural afferent impulse known as nociception. Noxious stimuli that can cause tissue damage is an extensive list: trauma, various disease states, catheters, drains, noninvasive ventilating devices, endotracheal tubes, airway suctioning, physical therapy, dressing changes, patient mobilization, prolonged immobility, and numerous others.[22,23] Understandably, any procedure can potentially cause pain, but in a large trial with more than 6,000 ICU patients, turning was identified as the most painful procedure in adult patients.[24]

Pain will propagate the stress response and a number of effects will be seen, including catecholamine release, sympathetic stimulation, mydriasis, anxiety, diaphoresis, catabolism, tachycardia, increased myocardial oxygen

Table 5–2 Common Sedation Scales[18-21]

Score	Description	Definition
Ramsay Sedation Scale		
1	Patient anxious or agitated, or both	
2	Patient cooperative, oriented, and tranquil	
3	Patient responds to commands only	
4	Brisk response to light, glabellar tap, or loud auditory stimulus	
5	Sluggish response to light, glabellar tap, or loud auditory stimulus	
6	No response to light, glabellar tap, or loud auditory stimulus	
Riker Sedation-Agitation Scale (SAS)		
7	Dangerous agitation	Pulling at endotracheal tube, trying to remove catheters, climbing over bedrail, striking at staff, thrashing side to side
6	Very agitated	Does not calm despite frequent verbal reminding of limits, requires physical restraints, biting endotracheal tube
5	Agitated	Anxious or mildly agitated, attempts to sit up, calms down to verbal instruction
4	Calm and cooperative	Calm, awakens easily, follows commands
3	Sedated	Difficult to arouse, awakens to verbal stimuli or gentle shaking but drifts off again, follows simple commands
2	Very sedated	Arouses to physical stimuli but does not communicate or follow commands, may move spontaneously
1	Unarousable	Minimal or no response to noxious stimuli, does not communicate or follow commands
Motor Activity Assessment Scale (MAAS)		
6	Dangerous agitation, uncooperative	No external stimulus is required to elicit movement; patient is uncooperative (pulling/thrashing/striking) and does not calm when asked

Table 5–2 Common Sedation Scales[18-21] (*continued*)

Score	Description	Definition
5	Agitated	No external stimulus is required to elicit movement; patient tries to sit up or climb out of bed and does not consistently follow commands
4	Restless and cooperative	No external stimulus is required to elicit movement; patient pulls at sheets or uncovers self, but follows commands
3	Calm and cooperative	No external stimulus is required to elicit movement; patient adjusts sheets or clothing purposefully and follows commands
2	Responsive to touch or name	Opens eyes, raises eyebrows, or turns head toward stimulus or moves limbs when touched or spoken to
1	Responsive only to noxious stimulus	Opens eyes, raises eyebrows, or turns head toward stimulus or moves limbs with noxious stimulus
0	Unresponsive	Does not move with noxious stimulus

Richmond Agitation and Sedation Scale (RASS)

Score	Description	Definition
+4	Combative	Overtly combative, violent, immediate danger to staff
+3	Very agitated	Pulls or removes tube(s) or catheter(s)
+2	Agitated	Frequent non-purposeful movement, fights ventilator
+1	Restless	Anxious but movements are not aggressive or vigorous
0	Alert and calm	
−1	Drowsy	Not fully alert, but has sustained awakening to voice (≥10 sec)
−2	Light sedation	Briefly awakens with eye contact to voice (<10 sec)
−3	Moderate sedation	Movement or eye opening to voice (but no eye contact)
−4	Deep sedation	No response to voice, but movement or eye opening to physical stimulation
−5	Unarousable	No response to voice or physical stimulation

demand, tachypnea, water retention, and others. If pain goes untreated and unrelieved, additional effects may be seen, such as desynchronized ventilation, disruption of sleep, immune suppression, inappropriate thrombus formation, and altered glucose control. Unrelieved pain can also impact tissue perfusion by altering hemodynamic parameters through the release of interleukin-6, interleukin-1, and tumor necrosis factors.[2]

Pain Receptor Pharmacology

A number of receptors are involved in the multifaceted neurotransmission of pain. The initial receptor responsible for sensing and initiating the pain signal is called the nociceptor. Following noxious stimuli and the initial signal of pain, a balance of excitatory and inhibitory receptors will either maintain or block the transmission of the signal. Excitatory receptors include neurokinins, tackykinins, and glutamate, and inhibitory receptors include serotonin, noradrenaline, and opioid. Research and pharmacologic management of pain has found the most significant receptors are the opioid receptors, the most common of which include delta, kappa, and mu receptors.[2] These receptors are presynaptic and primarily located in the periphery, dorsal root ganglia, spinal cord, and select supraspinal areas.[25]

Stimulation of opioid receptors and subsequent coupling with G-protein cause potassium channels to open, allowing an efflux of the cation. Inhibition of calcium influx is also seen with stimulation of an opioid receptor. With a relative decrease in intracellular positively charged ions (i.e., potassium and calcium), the cell becomes hyperpolarized or less excitable; therefore, stimulation of the nociceptor cannot cause enough depolarization to transmit a signal of pain.[25] The stimulation of opioid receptors is also thought to decrease the release of the excitatory neurotransmitter tachykinin, but the significance of this mechanism has not been established.[26] Amnestic effects have been described with stimulation of the opioid receptors, but these effects are not dependable.[5]

Of the opioid receptors, mu is the most common target for opiate medications such as morphine and fentanyl. While binding to the mu-1 receptor produces the desired effect of analgesia, mu-2 receptors are responsible for the adverse effects of reduced gastric motility and constipation, as well as respiratory depression, sedation, and euphoria.[2,5] Kappa receptors are stimulated by the analgesic agents butorphanol and naloxone. Adverse effects from kappa stimulation are typically dysphoria, sedation, and miosis; these adverse effects may be reduced if the kappa agonist is selective to peripheral kappa receptors. Currently there are no medications on the market that stimulate gamma, but gamma agonists are actively being studied given the minimal effects seen on the respiratory and gastrointestinal system. There is also less potential for opioid abuse with a gamma agonist.[2,5,25]

Analgesic Agents

Morphine, fentanyl, and hydromorphone are the most common analgesic agents used in critical care.[4] Acetaminophen, ketorolac, remifentanil, and meperidine are other analgesic agents that can be used. Head-to-head trials of analgesics have not been performed in the setting of critically ill patients. Selection between analgesic agents is primarily based on the pharmacokinetic and pharmacodynamic properties of the agent, type of pain, co-morbid disease states, and clinician or patient preference. Dosing of analgesic agents should be based on several factors: acute vs. chronic pain, invasive vs. noninvasive ventilation, severity of pain, and opioid-naïve vs. opioid-tolerant patients.[2] Scheduled or continuous infusions have been recommended over intermittent, "as needed" regimens by clinical guidelines. It is also apparent that using analgesia for prevention of pain is more effective than treatment of existing pain.[4] With selection and administration of an analgesic agent, nonpharmacologic interventions should also be considered in order to increase patient comfort. Table 5–3 summarizes the properties of the narcotic analgesics.[2,4,5,23,25,27,34]

Opioid Analgesics

Morphine Morphine, named after Morpheus, the Greek god of dreams, is the oldest opioid and has classically been the drug of choice for analgesia in the ICU.[26,27] Due to morphine's hydrophilic properties, a long onset of action is observed.[5] Intermittent therapy is recommended, since morphine has a longer half-life and duration of effect.[4] Morphine undergoes glucuronidation in the liver and is metabolized to 80% morphine-3-glucuronide and 20% morphine-6-glucuronide. Morphine-3-glucuronide has no analgesic effect, but morphine-6-glucuronide has 20 to 40 times the activity of its parent compound.[28] Both metabolites are eliminated by the kidney, and so administration of morphine in the setting of renal insufficiency leads to accumulation of metabolites and, subsequently, an increased risk of adverse effects.[27] All opioids can potentially cause hypotension through reduction in sympathetic tone, and therefore decrease heart rate and systemic vascular resistance. Morphine, in particular, has additional hypotensive effects caused by increased venous capacitance that leads to reduced venous return as well as a histamine release.[2,5] Morphine is, therefore, considered the preferred analgesic agent in acute

Table 5-3 Analgesic Agents[2,4,5,23,25,27,34]

Drug	MOA	Onset (min)	Duration (hrs)	Starting IV Dose	IV Equianalgesic Dose	Metabolism	Active Metabolites	Ellimination	Comment
Fentanyl	mu receptor agonist	5	1-2	25-50 mcg	100 mcg	Oxidation	None	Renal	Fast onset. Repeated doses may accumulate
Hydromorphone	mu receptor agonist	5-8	2-3	0.2-0.6 mg	1.5 mg	Glucuronidation	None	Renal	High potency
Morphine	mu receptor agonist	30	3-5	2-5 mg	10 mg	Glucuronidation	morphine-3-glucuronide, morphine-6-glucuronide	Renal	Avoid in renal impairment & hemodynamic instability
Remifentanil	mu receptor agonist	1.5	≈5 min	0.05-0.15 mcg/kg/min		Plasma esterase	remifentanil acid	N/A	Requires continuous infusion

myocardial infarctions. In the setting of euvolemia, hemodynamic effects are usually transient and cause minimal complications.[29] However, the use of morphine should be avoided in patients who are hemodynamically unstable, with renal insufficiency, or who have a morphine allergy. The release of histamine by morphine may cause pruritus or a mild rash, which typically resolves in 5 to 7 days.[2] Some clinicians believe that, at normal doses, histamine release is rarely of clinical importance.[27,29]

Hydromorphone   Hydromorphone is a potent opioid with a quick onset of action (5 to 8 minutes) and duration of action similar to that of morphine (~3 hours). Metabolism and elimination are also similar to morphine, which requires the liver to degrade the molecule and the kidneys to excrete the metabolites. Hydromorphone has several distinct advantages over morphine. First, it lacks clinically significant active metabolites, so even in renal insufficiency an accumulation of metabolites should not increase adverse events. Second, hydromorphone has no significant histamine release, leading to fewer alterations in hemodynamic parameters. Third, the intravenous formulation of hydromorphone is seven times more potent than morphine. With a ratio of 1:7 for intravenous hydromorphone:morphine, a prescribed dose of hydromorphone 1 mg IV would be equal to 7 mg IV of morphine. Caution should be used with doses greater than 1 mg in opioid naïve patients. Hydromorphone is recommended for patients with hemodynamic instability or renal insufficiency.[2] Due to hydromorphone's structural similarity to morphine, cross sensitivity is possible, and consequently, use of hydromorphone should be avoided when patients have a true morphine allergy.

Fentanyl   Fentanyl has the most rapid onset and shortest half-life of the commonly-used opioids, which is due to the lipophilic nature of the medication. The lipophilic properties also increase the risk of accumulation with prolonged infusions and potentially delay recovery.[27] This highly-potent opioid has fewer hemodynamic effects than any other opioid.[2] Fentanyl is often considered the preferred agent for acute pain in the ICU. It is metabolized to inactive metabolites that are then excreted via renal elimination, which makes it an attractive agent in the setting of renal insufficiency, and clinical guidelines currently recommend fentanyl over all other analgesic agents in the setting of renal insufficiency.[4]

Fentanyl patch formulations should be used with caution, if used at all, in the ICU. First, with concomitant use of vasopressors, peripheral vasoconstriction may lead to decreased subcutaneous absorption. Second, patch formulations are not easily titrated to desirable effects and may result in prolonged duration to peak effect and time to elimination after discontinuation. Third, ICU patients frequently have fevers, which may affect absorption of a patch formulation. Finally, the acute nature and rapid changes of type and intensity of most pain in the ICU make transdermal formulations particularly difficult to manage.

Overall, fentanyl has been shown to be the preferred agent in hemodynamically unstable patients and those with renal insufficiency or severe acute pain, and it may be used in patients with morphine allergies because it is a synthetic compound. However, its use should be avoided in those with an allergy to fentanyl.

Remifentanil Due to a limited number of studies in the ICU and its cost, remifentanil is not widely used at this time. Its properties are intriguing and potentially advantageous for critically ill patients. Remifentanil is a derivative of fentanyl and has an ultra-short half-life that requires administration as a continuous infusion.[30] The metabolism of remifentanil is unique to that of the opioid class; other opioids, such as fentanyl, require hepatic biotransformation followed by renal elimination, whereas remifentanil is metabolized by nonspecific tissue and plasma esterases.[27,31] The metabolite remifentanil acid is active but significantly less potent than the parent compound (800 to 2000 times less).[31] Volume of distribution is approximately one-tenth that of fentanyl, so accumulation and delayed recovery are not complications of remifentanil even with prolonged infusion as the half-life remains consistent at 3.2 minutes. Pharmacokinetic properties of remifentanil are not affected by any degree of renal or hepatic insufficiency. The adverse effects profile is similar to that of all other opioids; of note, chest wall rigidity is common after bolus doses.[31] When comparing remifentanil to fentanyl in postoperative ICU patients, both agents were found to be safe and equally efficacious,[32] but when comparing remifentanil to a morphine-based regimen, a significantly reduced mechanical ventilation time was observed in the remifentanil arm.[33] The use of remifentanil analgosedation (analgesia-based sedation), as compared to midazolam plus fentanyl or morphine (sedative-based sedation), found significantly shorter mechanical ventilation time and shorter ICU length of stay.[34] Infusions of remifentanil lasting longer than three days should be avoided due to limited data in long term use of the medication. With growing data about remifentanil's safety and efficacy, as well as improved outcomes with use of analgesia before sedation, perhaps a trend may be seen toward analgosedation with use of remifentanil or other narcotics over current sedation and analgesia regimens.

Opioid Adverse Effects

Major adverse effects of nausea and vomiting, euphoria, respiratory depression, and reduced gastric motility are concerns with any opioid receptor agonist. Stimulation of chemoreceptors, the vestibular apparatus, and the gastrointestinal system all contribute to the adverse effect of nausea and vomiting. However, as treatment continues, tolerance to nausea and vomiting may develop.[2]

Opioids are well known to interact with the dopaminergic system, often producing euphoria or mood alterations, but the exact mechanism of central nervous system (CNS) adverse effects is unknown. Miosis or pinpoint pupils may be observed after opioid administration due to stimulation of the parasympathetic system. In a dose-dependent fashion, respiratory depression is likely due to reduced responsiveness to carbon dioxide in the brainstem respiratory centers.[26] An increase in respiratory depression may be seen if opioids are given in conjunction with benzodiazepines.[27] Respiratory rate, minute volume, and tidal exchange can all be affected by opioid administration.[26] The ventilation response to hypoxia may be blunted, and if this occurs a right shift in the CO_2 response curve will be observed. Lipophilic agents will reach maximal respiratory depression more rapidly than hydrophilic agents; the maximal effect on respiratory drive can be observed in 5 to 10 minutes after intravenous administration of morphine. With standard opioid doses and normal elimination, respiratory depression rarely occurs.[26]

Unfortunately, patients do not develop tolerance to constipation or reduced gastric motility. Stimulant medications and stool softeners should be administered while on opioid therapy.[2]

Opioid withdrawal may occur in more than 30% of ICU patients who receive analgesic therapy for greater than seven days. Opioid withdrawal may appear in a wide array of signs, such as diaphoresis, hypertension, tachypnea, tachycardia, piloerection, vomiting, or diarrhea. Symptoms may include hypersensitivity to pain, anxiety, restlessness, opioid craving, irritability, etc., and may arise within 12 hours of opiate discontinuation.[35] To prevent signs and symptoms of withdrawal, guidelines recommend gradual tapering, with daily dose decreases of 5–10%.[2]

Opioid agents described thus far have been parenteral agents. It is important to remember that oral opioid analgesics such as oxycodone or hydrocodone/acetaminophen are excellent alternatives to intravenous medications if the patient is able to swallow tablets, or has other enteral access, and has a functional gastrointestinal system.

Other Analgesics

There are other analgesic agents available for use in the ICU, which in certain situations may prove beneficial over the commonly used intravenous opioid agents. Acetaminophen is a common analgesic agent used in intensive care units; primarily used for its antipyretic properties, when used in combination with an opioid, it often produces a greater analgesic effect than the opioid alone.[4] It is available in multiple formulations, including the recently approved IV formulation marketed as Ofirmev. Practitioners should be cognizant of the amount of acetaminophen used so as not to exceed 3 grams (4 grams at most) in a 24-hour period or 2 grams with patients who have a history of significant alcohol use.[36] Caution should also be taken to prevent excessive acetaminophen use or avoid use altogether in individuals with depleted glutathione stores caused by hepatic dysfunction or malnutrition.[4]

Ketorolac is a nonsteroidal anti-inflammatory with opioid-like analgesic effects and minimal anti-inflammatory effect. The analgesic effect may not be enough for ketorolac to be used alone, but its use may decrease narcotic analgesic requirements.[37] No respiratory depression or drug dependence is seen with ketorolac, but five or more days of ketorolac therapy may increase the risk of gastrointestinal bleeding and more than doubles the risk of acute renal failure.[38-40] In select high-risk patients with a history of chronic renal insufficiency, volume depletion, or other significant risk factors for kidney injury, even one dose can cause acute kidney injury.

Similar to the other opioid agents, meperidine is metabolized by the liver and excreted by the kidneys.[5] Meperidine has a more rapid onset of action (3 to 5 min) compared to morphine due to its more lipophilic properties, has a shorter duration of action, and is much less potent. The metabolite normeperidine has significant CNS toxicities including apprehension, tremors, delirium, and seizures.[41] Due to its similar structure to atropine, meperidine may also cause tachycardia.[29] Meperidine has significant drug–drug interactions with monoamine oxidase inhibitors (MOAIs) as well as selective serotonin reuptake inhibitors (SSRIs); therefore, these combinations should be avoided.[4] Use of meperidine should be avoided in most settings, with the exception of some benefit as a onetime dose to treat shivering secondary to induced hypothermia, amphotericin B administration, or postoperative shivering. In fact, many institutions have removed meperidine from their formulary or significantly restrict its use.

SEDATION

One of the primary goals of treating any patient is to provide comfort and rest. While pain is one of the most common causes of discomfort, numerous other factors may contribute. Inability to communicate, constant noise, ambient light, overstimulation, lack of mobility, temperature, sleep deprivation, and physiologic disturbances, among other elements, could all lead to discomfort.[4] Eventually, these factors produce feelings of anxiety often resulting in agitation, but some patients may exhibit fear or become withdrawn.[4] The incidence of agitation in the ICU has been estimated at 71% of all ICU patients, with the majority (97%) of etiology being multifactoral.[42] Untreated anxiety and agitation could lead to ventilator dysynchrony, increased oxygen consumption, and unintentional removal of devices and catheters.[4] The use of sedative agents reduces the stress response and increases patient tolerance to routine ICU care.[43]

The use of sedative agents to provide comfort and rest comes with a price of several adverse effects that may cause additional complications in care or delay recovery. These adverse effects differ depending on the selected sedative agent. Selection of sedative agent may be made in order to avoid an adverse effect of another agent, but may also be made based on certain properties of a particular agent. As with the selection of analgesics, no single agent works for all situations; the advantages and disadvantages must be considered with each agent. Table 5–4 lists common sedatives and basic information for each.[4,5,27,29,39]

Gamma-Aminobutyric Acid Stimulants

Gamma-aminobutyric acid (GABA) is an inhibitory neuroreceptor that, when stimulated, causes CNS depression. The GABA receptors are a counterbalance to the excitatory neurotransmitters.[27] Stimulation of the GABA receptor causes an influx of chloride ions, thus producing a hyperpolarized state and reducing the neurons' ability to propagate an action potential.[29] This mechanism of action is depicted in Figure 5–1.[44] Commonly used GABA stimulants include benzodiazepines as well as propofol.

Benzodiazepines

All benzodiazepines produce a dose-dependent depression of the CNS, ranging from mild depression of responsiveness to complete obtundation. Benzodiazepines are lipophilic agents and distribute widely into fat tissue and, therefore, have a large volume of distribution. Distribution into the peripheral tissues has no clinical effect.[29] To reach full clinical effect, a saturation of tissues may be necessary, which may require large doses in the setting of obesity.

Administration of midazolam or lorazepam can achieve sedation through intermittent dosing or continuous infusions.[45] With prolonged continuous infusions of benzodiazepines, these lipid-soluble drugs accumulate in the peripheral tissues. Upon discontinuation of the infusions, a redistribution of the peripheral stores produces a prolonged sedative

Table 5-4 Sedative Agents[4,5,27,29,39]

Drug	Mechanism of action	Onset (min)	Duration	Half-life (hrs)	Starting Dose	Metabolism	Excretion	Comment
Midazolam	GABA stimulation	3–5	30–80 min	1.8–6.4*	Intermitent: 1–4mg q1hr prn Infusion: 0.C2–0.1 mg/kg/hr	Liver	Renal	Amnesic properties
Lorazepam	GABA stimulation	5–20	6–8 hrs	12	Intermitent: 1–4mg q1–6hr prn Infusion: 1–4 mg/hr	Liver	Renal	Propylene glycol (PEG) accumulation with prolonged use
Propofol	GABA stimulation	1–2	3–10 min	1.5–12.4 min	5 mcg/kg/min	Liver	Renal	Formulated in a lipid emulsion
Dexmedetomidine	alpha-2 agonist	1–2	4 hrs	2–2.67	0.2 mcg/kg/hr	Liver	Renal	Loading dose not commonly recommended
Ketamine	NMDA antagonist	<1	5–10 min	2–3	Bolus: 0.2–0.75 mg/kg Infusion: 5–20 mcg/kg/min	Liver	Renal	
Pentobarbital	GABA stimulation	<5	Varies	15–48	Bolus: 10 mg/kg over 30 min, then 5 mg/kg q1hr x 3 hrs Infusion: 1 ng/kg/hr	Liver	Renal	Primary use is to decrease intracranial pressure. Requires frequent monitoring
Thiopental	GABA stimulation	<1	10–30 min	3–18	1.5–3.5 mg/kg	Liver	Renal	Decreases intracranial pressure

*Half-life in renal failure patients may increase 1.5–2 fold

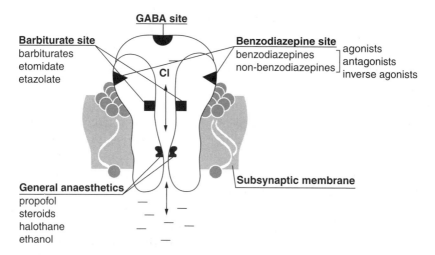

Figure 5-1 GABA receptor mechanism of action

Source: Reproduced from Richards G, Schoch P, Haefely W. Benzodiazepine receptors: new vistas. *Seminars in Neuroscience*. 1991;3:191–203.

effect that will unpredictably delay awakening times.[4,46,47] Clinical recovery from benzodiazepine accumulation may take hours to days.[47] Risk of accumulation increases in several clinical settings, including obese or elderly patients, as well as those with hepatic and/or renal insufficiency.[29] Use of the lowest effective dose, daily sedative interruptions, frequent reassessment of sedation requirements, and active tapering can reduce the risk of accumulation.[4,16,29]

There are numerous other characteristics shared by all benzodiazepines. Twenty percent receptor occupancy by benzodiazepines provides anxiolysis, 30% to 50% occupancy provides sedation, and 60% occupancy is needed to induce hypnosis.[48] Benzodiazepines produce anterograde amnesia or amnesia of current events, but induction of retrograde amnesia is not perceived.[4] In addition to amnesia, benzodiazepines have anxiolytic properties and at high-enough doses, can produce hypnosis.[29] An opioid sparing effect may be seen with appropriate use of benzodiazepines.[45] All benzodiazepines have anticonvulsant properties and are drugs of choice in the treatment of active seizures.[50] A dose-dependent, centrally mediated respiratory depression can be observed with any benzodiazepine. Respiratory depression is only moderate in healthy individuals but is enhanced in those with chronic respiratory disease.[27] The respiratory depression characteristics are different from that of opioids and presents as a decrease in tidal volume, increase in respiratory rate, and elimination of ventilatory response to hypoxia. The respiratory depression may not be as profound as from opioids, but a synergistic effect has been observed when using benzodiazepines and opioids together. Effects on the cardiovascular system are typically a decrease in blood pressure without a change in heart rate, but this is rarely seen in the setting of euvolemia.[29] Paradoxical agitation with use of benzodiazepines is not well understood, though a hypothesis of drug-induced disorientation from light sedation has been proposed to cause this inconsistent agitation.[4] Benzodiazepines, in particular lorazepam, are independent risk factors for the development of delirium.[51] Benzodiazepine-induced delirium will be further discussed later in this chapter.

Midazolam and lorazepam are the most frequently used benzodiazepines for sedation. Midazolam has a rapid onset of action (3 to 5 min) and a short duration of action (30 to 80 min). These parameters make midazolam a preferred agent for acute agitation.[4] Midazolam is extensively metabolized via oxidation by the CYP450 enzyme system in the liver. The primary metabolite, alpha-hydroxymethylmidazolam, is an active metabolite which is excreted by the kidneys.[27] Therefore, use of midazolam in renal insufficiency increases the risk of accumulation. Accumulation may also be seen in the obese and patients with low albumin.[52-54] The metabolism of midazolam may be inhibited by propofol, diltiazem, macrolide antibiotics, and other inhibitors of the CYP450 enzyme system, therefore causing prolonged sedative effects.[55-57]

Lorazepam's onset of action is 5 to 20 minutes, as it takes longer to cross the blood–brain barrier in comparison to midazolam. The duration of action is 6 to 8 hours and is relative to the dose given.[29] Metabolism of lorazepam goes through hepatic glucuronidation to inactive metabolites, which are then excreted via renal elimination.[5] Lorazepam requires a diluent of propylene glycol (1,2-propanediol) vehicle in order to dissolve into a solution. This is a common diluent used for many other medications, such as etomidate, diazepam, nitroglycerin, and phenytoin; however, lorazepam requires the highest concentration (830 mg/ml) to produce a solution.[58]

Despite the fact that the Food and Drug Administration (FDA) has determined propylene glycol to be safe as a vehicle for IV medication, adverse effects have been reported. These adverse effects include hyperosmolarity, hemolysis, cardiac arrhythmias, seizure, coma, and agitation. Propylene glycol toxicity can present much like systemic inflammatory response syndrome (SIRS) with lactic acidosis, hypotension, and multi-organ dysfunction.[59] Assays to measure propylene glycol concentrations typically are unavailable at most institutions, so osmolar gap may be a surrogate marker for propylene glycol toxicity. For patients receiving 1 mg/kg/day or greater doses of lorazepam, a correlation to osmol gap was found.[58] An osmol gap of 10 or greater had a high predictive value for propylene glycol toxicity.[60] Additionally, an osmol gap of 12 or greater predicted the development of acute kidney injury or metabolic acidosis, which are clinical markers of propylene glycol toxicity. If a propylene glycol assay is done, concentrations of greater than 18 mg/dl are associated with acute kidney injury and/or metabolic acidosis that may be representative of propylene glycol toxicity, although it should be noted that toxicity has been found with concentrations as low as 12 mg/dl.[58] The incidence of propylene glycol toxicity in patients receiving lorazepam for sedation was suggested in a small trial to be about 19%.[59]

In a direct comparison of midazolam vs. lorazepam for sedation, lorazepam was found to be more potent and have a longer duration of action, which may correlate to longer delays in recovery time.[61] In this trial, lorazepam was found to maintain optimal sedation goals 49% of the time, where midazolam met goals 69% of the time. Deep sedation was seen more often with lorazepam than midazolam. The average awakening time with lorazepam was 8.7 hours, compared to 3 hours for midazolam. Similarly, time to extubation after drug discontinuation was longer with lorazepam (21.2 hours) than midazolam (5.4 hours).

Overall, benzodiazepines are preferred in cases of seizures, alcohol withdrawal, deep or prolonged sedation, asthma and ARDS (if respiratory depression is desired), and in end-of-life care. Lorazepam should be avoided in patients with hepatic insufficiency, whereas midazolam should be avoided in patients with renal insufficiency. The benzodiazepines should also be avoided in individuals who require frequent neurological checks.

Propofol

Propofol (2,6 diisopropylphenol) is a sterically hindered phenol and has a similar mechanism of action to benzodiazepines, in that it stimulates the GABA receptors. It should be noted that the binding site for propofol on the GABA receptor is different than that of benzodiazepines; it is this alternative binding site that gives propofol the ability to produce sedation or hypnosis, as well as work as a general anesthetic.[4,27] Propofol has a significantly shorter onset (1 to 2 minutes) and duration of action when compared to benzodiazepines, primarily based on its lipophilic properties that allow rapid crossing of the blood–brain barrier. The depth of sedation and duration of action is dose dependent. Upon discontinuation of propofol infusion, the drug redistributes into the periphery, where it is inactive, and this results in a rapid emergence from sedation.[5] It appears that propofol may have shorter extubation times than midazolam-based sedation regimens. Oxidation in the liver metabolizes propofol to inactive metabolites, which are then excreted by the kidneys. Unlike benzodiazepines, propofol pharmacokinetics are not affected by hepatic or renal insufficiency.[27] Propofol has anxiolytic and amnesic properties but no analgesic effects.[5] Although somewhat controversial, propofol may be an effective anticonvulsant.[62,63] The adverse effect profile of propofol includes bradycardia, hypotension (particularly with bolus doses and rare in euvolemia), and significant respiratory depression with a decrease in tidal volume and respiratory rate. Injection site pain may occur in up to two-thirds of patients if a peripheral vein is used for infusions.[27]

Propofol is highly hydrophobic and therefore requires a formulation of oil-in-water emulsion in order to produce a solution. This 10% lipid emulsion provides 1.1 kcal/ml and should be accounted for as part of caloric intake. Extended infusions or high doses of propofol have been associated with causing hypertriglyceridemia and pancreatitis.[4] While reports are conflicting, it is estimated 31% of patients on propofol experience one elevated triglyceride level and 18% develop hypertrigylceridemia. Of the patients who develop hypertriglyceridemia, 10% will develop pancreatitis. Due to the risk of hypertriglyceridemia and pancreatitis, it is recommended to check serum triglycerides for any patient receiving more than two days of therapy, especially in individuals requiring infusions of 50 mcg/kg/min or greater.[64] Anecdotally, triglycerides should also be closely monitored in obese patients. When hypertriglyceridemia is detected, alternative sedative therapy should be considered.

Propofol infusion syndrome is a potentially life-threatening adverse effect. Complications from propofol infusions were first identified in pediatric patients, and the syndrome was then later defined by Bray in 1998.[65] Subsequently in 2000, Perrier et al. [66] reported the first case of death related to propofol infusion in an adult, and in 2001, Cremer et al.,[67] in a retrospective analysis, identified seven adult patients determined to have died from propofol infusion syndrome.

Propofol infusion syndrome is defined as: (1) the sudden onset of marked bradycardia resistant to treatment, with progression to asystole; (2) the presence of lipemia; (3) a clinically enlarged liver secondary to fatty infiltration; (4) the presence of severe metabolic acidosis; and (5) the presence of muscle involvement with evidence of rhabdomyolysis or myoglobinuria. A positive diagnosis requires the presence of bradycardia and at least one sign of lipemia, enlarged liver, metabolic acidosis, or rhabdomyolysis.[65] Other clinical features include: hypotension, increased serum creatine kinase, hyperkalemia, increased triglycerides, and renal and cardiac failure.[63,68,69]

Several mechanisms have been proposed that may contribute to propofol infusion syndrome. Propofol inhibits the mitochondria's ability to uptake long chain free fatty acids and uncouples oxidative phosphorylation, which inhibits short and medium chain free fatty acids from mitochondria utilization, ultimately reducing energy production and causing cardiac and peripheral muscle necrosis. Other possible contributory mechanisms include impairment of oxygen utilization, inhibition of electron flow, reduction of ventricular performance, beta receptor antagonism, and diminished cardiac contractility.[68]

An unexplained metabolic acidosis may trigger clinical suspicion of propofol infusion syndrome.[4] Metabolic acidosis may develop due to the conversion of fatty acids to ketone bodies by the liver. It may also be caused by hypoperfusion secondary to propofol induced bradycardia.[69] The most common aspect of case reports found infusions of longer than 48 hours with sustained rates of greater than 75 mcg/kg/min.[63] While it appears high infusion rates for extended periods of time produce most cases, Merz et al.[70] reported a fatal case of propofol infusion syndrome in an adult with a maximum infusion rate of about 40 mcg/kg/min. Other potential risk factors for developing propofol infusion syndrome include sepsis, systemic inflammatory response syndrome, catecholamine therapy, corticosteroid therapy, and brain injury.[68,69] There is a growing body of literature surrounding propofol infusion syndrome, and clinicians are encouraged to monitor for this potential life-threatening adverse effect.

Overall, propofol is a preferred sedative agent for patients with a history of asthma, severe ARDS, or seizure activity, as well as those who need frequent neurologic exams or require deep sedation. Propofol should be avoided in patients who experience bradycardia and those with an allergy to eggs.

Dexmedetomidine

Dexmedetomidine is a central alpha-2-adrenoceptor agonist that has sedative, anxiolytic, and analgesic effects. Stimulation of the presynaptic alpha-2-receptor causes a negative feedback mechanism that inhibits the release of norepinephrine, thus inhibiting sympathetic activity. This produces sedation as well as causing a termination of pain signal propagation as illustrated in Figure 5–2. One of the highest densities of alpha-2-adrenoceptor in the body and the primary site of action for dexmedetomidine is the locus ceruleus. The locus ceruleus is the predominant noradrenergic nucleus in the brain and a modulator of alertness and nociceptive neurotransmission.[71]

Sedation with dexmedetomidine is thought to mimic a more natural sleep pattern compared to GABA receptor stimulators. Alpha-2-agonists produce sleep by reduction of norepinephrine release from the locus ceruleus, triggering the release of inhibitory neurotransmitters GABA and galanin, and suppression of histamine, inducing a hypnotic state. This mechanism for inducing sleep is similar to that of natural sleep. Compared to GABA receptor agonists, neurons in the locus ceruleus maintain wakeful activity, and

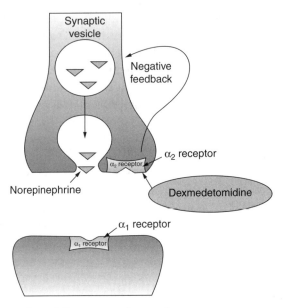

Figure 5-2 Dexmedetomidine receptor interaction

Source: Reproduced from Gertler R, Brown C, Mitchell D, Silvius E. Dexmedetomidine: a novel sedative-analgesic agent. *BUMC Proceedings*. 2001;14:13–21 with permission.

hypnosis is produced by mimicking GABA release from the ventrolateral preoptic nucleus, essentially inducing sleep at the second step of the natural sleep pattern. The difference in origin of hypnosis produced by dexmedetomidine vs. benzodiazepines/propofol may explain the qualitative difference in sedation/hypnosis.[3]

Dexmedetomidine is closely related to clonidine with eight times the potency and a much higher affinity for alpha-2 to alpha-1 (ratios of alpha-2: alpha-1 activity: 1620:1 for dexmedetomidine, 220:1 for clonidine). With a distribution half-life of about 6 minutes, dexmedetomidine has a rapid onset.[72] Metabolism of dexmedetomidine is biotransformation through glucoronidation and hydroxylation mediated by CYP2A6, therefore pharmacokinetics are affected in severe liver insufficiency.[73] Metabolites are eliminated by the kidneys.

Currently, FDA approved dosing recommends a loading dose of 1 mcg/kg over 10 minutes followed by a continuous infusion of 0.2 to 0.7 mcg/kg/hr for short term sedation (<24 hours).[74] Due to hemodynamic effects (primarily bradycardia) of a large initial dose, most clinicians avoid utilization of the loading dose or instead infuse over a longer time period.[73] Several trials have safely and effectively used infusions greater than 0.7 mcg/kg/hr for a duration of greater than 24 hours.[75-79] In a large clinical trial, Riker and colleagues[75] demonstrated safety and efficacy with infusions up to 1.4 mcg/ kg/hr. Additionally, 61% of patients required more than the FDA-approved maximum dose of 0.7 mcg/kg/hr, and 80% of infusions ran longer than 24 hours. Dexmedetomidine has been used for the management of alcohol withdrawal symptoms, however, data are currently limited to case reports.

The adverse effect profile for dexmedetomidine shares some similarities to that of benzodiazepines and propofol. Bradycardia is a dose-dependent effect mediated by a decrease in sympathetic tone and enhanced vagal activity.[76] Significant bradycardia may be avoided with omission or lengthened infusion of the loading dose. A biphasic dose-dependent blood pressure response may be observed with dexmedetomidine. At high doses, a transient hypertension is produced due to stimulation of peripheral alpha-2b-receptors, which could cause vasoconstriction. With stimulation of central alpha-2a-receptors at lower doses, dexmedetomidine decreases sympathetic outflow, causing vasodilatation that can lead to hypotension.[77] Other adverse effects may include nausea and dry mouth.[74]

The adverse effect profile of dexmedetomidine does not include respiratory depression, and there is no impact on oxygen saturation, respiratory rate, arterial pH, and partial pressure of carbon dioxide in arterial blood ($PaCO_2$).[79] In fact, dexmedetomidine has shown statistically significant higher ratio of partial pressure of oxygen in arterial blood to fraction of inspired oxygen ($PaO_2:FiO_2$) when compared to placebo.[78] When directly comparing mean extubation times, Riker et al.[75] observed a statistically significant shorter duration of mechanical ventilation for patients on dexmedetomidine vs. midazolam (3.7 days [95% CI, 3.1 to 4.0] vs. 5.6 days [95% CI, 4.6 to 5.9]; $p = 0.01$). The ICU length of stay was similar between the groups (5.9 days [95% CI, 5.7 to 7.0] vs. 7.6 days [95% CI, 6.7 to 8.6]; $p = 0.24$).

Avoidance or reduced incidence of delirium has been demonstrated in two trials which directly compare dexmedetomidine to benzodiazepines. In the MENDS trial,[79] mechanically ventilated patients were sedated with dexmedetomidine or lorazepam and had individual sedation targets. Researchers found patients in the dexmedetomidine group spent more time within target sedation (median percentage of days: 80% vs. 67%; $p = 0.04$), more days alive without delirium or coma (median days: 7.0 vs. 3.0; $p = 0.01$), and a lower prevalence of coma (63% vs. 92%; $p < 0.001$) than sedation with lorazepam. A similar result was found in the SEDCOM trial[75] comparing dexmedetomidine vs. midazolam for mechanically ventilated patients. Sedation targets were standardized for all patients with a goal RASS of –2 to +1. The prevalence of delirium during treatment was 54% in the dexmedetomidine arm vs. 76.6% in the midazolam arm (absolute difference, 22.6% [95% CI, 14% to 33%]; $p < 0.001$).

Dexmedetomidine is preferred for individuals who require frequent neurologic exams, those with delirium, and patients in septic shock.[80] Dexmedetomidine should be avoided in patients with bradycardia, heart block, those requiring deep sedation (i.e., therapeutic paralysis), and patients with poor left ventricular function, as there are limited studies evaluating this group of patients.

Sedation Holiday/Daily Interruption

In the late 1990s, continuous intravenous sedation was found to prolong mechanical ventilation when compared to patients who received either bolus sedatives or no sedation (185 ± 190 hrs vs. 55.6 ± 75.6 hrs; $p < 0.001$). Similarly, the lengths of intensive care (13.5 ± 33.7 days vs. 4.8 ± 4.1 days; $p < 0.001$) and hospitalization (21.0 ± 25.1 days vs. 12.8 ± 14.1 days; $p < 0.001$) were statistically longer among patients receiving continuous intravenous sedation.[81]

In a follow-up landmark trial, Kress and colleagues[82] tested continuous intravenous sedation with interruption only at the discretion of the clinicians (control group) vs. scheduled daily interruption of sedation (intervention group). After daily interruption, sedation and analgesia were reinitiated at half the previous rate and titrated as needed. The mean duration of mechanical ventilation was 2.4 days shorter in the intervention group vs. the control group. A significantly shorter (3.5 days) median length of ICU stay was also observed in the intervention group. Based on this and subsequent studies, daily sedative interruptions or frequent sedation holidays are now considered standard practice and highly recommended by clinical guidelines.[4]

Analgosedation

The concept of analgosedation, otherwise known as analgesia first or analgesia-based sedation, has been attracting more attention and has potential benefits over the traditional sedation regimens. One example is that the use of ultra-short-acting remifentanil alone without sedative/hypnotic agents has been shown to be safe and effective. Thirty-seven percent of patients can be managed with remifentanil alone, while the remaining patients had a significant reduction in the use of sedative/hypnotic agents when remifentanil was used as the primary analgesic/sedative agent. Additionally, the use of analgesia-based sedation had a greater percentage of time within satisfactory sedation levels defined as awake or easily arousable (median 19% vs. 50%, $p < 0.001$).[83] In an open-label comparison of a remifentanil-based regimen with propofol vs. traditional sedation regimen (sedation plus analgesia), researchers found a non-significant reduction in mechanical ventilation (3.9 vs. 5.1 days). However, remifentanil-based regimens reduced median weaning times by 18.9 hours (p = 0.0001). Median ICU length of stay was 5.9 days in the intervention group vs. 7.9 days in the control group, but was a statistically non-significant finding. Sedation–agitation scores were significantly and consistently better with remifentanil-based regimens (p < 0.0001).[84] The success of these early trials should lead to additional confirmatory trials and cost–benefit trials to determine if analgosedation regimens become recommended therapy.

DELIRIUM

Clinical guidelines define delirium as acutely changing or fluctuating mental status, inattention, disorganized thinking, and an altered level of consciousness that may or may not be accompanied by agitation.[4] The Diagnostic and Statistical Manual of Mental Disorders, fourth edition (DSM-IV) criteria for the diagnosis of delirium are as follows: (1) disturbance of consciousness with reduced ability to focus, sustain, or shift attention; (2) a change in cognition or the development of a perceptual disturbance that is not better accounted for by a pre-existing dementia; (3) the disturbance develops after a short period of time and tends to fluctuate; and (4) evidence from history, physical examination, or laboratory findings that the disturbance is caused by the physiologic consequences of a general medical condition.[85] It is estimated that up to 87% of ICU patients may suffer from delirium.[86] Delirium can be further categorized in motor subtypes: hypoactive, hyperactive, or mixed.[87] Hypoactive delirium is observed as a calm appearance, inattention, decreased mobility, and obtundation. Hyperactive delirium is more easily recognized and is characterized by agitation, combative behaviors, lack of orientation, and progressive confusion; and mixed delirium involves manifestations of both hypoactive and hyperactive delirium at different times.

Delirium in the critically ill patient is associated with increased length of stay, higher mortality, and more adverse outcomes.[86] Therefore, the assessment for ICU delirium and treatment has become a major focal point in caring for patients. The Confusion Assessment Method for the Intensive Care Unit (CAM-ICU) was designed for nonverbal, mechanically ventilated, or restrained patients in ICU settings. The CAM-ICU is an abbreviated version of the Cognitive Test for Delirium. The four features assessed in CAM-ICU include: (1) acute onset and fluctuating course; (2) inattention; (3) disorganized thinking; and (4) altered level of consciousness. Delirium is considered present if 1 and 2 are present, plus either 3 or 4. The CAM-ICU was validated in a large cohort study[88,89] of patients in the ICU patients against delirium expert assessments. It had a sensitivity of 95% to 100%, a specificity of 89% to 93%, and high inter-observer reliability. Clinical guidelines recommend routine assessment delirium with tools such as the CAM-ICU.[4]

Delirium is particularly common in the ICU due to numerous factors contributing to cycles of anxiety, agitation, and ultimately delirium, as illustrated in Figure 5-3.[3] Other contributory factors include advanced age, critical illness, medical procedures and interventions, interaction between host factors, acute illness, and iatrogenic or environmental factors. Delirium is the leading complication of hospitalization in elderly patients. Benzodiazepines, narcotics, and other psychoactive drugs have demonstrated a 3 to 11 fold increase in the relative risk for the development of delirium.[82] Benzodiazepines, in particular lorazepam, have been identified as an independent risk factor for development of delirium. In an *a priori* design, lorazepam had an odds ratio of 1.2 for risk of daily transition to delirium (p = 0.003).[90] Four other medications were also associated with trends towards significance, including midazolam (OR 1.7; p = 0.09), fentanyl (OR 1.2; p = 0.09), morphine (OR 1.1; p = 0.24), and propofol (OR 1.2; p = 0.18). This trial further identified that the

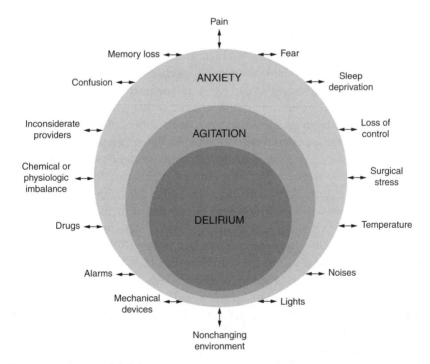

Figure 5-3 Causes of delirium

Source: Reproduced from Peruzzi, W. Sleep in the Intensive Care Unit. *Pharmacotherapy*. 2005; 25(5 Pt 2):34S–39S with permission.

probability of transitioning to delirium increased with increasing lorazepam dose. At 20 mg per day, the probability of developing delirium was 100%.

The management of delirium in the ICU can be divided into prevention, treatment of the underlying disorder, and pharmacologic management.[86] Some strategies to help prevent delirium include repeated orientation of the patient, cognitively stimulating activities, sleep protocol to enhance normalization of sleep/wake cycles, early mobilization and range of motion activities, timely removal of catheters and physical restraints, use of eyeglasses, and early correction of dehydration. When these strategies are utilized, a 40% reduction in incidence of delirium was observed.[91]

Standard practices should be followed in order to quickly diagnose and treat patients effectively. Treatment of underlying disorders can aid in resolution of delirium or reveal the actual cause of delirium. Often, pharmacologic treatment is needed to prevent the patient from doing harm to oneself or medical personnel. Neuroleptic agents are thought to treat the symptoms of delirium by exerting a stabilizing effect on cerebral function via antagonizing dopamine-mediated neurotransmission at the cerebral synapses and basal ganglia. Goals of neuroleptic therapy include: faster resolution of delirium, fewer acute agitation events, less sedation therapy, shorter hospital stay, and fewer adverse effects. The most commonly used neuroleptic for delirium is haloperidol because it is highly potent, minimally sedative, and has numerous dosage forms. In order to avoid potential side effects of haloperidol, atypical antipsychotics may also be used for delirium. Delirium usually resolves within 7 to 10 days; therefore, neuroleptic therapy is rarely needed for more than 2 weeks.[92]

Haloperidol

Haloperidol is a butyrophenone, which produces a tranquil state through a mechanism that has not been fully identified; however, a proposed mechanism is that it works via the antagonism of dopamine, primarily in the basal ganglia. Administration of haloperidol may cause a detached effect or even demonstrate a cataleptic, immobilized state. Haloperidol has insignificant analgesic, amnesic, or anticonvulsant properties, as well as minimal respiratory effects.[5,29] An initial dose of haloperidol will have an onset of action within 2 to 5 minutes and a dose dependent half-life of 18 to 54 hours. Haloperidol is metabolized by the liver.[29] An optimal dosing regimen for haloperidol has yet to be defined, but it is typically given intravenously every 15 to 20 minutes as needed at doses of 1 mg to 10 mg initially, then titrated to goal effect.[4,5] Continuous infusions of haloperidol (3 to 25 mg/hour) have been used.[93]

Haloperidol may cause a mild hypotensive effect as a result of peripheral alpha-1-antagonism.[5] A dose dependent electrocardiogram (ECG) QTc prolongation may lead to increase risk of ventricular arrhythmias, with cumulative doses of greater than 35 mg in a 24-hour period demonstrating a significantly higher incidence of torsades de pointes.[94] Haloperidol should be used with caution in patients with prolonged baseline QTc intervals, electrolyte abnormalities, or receiving other QTc prolonging medications.[5] Extrapyramidal effects are occasionally seen but are much less common with intravenous than with oral haloperidol.[95]

Atypical Antipsychotics

The use of atypical antipsychotics for ICU delirium is a relatively new concept. Open label studies of risperidone,[96] quetiapine,[97] and olanzapine[98] have shown reduced duration of delirium. These trials also demonstrated minimal adverse effects and a high degree of safety. When comparing low-dose atypical antipsychotics to low-dose haloperidol, these agents can be considered equally efficacious. These trials are limited by sample size, lower atypical antipsychotic doses than for other indications, and some by retrospective design. With no clear difference between atypical antipsychotics and haloperidol and no trials directly comparing two atypical antipsychotics, the choice between agents becomes a matter of avoidance of adverse effects and clinician preference.

Adverse effects of a particular agent may be associated with the relative affinity it has for a particular receptor.[92] The higher ratio of serotonergic 5-HT2:dopaminergic D2 receptor blockade shown with atypical antipsychotics correlates with less extrapyramidal symptoms (EPS) such as dystonia, parkinsonism, and akathisia.[99] Of the antipsychotics, olanzapine has the least amount of EPS. Hypotensive effects, mediated by alpha-1-antagonism, are a potential effect by atypical antipsychotics but are considered a lower risk than haloperidol. Risk of hypotension has been stratified in decreasing frequency: clozapine, quetiapine, risperidone, and olanzapine.[92] All antipsychotics can produce sedation through histamine receptor blockade; this is a dose-dependent effect, with clozapine and quetiapine producing the most sedation.[100] Anticholinergic effects of dry mouth, tachycardia, constipation, urinary retention, and blurred vision are most commonly seen with olanzapine and quetiapine. Prolongation of the QTc interval with atypical antipsychotics is thought to be less than with haloperidol, but this could be related to lack of evaluation. Ziprasidone is the most prominent offender of QTc prolongation.[92] Neuroleptic malignant syndrome is very rare with any of these agents.[100]

Product formulation may also guide therapy. Risperidone and aripiprazole are available in liquid formulation and may be administered through feeding tubes; olanzapine, risperidone, and aripiprazole are available as orally dissolving tablets; ziprasidone may be given intravenously; and olanzapine has an intramuscular route of administration. However, IV ziprasidone and IM olanzapine have limited data for use in ICU delirium.[92]

Recommended starting doses for atypical antipsychotics are as follows: Olanzapine should be started at 2.5 to 5 mg once/day at bedtime and increased as needed; quetiapine should be started at 25 mg once or twice/day and titrated in increments of 25 mg/dose every 2 days; and risperidone should be started at 0.5 mg once or twice/day and increased in increments of 0.5 mg/day every 2 to 3 days.[92]

NEUROMUSCULAR BLOCKERS

Neuromuscular blockers (NMBs) should be considered a last resort therapy for indications of the facilitation of mechanical ventilation, management of intracranial pressure (ICP), and need for decreased oxygen consumption. Some protocols for hypothermia use NMBs as first line therapy for shivering, while others use NMBs for refractory shivering.

Neuromuscular blockers can be categorized either by mechanism of action (depolarizing or nondepolarizing) or by duration of action (ultra-short, short, intermediate, or long). All NMBs act on the neuromuscular junction. When a nerve impulse arrives at the junction, the synaptic vesicles release the neurotransmitter acetylcholine. Acetylcholine then binds to specialized ligand-gated, nicotinic acetylcholine receptors (nAChRs) on the post synaptic motor endplate. Stimulation of these receptors allows ions to flow intracellularly and depolarizes the end plate, thus causing muscle contraction. Acetylcholine is then rapidly broken down by the enzyme acetylcholinesterase. Depolarizing NMBs physically resemble acetylcholine and bind to the alpha subunit producing a contraction called fasciculation. Persistent depolarization ensues since the depolarizing NMBs agent is not broken down by acetylcholinesterase and neuromuscular blockade is produced. A nondepolarizing NMB, on the other hand, competitively antagonizes acetylcholine receptors, subsequently inhibiting depolarization of the motor endplate and resulting in flaccid muscles.[6,101]

Depolarizing Neuromuscular Blockers

Currently, the only depolarizing NMBs available is succinylcholine. Structurally, it is similar to two acetylcholine molecules. Neuromuscular blockade onset is about one minute and duration of action is only seven to eight minutes. This characteristic makes succinylcholine an ideal agent for rapid sequence intubation but is not indicated for long term use. Plasma cholinesterases metabolize this depolarizing NMB agent. Adverse effects from succinylcholine include muscle pain, hyperkalemia, and increased intraocular and intragastric pressure, as well as it being a potential trigger for malignant hyperthermia.

Nondepolarizing Neuromuscular Blockers

Nondepolarizing NMBs can be subdivided into aminosteroidal compounds and benzylisoquinolinium compounds. Amionsteroidal compounds include pancuronium, pipecuronium, vecuronium, and rocuronium. Benzylisoquinolinium compounds include D-tubocurarine, atracurium, cisatracurium, doxacurium, and mivacurium. The onset of action of nondepolarizing NMB agents is relatively longer than succinylcholine, and the longer duration of action makes these agents more suitable for maintaining neuromuscular blockade when indicated. The specific pharmacokinetic parameters, dosing, and specific comments of each of these agents is briefly reviewed in Table 5–5.[6]

The selection of neuromuscular agents is chiefly made based on pharmacokinetic properties and specific clinical situations. Patients with renal impairment may have prolonged neuromuscular blockade if pancuronium, tubocurarine, pipecuronium, doxacurium, or vecuronium are used. Atracurium and cisatracurium undergo Hofmann elimination; therefore, the pharmacokinetics are not altered in chronic renal insufficiency and should be considered in these patients. Most nondepolarizing neuromuscular blockers have at least some biliary excretion, so for patients with extrahepatic biliary obstruction, atracurium, cisatracurium, or doxacurium are considered first line NMBs.[101]

Nondepolarizing NMBs have the potential of causing hypertension or tachycardia mediated by muscarinic blockade. Atracurium, cisatracurium, and vecuronium have no direct cardiovascular effects. Nondepolarizing NMBs may also cause the release of histamine and lead to vasodilatation, hypotension, and compensatory tachycardia.[101]

Assessment of pain and sedation becomes more difficult when neuromuscular blockers are used. In order to ensure patient comfort while on NMBs, continuous sedation and analgesia are required. Clinical guidelines recommend increasing sedation and analgesia until the patient does not appear to be conscious, at which point the NMBs may be started.[6] Some clinicians utilize the bispectral index (BIS) monitor to measure levels of sedation.

Table 5-5 Neuromuscular Blockers[6,34]

Duration/ Category	Drug	Bolus (mg/kg)	Maintenance (mg/kg)	Infusion (mcg/kg/min)	Onset (min)	Duration (min)	Metabolism	Excretion	Comments
Depolarizing:									
Ultra Short	Succinylcholine	1–2	N/A	N/A	<1	5–10	Hydrolysis	Minimal Renal	Used for RSI, not for long term use
Non-depolarizing:									
Short	Mivacurium	0.15–0.25	0.1	9–10	2–6	20–30	Hydrolysis	Minimal Renal	Limited data for continuous infusions
Intermediate	Atracurium	0.5	0.08–0.1	5–9	3–5	35–70	Hofmann elimination	Renal	May precipitate seizure activity
	Cisatracurium	0.15	0.03	1–2	2	30–90	Hofmann elimination	Renal/Hepatic	Less cardiac effects than Atracurium
	Rocuronium	0.6	0.1–0.25	10–12	1–2	20–90	Minimal Hepatic	Bilary	Mildly active metabolite
	Vecuronium	0.075–0.1	0.01–0.015	1	2–4	30–40	Hepatic	Bilary > Renal	Caution in renal/ hepatic failure
Long	Pancuronium	0.04–0.1	0.01–0.06	N/A	2–3	45–60	Minimal Hepatic	Renal > Bilary	Caution in renal/ hepatic failure, Vagolytic

The BIS monitor uses electroencephalogram readings from frontal leads and converts those readings to a number between 0 and 100 with 0 being no activity (deep sedation) and 100 being wide awake. Guidelines also recommend monitoring the use of NMBs both clinically and with the train-of-four. Clinicians should monitor skeletal muscle movement and respiratory effort. Train-of-four monitoring uses a peripheral nerve stimulator (PNS), which transcutaneously delivers an electric current in four pulses, causing twitching. A goal of one to two twitches out of four is typically recommended for adequate neuromuscular blockade. After the administration of a nondepolarizing drug, the height of each successive electrical stimulation response decreases. Clinically, the use of PNS for assessment of NMBs has resulted in a significantly lower total dose and lower mean infusion rate of NMBs.

SUMMARY

Providing adequate relief of pain, anxiety, and delirium may minimize the duration of mechanical ventilation, shorten the ICU length of stay, and reduce mortality. Effective management of analgesic, sedative, and neuroleptic agents is key to achieving this goal. Medication selection based on pharmacokinetic and pharmacodynamic properties in each unique patient case plays an important role in promoting patient comfort. Sedation scales, pain scales, delirium assessments, sedation protocols, and daily interruption of sedatives will aid to diminish deleterious effects from these agents. Clinicians are encouraged to continue to strive for the optimal sedation and analgesic regimen for each patient. These topics will likely continue to grow exponentially, with research stimulating new and exciting concepts in treatment of the critically ill patient.

KEY POINTS

- Management of pain, sedation, and delirium in the critically ill is an important, complex, and challenging process.
- Multiple medications are effective for treating pain in the critically ill, with narcotics being the most common agents used.
- If analgesia alone is not adequate to alleviate anxiety or agitation symptoms, sedative agents are used.
- The individual properties of the common analgesics and sedatives should be considered when determining optimal medication regimens.
- Delirium is a challenging complication in the critically ill and is associated with increased mortality.

- Neuromuscular blockade should only be used when analgesia and sedation are unable to attain the goals of therapy, and they should be closely monitored and used for the shortest time possible.

SELECTED SUGGESTED READING

- Society of Critical Care Medicine and American Society of Health-System Pharmacists: Clinical practice guidelines for the sustained use of sedatives and analgesics in the critically ill adult. *Am J Health-Syst Pharm.* 2002;59:150–158. (Editor's note: guideline statement due for update by 2012.)
- Brush D, Kress J. Sedation and analgesia for the mechanically ventilated patient. *Clin Chest Med.* 2009;30:131–141.
- Society of Critical Care Medicine, American Society of Health-System Pharmacists: Clinical practice guidelines for sustained neuromuscular blockade in the adult critically ill patient. *Crit Care Med.* 2002; 30:142–156.
- Peruzzi, W. Sleep in the Intensive Care Unit. *Pharmacotherapy.* 2005;25(5 Pt 2):34S–39S.

REFERENCES

1. Epstein J, Breslow M. The stress response of critical illness. *Crit Care Clin.* 1999;15(1):17–23.
2. Mularski R. Pain management in the intensive care unit. *Crit Care Clin.* 2004;20:381–401.
3. Peruzzi W. Sleep in the Intensive Care Unit. *Pharmacotherapy.* 2005;25 (5 Pt 2):34S–39S.
4. Society of Critical Care Medicine and American Society of Health-System Pharmacists: Clinical practice guidelines for the sustained use of sedatives and analgesics in the critically ill adult. *Am J Health-Syst Pharm.* 2002;59:150–178.
5. Brush D, Kress J. Sedation and analgesia for the mechanically ventilated patient. *Clin Chest Med.* 2009;30:131–141.
6. Society of Critical Care Medicine, American Society of Health-System Pharmacists: Clinical practice guidelines for sustained neuromuscular blockade in the adult critically ill patient. *Crit Care Med.* 2002; 30:142–156.
7. Bernard SA, Gray TW, Buist MD, et al. Treatment of comatose survivors of out-of-hospital cardiac arrest with induced hypothermia. *N Engl J Med.* 2002;346:557–563.
8. Gordon M, Greenfield E, Marvin J, Hester C, Lauterach S. Use of pain assessment tools: is there a preference? *J Burn Care Rehab.* 1998;19:451–454.
9. Desbiens NA, Mueller-Rizner N. How well do surrogates assess the pain of seriously ill patients? *Crit Care Med.* 2000;28:1347–1352.

10. Terai T, Yukioka H, Asada A. Pain evaluation in the intensive care unit: observer reported faces scale compared with self reported visual analog scale. *Reg Anesth Pain Med.* 1998;23:147–151.

11. Mateo OM, Krenzischek DA. A pilot study to assess the relationship between behavioral manifestations of pain and self-report of pain in post anesthesia care unit patients. *J Post Anesth Nurs.* 1992;7:15–21.

12. Odhner M, Wegman D, Freeland N, Steinmetz A, Ingersoll G. Assessing pain control in nonverbal critically ill adults. *Dimens Crit Care Nurs.* 2003;22(6):260–267.

13. Pasero C, McCafferty M. When patients can't report pain. *Am J Nurs.* 2000;100(9):22–23.

14. Campbell J. Past Presidents' Perspectives. American Pain Society. APS Bulletin Volume 17, Number 1, 2007. http://www.ampainsoc.org. Accessed July 24, 2010.

15. Chanques G, Jaber S, Barbotte E, et al. Impact of a systematic evaluation of pain and agitation in an intensive care unit. *Crit Care Med.* 2006;34(6):1691–1699.

16. Brook A, Ahrens T, Schaiff R, Prentice D, Sherman G, Shannon W, Kollef M. Effect of a nursing-implemented sedation protocol on the duration of mechanical ventilation. *Crit Care Med.* 1999;27(12):2609–2615.

17. DeJonghe B, Cook D, Appere-De-Vecchi C, et al. Using and understanding sedation scoring systems: a systematic review. *Intensive Care Med.* 2000;26:275–285.

18. Ramsay MAE, Savege TM, Simpson BRJ, Goodwin R. Controlled sedation with Alphaxalone-Alphadolone. *BMJ.* 1974;2.656–659.

19. Riker RR, Picard JT, Fraser GL. Prospective evaluation of the Sedation-Agitation Scale for adult critically ill patients. *Crit Care Med.* 1999 Jul;27(7):1325–1329.

20. Devlin JW, Boleski G, Mlynarek M, et al. Motor Activity Assessment Scale: a valid and reliable sedation scale for use with mechanically ventilated patients in an adult surgical intensive care unit. *Crit Care Med.* 1999 Jul;27(7):1271–1275.

21. Sessler CN, Gosnell MS, Grap MJ, et al. The Richmond Agitation-Sedation Scale: validity and reliability in adult intensive care unit patients. *Am J Respir Crit Care Med.* 2002 Nov 15;166(10):1338–1344.

22. Novaes M, Knobel E, Bork A, et al. Stressors in ICU: perception of the patient, relatives and healthcare team. *Intensive Care Med.* 1999;25:1421–1426.

23. Desbiens N, Wu A, Broste S, et al. Pain and satisfaction with pain control in seriously ill hospitalized adults: findings from the SUPPORT research investigators. *Crit Care Med.* 1996;24:1953–1961.

24. Puntillo K, et al. Patients' perceptions and responses to procedural pain: results from Thunder Project II. *Am J Crit Care.* 2001;10(4):238–251.

25. Vanderah T. Delta and kappa opioid receptors as suitable drug targets for pain. *Clin J Pain.* 2010;26:S10–S15.

26. Hardman J, Limbird L. *Goodman & Gilman's: the pharmacological basis of therapeutics.* New York: McGraw-Hill; 2001.

27. Gommers D, Bakker J. Medications for analgesia and sedation in the intensive care unit: an overview. *Crit Care.* 2008;12(Suppl 3):S4.

28. Pasternak GW, Bodnar RJ, Clark JA, et al. Morphine-6-glucuronide, a potent mu agonist. *Life Sci.* 1987;41(26):2845–2849.

29. Gehlbach B, Kress J. Sedation in the intensive care unit. *Curr Opin Crit Care.* 2002;8:290–298.

30. Tipps L, Coplin W, Murry K, Rhoney D. Safety and feasibility of continuous infusion of remifentanil in the neurosurgical intensive care unit. *Neurosurgery.* 2000;46(3):596–602.

31. Beers R, Camporesi E. Remifentanil update: clinical science and utility. *CNS Drugs.* 2004;18(15):1085–1104.

32. Muellejans B, Lopez A, Cross MH, Bonome C, Morrison L, Kirkham AJ. Remifentanil versus fentanyl for analgesia based sedation to provide patient comfort in the intensive care unit: a randomized, double-blind controlled trial. *Crit Care.* 2004;8:R1–R11.

33. Dahaba AA, Grabner T, Rehak PH, List WF, Metzler H. Remifentanil versus morphine analgesia and sedation for mechanically ventilated critically ill patients: a randomized double-blind study. *Anesthesiology.* 2004;101:640–646.

34. Bakker J, Mulder P. Remifentanil shortens duration of mechanical ventilation and ICU stay. *Intensive Care Med.* 2006;32(Suppl.):S85.

35. Cammarano W, Pittet J, Weitz S, Schlobohm R, Marks J. Acute withdrawal syndrome related to the administration of analgesic and sedative medications in adult intensive care unit patients. *Crit Care Med.* 1998;26:676–684.

36. Zimmerman HJ, Maddrey W. Acetaminophen hepatotoxicity with regular intake of alcohol. Analysis of instances of therapeutic misadventure. *Hepatology.* 1995;22:767–773.

37. Parker RK, Holtmann B, Smith I, et al. Use of ketorolac after lower abdominal surgery. *Anesthesiology.* 1994;80:6–12.

38. Feldman H, Kinman J, Berlin J, et al. Parenteral ketorolac: the risk for acute renal failure. *Ann Intern Med.* 1997;126:193–199.

39. Micromedex® Healthcare Series Intranet. Thomson Reuters (Healthcare) Inc. Version 5.1.

40. Strom BL, Berlin JA, Kinman JL, et al. Parenteral ketorolac and risk of gastrointestinal and operative site bleeding. *JAMA.* 1996;275:376–382.

41. Goetting M, Thirman M. Neurotoxicity of meperidine. *Ann Emerg Med.* 1985;14(10):1007–1009.

42. Fraser GL, Prato S, Berthiaume D, et al. Evaluation of agitation in ICU patients: incidence, severity, and treatment in the young versus the elderly. *Pharmacotherapy.* 2000;20:75–82.

43. Cohen D, Horiuchi K, Kemper M, et al. Modulating effects of propofol on metabolic and cardiopulmonary responses to stressful intensive care unit procedures. *Crit Care Med.* 1996;24:612–617.

44. Richards G, Schoch P, Haefely W. Benzodiazepine receptors: new vistas. *Seminars in Neuroscience.* 1991;3:191–203.

45. Watling SM, Johnson M, Yanos J. A method to produce sedation in critically ill patients. *Ann Pharmacother.* 1996;30:1227–1231.

46. Bauer T, Ritz R, Haberthur C, Riem Ha H, Hukeler W, Sleight A, Scollo-Lavizzari G, Haefeli W. Prolonged sedation due to accumulation of conjugated metabolites of midazolam. *Lancet.* 1995;346:145–147.

47. Byatt CM, Lewis LD, Dawling S, Cochrane GM. Accumulation of midazolam after repeated dosage in patients receiving mechanical ventilation in an intensive care unit. *BMJ.* 1984;289:799–800.

48. Amrein R, Hetzel W, Hartmann D, Lorscheid T. Clinical pharmacology of flumazenil. *Eur J Anaesthesiol Suppl.* 1988;2:65–80.

49. Gilliland HE, Prasad BK, Mirakhur RK, et al. An investigation of the potential morphine sparing effect of midazolam. *Anaesthesia.* 1996;51:808–811.

50. Treiman DM: The role of benzodiazepines in the management of status epilepticus. *Neurology.* 1990;40:32–42.

51. Pandharipande P, Shintani A, Peterson J, et al. Lorazepam is an independent risk factor for transitioning to delirium in intensive care unit patients. *Anesthesiology.* 2006;104(1):21–26.

52. Vree TB, Shimoda M, Driessen JJ, et al. Decreased plasma albumin concentration results in increased volume of distribution and decreased elimination of midazolam in intensive care patients. *Clin Pharmacol Ther.* 1989;46:537–544.

53. Driessen JJ, Vree TB, Guelen PJ. The effects of acute changes in renal function on the pharmacokinetics of midazolam during long-term infusion in ICU patients. *Acta Anaesthesiol Belg.* 1991;42:149–155.

54. Greenblatt DJ, Abernethy DR, Locniskar A, et al. Effect of age, gender, and obesity on midazolam kinetics. *Anesthesiology.* 1984;61:27–35.

55. Hamaoka N, Oda Y, Hase I, et al. Propofol decreases the clearance of midazolam by inhibiting CYP3A4: an in vivo and in vitro study. *Clin Pharmacol Ther.* 1999;66:110–117.

56. Gorski JC, Jones DR, Haehner-Daniels BD, et al. The contribution of intestinal and hepatic CYP3A to the interaction between midazolam and clarithromycin. *Clin Pharmacol Ther.* 1998;64:133–143.

57. Michalets EL. Update: clinically significant cytochrome P-450 drug interactions. *Pharmacotherapy.* 1999;18:84–112.

58. Yahwak J, Riker R, Fraser G, Subak-Sharpe S. Determination of a lorazepam dose threshold for using the osmol gap to monitor for propylene glycol toxicity. *Pharmacotherapy.* 2008;28(8):984–991.

59. Wilson KC, Reardon C, Theodore AC, Farber HW. Propylene glycol toxicity: a severe iatrogenic illness in ICU patients receiving IV benzodiazepines. *Chest.* 2005;128:1674–1681.

60. Barnes BJ, Gerst C, Smith JR, Terrell AR, Mullins ME. Osmol gap as a surrogate marker for serum propylene glycol concentrations in patients receiving lorazepam for sedation. *Pharmacotherapy.* 2006;26:23–33.

61. Barr J, Zomorodi K, Bertaccini EJ, et al. A double-blind, randomized comparison of i.v. lorazepam versus midazolam for sedation of ICU patients via a pharmacologic model. *Anesthesiology.* 2001;95(2):324–333.

62. Marik PE, Varon J. The management of status epilepticus. *Chest.* 2004;126(2):582–591.

63. Riker R, Fraser G. Adverse events associated with sedatives, analgesics, and other drugs that provide patient comfort in the intensive care unit. *Pharmacotherapy.* 2005;25(5 Pt 2):8S–18S.

64. Devlin JW, Lau AK, Tanios MA. Propofol associated hypertriglyceridemia and pancreatitis in the intensive care unit: an analysis of frequency and risk factors. *Pharmacotherapy.* 2005;25(10):1348–1352.

65. Bray R. Propofol infusion syndrome in children. *Paed Anaesth.* 1998;8: 491–499.
66. Perrier ND, Baerga-Varela Y, Murray MJ. Death related to propofol use in an adult patient. *Crit Care Med.* 2000;28:3071– 3074.
67. Cremer O, Moons K, Bouman E, Kruijswijk J, de Smet A, Kalkman C. Long-term propofol infusion and cardiac failure in adult head-injured patients. *Lancet.* 2001;357:117–118.
68. Vasile B, Rasulo F, Candiani A, Latronico N. The pathophysiology of propofol infusion syndrome: a simple name for a complex syndrome. *Intensive Care Med.* 2003;29:1417–1425.
69. Kang TM. Propofol infusion syndrome in critically ill patients. *Ann Pharmacother.* 2002;36:1453–1456.
70. Merz T, Regli B, Rothen H. Propofol infusion syndrome – a fatal case at a low infusion rate. *Anesth Analg.* 2006;103(4):1050.
71. Gertler R, Brown C, Mitchell D, Silvius E. Dexmedetomidine: a novel sedative-analgesic agent. *BUMC Proc.* 2001;14:13–21.
72. Venn RM, Karol MD, Grounds RM. Pharmacokinetics of dexmedetomidine infusions for sedation of postoperative patients requiring intensive care. *Br J Anaesth.* 2002;88(5):669–675.
73. Lam S, Alexander E. Dexmedetomidine use in critical care. *AACN Adv Crit Care.* 2008;19(2):113–120.
74. Precedex (Dexmedetomidine). Lake Forest, IL: Hospira. April 2004.
75. Riker R, Shehabi Y, Bokesch P, et al. Dexmedetomidine vs midazolam for sedation of critically ill patients: a randomized trial. *JAMA.* 2009:301(5): 489–499.
76. Penttila J, Helminen A, Anttila M, Hinkka S, Scheinin H. Cardiovascular and parasympathetic effects of dexmedetomidine in healthy subjects. *Can J Physiol Pharmacol.* 2004;82(5):359–362.
77. Paris A, Tonner PH. Dexmedetomidine in anaesthesia. *Curr Opin Anaesthesiol.* 2005;18(4):412–418.
78. Venn R, Hell J, Grounds M. Respiratory effects of dexmedetomidine in the surgical patient requiring intensive care. *Crit Care.* 2000;4:302–308.
79. Pandharipande P, Pun B, Herr D, et al. Effect of sedation with dexmedetomidine vs lorazepam on acute brain dysfunction in mechanically ventilated patients: the MENDS randomized controlled trial. *JAMA.* 2007;298(22): 2644–2653.
80. Pandharipande P, Sanders R, Girard T, et al. Effect of dexmedetomidine versus lorazepam on outcome in patients with sepsis: an *a priroi*-designed analysis of the MENDS randomized controlled trial. *Crit Care.* 2010;14:R38.
81. Kollef MH, Levy NT, Ahrens TS, Schaiff R, Prentice D, Sherman G. The use of continuous i.v. sedation is associated with prolongation of mechanical ventilation. *Chest.* 1998;114:541–548.
82. Kress J, Pohlman A, O'Connor M, Hall J. Daily interruption of sedative infusions in critically ill patients undergoing mechanical ventilation. *N Engl J Med.* 2000;342:1471–1477.

83. Park G, Lane M, Rogers S, Bassett P. A comparison of hypnotic and analgesic based sedation in a general intensive care unit. *Br J Anaesth.* 2007;98(1):76–82.

84. Rozendaal F, Spronk P, Snellen F, Schoen A, et al. Remifentanil-propofol analgo-sedation shortens duration of ventilation and length of ICU stay compared to a conventional regimen: a centre randomized, cross-over, open-label study in the Netherlands. *Intensive Care Med.* 2009;35:291–298.

85. American Psychiatric Association. Diagnostic and statistical manual of mental disorders (Revised 4th ed.). Washington, DC: Author; 2000.

86. Pisani MA, McNicoll L, Inouye SK. Cognitive impairment in the intensive care unit. *Clin Chest Med.* 2003;24:727–737.

87. Meagher DJ, Trzepacz PT. Motoric subtypes of delirium. *Semin Clin Neuropsychiatry.* 2000;5:75–85.

88. Ely EW, Margolin R, Francis J, et al. Evaluation of delirium in critically ill patients: validation of the Confusion Assessment Method for the Intensive Care Unit (CAM-ICU). *Crit Care Med.* 2001;29(7):1370–1379.

89. Ely EW, Inouye SK, Bernard GR, et al. Delirium in mechanically ventilated patients: validity and reliability of the confusion assessment method for the intensive care unit (CAM-ICU). *JAMA.* 2001;286(21):2703–2710.

90. Pandharipande P, Shintani A, Peterson J, et al. Lorazepam is an independent risk factor for transitioning to delirium in intensive care unit patients. *Anesthesiology.* 2006;104:21–26.

91. Inouye SK. Prevention of delirium in hospitalized older patients: risk factors and targeted intervention strategies. *Ann Med.* 2000;32(4):257–263.

92. Rea R, Battistone S, Fong J, Devlin J. Atypical antipsychotics versus haloperidol for treatment of delirium in acutely ill patients. *Pharmacotherapy.* 2007;27(4):588–594.

93. Seneff MG, Mathews RA. Use of haloperidol infusions to control delirium in critically ill adults. *Ann Pharmacother.* 1995;29:690–693.

94. Sharma ND, Rosman HS, Padhi D, et al. Torsades de pointes associated with intravenous haloperidol in critically ill patients. *Am J Cardiol.* 1998;81:238–240.

95. Menza MA, Murray GB, Holmes VF, et al. Decreased extrapyramidal symptoms with intravenous haloperidol. *J Clin Psychiatry.* 1987;48:278–280.

96. Parellada E, Baeza I, Pablo J, et al. Risperidone in the treatment of patients with delirium. *J Clin Psychiatry.* 2004;65:348–353.

97. Kim KY, Bader GM, Kotlyar V, et al. Treatment of delirium in older adults with quetiapine. *J Geriatr Psychiatry Neurol.* 2003;16:29–31.

98. Kim K, Pae C, Chae J, et al. An open pilot trial of olanzapine for delirium in the Korean population. *Psychiatry Clin Neurosci.* 2001;55:515–519.

99. Markowitz JS, Brown CS, Moore TR. Atypical antipsychotics. Part I: pharmacology, pharmacokinetics, and efficacy. *Ann Pharmacother.* 1999;33:73–85.

100. Brown CS, Markowitz JS, Moore TR, et al. Atypical antipsychotics. Part II: adverse effects, drug interactions, and costs. *Ann Pharmacother.* 1999;33:210–217.

101. Hunter J. New neuromuscular blocking drugs. *Drug Therapy.* 1995;332(25): 1691–1699.

Chapter 6

Acid–Base Fundamentals

Thomas Johnson and David Kovaleski

LEARNING OBJECTIVES

1. Describe the common fundamental acid–base disorders in critically ill patients.
2. Differentiate the common causes of acid–base abnormalities in the critically ill.
3. Develop appropriate treatment recommendations for patients with acid–base disorders.
4. List the primary adverse events associated with the treatment of acid-base disorders.

INTRODUCTION

Acid-base disorders are common in critically ill patients and can influence or be significantly influenced by pharmacologic therapy. Medications can be a cause of the abnormality or serve as a treatment.[1] Acid-base disorders can affect the action, elimination, and clearance of certain medications. Any pharmacist practicing in critical care medicine must have a fundamental working knowledge of acid-base disorders. They must be able to assist in appropriately determining causes and design treatment regimens that either directly affect acid-base balance or account for the acid-base disorder to maximize the effectiveness of other medications.

ACID–BASE PHYSIOLOGY

Human cellular function is optimal at a fairly neutral pH (ranging from 7.35 to 7.45) and the body is designed to maintain blood and most tissue pH at this point through the use of a buffer system that is described by the Henderson–Hasselbalch equation.[2]

$$pH = 6.1 + log([HCO_3^-]/(0.03 \times pCO_2))$$

Practice by entering normal values for HCO_3^- (24) and pCO_2 (40) into the equation. Did you get 7.4? Now change the values to $HCO_3^- = 20$ and $pCO_2 = 33$. Do you still get 7.4? Note that the pH is determined primarily based upon the ratio of bicarbonate (HCO_3) to carbon dioxide (CO_2). The association of HCO_3 to CO_2 is further described by the following equation.[3]

$$CO_2 + H_2O \rightleftharpoons H_2CO_3 \rightleftharpoons HCO_3^- + H^+$$

The lungs and the kidneys are the primary organs involved in the regulation of acid–base, although the gastrointestinal tract can also have a significant effect, particularly with the abnormal loss of fluids.[4] The lungs control the partial pressure of CO_2 dissolved in the blood stream (pCO_2 or $PaCO_2$) through the rate of elimination. Bicarbonate is controlled by the kidneys primarily through the elimination of hydrogen ions as ammonia and the reabsorption of bicarbonate from the tubules.[2]

A serum pH value of 7.35 to 7.45 is typically considered to be within the normal range. If the pH is less than 7.35, the patient is considered acidemic, and if the pH is more than 7.45, then the patient is considered to be alkalemic. However, simply being within the normal range does not infer that the patient does not have any underlying acid–base balance abnormalities. Since the body has buffer systems to maintain pH at an optimal level, serious imbalances may still be present, though compensated. The process that leads to acidemia is called acidosis and the process that leads to an alkalemia is known as alkalosis. Significant acidemia or alkalemia can have several detrimental effects in the critically ill patient.

Acidosis

Acidosis is more commonly identified in critically ill patients than alkalosis, and severe acidemia (pH <7.2) is associated with several deleterious effects. Acidemia can cause hypotension, changes in cardiac output, insulin resistance, hyperkalemia, and metabolic changes.[5] Acidemia will also alter the respiratory drive because the body is trying to increase excretion of carbon dioxide. This increased respiratory drive can lead to diaphragm muscle fatigue and weakness, which can necessitate either intubation and mechanical ventilation or delaying liberation from the mechanical ventilator. Factors and cofactors involved in coagulation are less active or do not work during severe acidemia, leading to difficulty in achieving hemostasis, or worse, triggering bleeding events.

Alkalosis

While alkalosis and the resultant alkalemia is much less common in the critically ill patient, there can still be significant adverse effects associated with the disorder. A pH value of >7.6 is associated with neurologic changes, seizures, arrhythmias, hypokalemia, and respiratory depression.[6] Respiratory depression due to even a mild alkalosis can delay liberation from the ventilator, which may lead to other adverse events.

ASSESSMENT OF ACID–BASE STATUS

Evaluation of the patient's acid–base status should be a routine part of evaluating any critically ill patient. Acid–base review can be helpful in determining the patient's severity of illness, daily progress, and response to therapy, or it can reveal an underlying confounding disease state. While the evaluation of acid–base status can be confusing and seem daunting, the majority of patients can be reviewed using a fairly simple approach if the patient has arterial blood gas (ABG) results available. This approach is detailed below and outlined in Figure 6–1.[2,7,8]

pH

First, begin with the pH. An elevated pH indicates alkalemia and decreased pH indicates acidemia. Remember that a normal pH does not indicate the absence of an underlying disorder, as compensation may have occurred. However, presence of an acidemia will indicate an acidosis and alkalemia will indicate the presence of an alkalosis.

Acid

Regardless of the pH value, the next step is to review the patient's pCO_2 level. Remember that CO_2 is an acid and eliminated through the lungs, with pCO_2 levels controlled by minute ventilation. Normal pCO_2 levels are usually 40 mmHg, and patients with pulmonary disorders or respiratory distress/failure will often have significantly increased levels of pCO_2. Based

1. Identify the most obvious disorder by evaluating pH, pCO_2 and HCO_3. If more than one abnormality is identified, just pick one as a starting point.

	pH	pCO_2	HCO_3
Metabolic Acidosis	↓	↓	↓
Metabolic Alkalosis	↑	↑	↑
Respiratory Acidosis	↓	↑	↑
Respiratory Alkalosis	↑	↓	↓

2. Apply the appropriate compensation formula.

For example: in metabolic disorders, HCO_3 is abnormal and the clinician needs to identify if the pCO_2 is compensated. If compensation is not complete or overcompensated, then perhaps a second or third disorder is present.

Metabolic acidosis: $pCO_2 = 1.5(HCO_3)+8$

Metabolic alkalosis: $pCO_2 = 40 + 0.7(HCO_{3\ measured} - HCO_{3\ normal})$

Respiratory Acidosis:

    Acute: HCO_3 ↑ by 1 mEq/L for every 10 mmHg ↑ in pCO_2

    Chronic: HCO_3 ↑ by 3.5 mEq/L for every 10 mmHg ↑ in pCO_2

Respiratory Alkalosis:

    Acute: HCO_3 ↓ by 2 mEq/L for every 10 mmHg ↓ in pCO_2

    Chronic: HCO_3 ↓ by 5 mEq/L for every 10 mmHg ↓ in pCO_2

3. Compare the predicted level of HCO_3 or pCO_2 to the actual level. More than minor difference may indicate mixed acid-base disorder

4. Calculate the Anion Gap (AG)

$$AG = Na^+ - (Cl^- + HCO_3^-)$$
$$\text{Normal} = 6\text{-}12$$

5. Calculate the degree of Anion Gap elevation
   a. If AG >20 then high AG acidosis is probably present
   b. If AG >30 then high AG acidosis is certainly present

6 If high AG acidosis, then evaluate serum creatinine, lactate, glucose, and osmolar gap to help determine cause

Figure 6–1 Acid-Base Algorithm[1,2]

on the Henderson–Hasselbalch equation, an increase in pCO_2 necessarily causes a shift in the buffer system and the body compensates by increasing the amount of HCO_3 in the blood stream. While it depends if the situation is acute or chronic, generally a change in pCO_2 by 10 mmHg will require a change in HCO_3 in the same direction of approximately 3 to 5 mEq/L to keep the pH balanced. Primary changes in pCO_2 levels leading to alterations in pH are referred to as respiratory acidosis or alkalosis. If the changes in pCO_2 are in response to a primarily metabolic disorder, then it will be referred to as respiratory compensation.

Base

The next step is to evaluate the HCO_3 level obtained from the ABG. Bicarbonate is alkaline and the normal serum HCO_3 level is approximately 24 mEq/L. Similar to the discussion of pCO_2, changes from this normal value have a predictable effect on pH. For every 10 mEq/L change in HCO_3, pCO_2 will need to change by about 15 to 20 mmHg in the same direction to maintain pH. Remember that HCO_3 is primarily controlled by the kidney and takes longer to equilibrate than pCO_2, which can be altered simply by altering the respiratory rate. Primary changes in HCO_3 leading to alterations of pH are commonly referred to as metabolic acidosis or alkalosis. If the change is in response to a primary respiratory disorder, then changes will be referred to as a metabolic compensation.

Base Deficit (or Excess)

The base deficit (BD) and base excess (BE) represent the same calculation expressed in opposite terms, and they are used to aid in describing metabolic acidoses and alkaloses. Simply stated, a patient with a metabolic acidosis would have a deficit of base present in the circulation, and a patient with a metabolic alkalosis would have an excess amount of base present in the circulation. The reported number represents the concentration of base (mEq/L) that would need to be added to (or removed from) the blood stream to bring the pH to 7.4. Because it is confusing to continually switch between BD and BE on a lab report, laboratories will report out only one of the two and use a negative (–) sign to describe changes. Therefore, if a patient has a metabolic acidosis and BE is reported, the number would be negative, while the same patient would have a BD reported as a positive number.

There are actually several different equations that can be used to calculate BE.[9] One common equation that is used is:

$$BE = (HCO_3^- - 24.4 + [2.3 \times Hb + 7.7] \times [pH - 7.4]) \times (1 - 0.023 \times Hb)$$

Both HCO_3^- and hemoglobin (Hb) are presented in mmol/L in this equation. In practice, manually calculating a BE is often not required, as the laboratory will report this number with certain lab panels.

Acidosis or Alkalosis

Once pH, pCO_2, HCO_3, and BE have all been reviewed and compared to normal levels, a picture of the acid–base disorder should begin to take shape. Further evaluation of the patient history and comparison to the acid–base profile will provide additional clarity. For example, a chronic obstructive pulmonary disease (COPD) patient with a pH of 7.32, a pCO_2 level of 60, and an HCO_3 level of 29 would be considered to have a respiratory acidosis that is partially compensated. Note that the patient has a respiratory condition and elevated pCO_2, which is consistent with the observed acidosis, yet the degree of acidosis is buffered by the increase in HCO_3.

It is possible for acid and alkali substances that may influence pH to not be completely accounted for in this fairly simplistic evaluation. Lactic acid is one of the common confounders that can be present. As an example, a patient is admitted to the intensive care unit (ICU) with a diagnosis of sepsis and respiratory failure, with arterial blood gases that reveal a pH of 7.2, pCO_2 of 35, HCO_3 of 14, and a BE of –13. In this particular case, with a known presentation of sepsis, which is commonly associated with elevated lactate concentrations due to the anaerobic metabolism in a patient with decreased tissue oxygenation, the clinician should review other available laboratory values to account for the degree of acidosis that is present, and in particular the lactate level. Upon review of the lactate level, if it is found to be elevated, it would be concluded that this patient has a metabolic lactic acidosis with minimal respiratory compensation.

While these two examples are relatively simple illustrations of the evaluation and review of acid–base balance, this approach is easy to use at the bedside and with practice allows for rapid review and evaluation of patients on a daily basis. It is important to remember that this system tends to describe the acid–base imbalance rather than identify the cause of an acid–base imbalance, and careful evaluation of the patient's history and laboratory values is very important.[9,10]

Alternative Assessment Approach of Acid–Base

As stated, the approach to acid–base interpretation listed previously does not always provide a solid indication of the underlying cause of the acid–base abnormality. Therefore, alternative assessment techniques have been developed. One of the most common approaches is called the physical-chemical approach, which uses calculation of strong ions and weak acids to interpret acid–base disorders.[8-16] A detailed description of this method will probably serve to confuse more than improve understanding of acid–base balance, but a summary of the approach to acid–base analysis with this method is provided in Figure 6–2.

First, calculate the Strong Ion Difference [SID] which is equal to the Sum of positive strong ions (cations) – sum of negative strong ions (anions).

$[SID] = (Na^+ + K^+ + Ca^{2+} + Mg^{2+}) - (Cl^- + \text{other strong ions} + \text{lactate})$

So in a "normal" patient:

$[SID] = (140 + 4 + 8 + 2.5) - (100 + {\sim}12 + 1)$

$= 154.5 - 113 = 41.5$

The [SID] is usually about 40 to 42 mEq/L in humans.

Once the [SID] is known, the principles of neutrality state that charges must balance, therefore weak anions must make up the remaining negative charge. This leads to the creation of a variable known as A_{TOT} which represents the weak acids present in the blood (mostly proteins, phosphate, and blood cell components). Because A_{TOT} takes proteins into account, changes in albumin can be accounted for in this model.

The remaining variable in the analysis is pCO_2. This theory holds that HCO_3 is not an important determinant of pH. Rather, other acids present within the bloodstream account for the changes. This method has been described as a more accurate method of identifying the underlying cause of the acid-base disorder.

Figure 6–2 Physical Chemical Approach to Acid-Base Analysis[8–16]

ANION GAP

Electrolytes can also affect acid–base balance, and one of the more common analyses related to electrolytes and acid–base evaluation is the anion gap. The anion gap is particularly useful when the presentation is not as straightforward as the two previous case examples. The anion gap is calculated by subtracting the negative ions of chloride and bicarbonate from the positive ion sodium.[5] The normal anion gap is 6 to 12 mmol/L.

$$\text{Anion gap} = Na^+ - (Cl^- + HCO_3^-)$$

An elevated anion gap is related to several common disorders, many involving medications or toxic substances. Diabetic ketoacidosis and lactic acidosis are the most common organic causes of an elevated anion gap.[3,5,17,18] Acute and chronic renal failure are also common causes. Of particular interest to the pharmacist, acute toxic ingestions of salicylates, methanol, ethylene glycol, and propylene glycol are common causes of an elevated anion gap metabolic acidosis. Investigation of ingestion of toxic substances should be part of the evaluation for a patient that presents with an elevated anion gap without other readily explainable reasons.

Further investigation of the osmolar gap is warranted in suspected poisoning with methanol or ethylene glycol.[9,17,19] The osmolar gap is simply the measured serum osmolarity minus the calculated serum osmolarity. A common equation for calculating serum osmolarity is:[9]

$$\text{Osmolarity} = 2[\text{Na}] + [\text{Glucose}]/18 + [\text{BUN}]/2.8$$

when glucose and BUN are measured in mg/dL. If all units are in mmol/L, then the equation is:[17]

$$\text{Osmolarity} = 2[\text{Na}] + \text{Glucose} + \text{Urea}$$

This equation can be further altered when specifically evaluating patients suspected of ingesting methanol or ethylene glycol concurrently with alcohol:[9,19]

$$\text{Osmolarity} = 2[\text{Na}] + [\text{Glucose}]/18 + [\text{BUN}]/2.8 + [\text{Ethanol}]/4.6$$

An elevated osmolar gap can be helpful to differentiate ingestion of methanol or ethylene glycol from other causes of acidosis. It should be noted that early on after ingestion of methanol or ethylene glycol, the osmolar gap will be elevated, but as the toxins are metabolized, the osmolar gap will decrease, and become normal or nearly normal.[19] Therefore, a clear knowledge of the patient's history is important.

A non-anion gap metabolic acidosis is also commonly referred to as hyperchloremic metabolic acidosis. While many causes exist, the most common include significant gastrointestinal fluid losses through diarrhea, large volumes of saline administration (particularly hypertonic saline), and several medications such as NSAIDS, ACE-I, and trimethoprim.[4,5,11] Hyperchloremic acidosis is also possible when parenteral nutrition formulas are not monitored and adjusted carefully.

Alkalosis is less common than acidosis in ICU patients, but it can be very difficult to manage. Metabolic alkaloses can be caused by a variety of disorders including significant upper gastrointestinal losses and medications such as loop diuretics (a so-called "contraction alkalosis").[4,6] Alkalosis can also occur when patients with chronic respiratory acidosis have pCO_2 levels corrected rapidly. Since HCO_3 does not change as rapidly as pCO_2, the compensatory elevation in HCO_3 now creates an alkalosis.

ACID–BASE MANAGEMENT

Treatment of acid–base abnormalities is primarily supportive and should be directed at the underlying cause. Definitive medication therapy for correction of acidosis or alkalosis is often not necessary, as correction of the underlying disorder (utilizing mechanical ventilation in the case of respiratory distress or the improvement of oxygenation in the septic patient) will lead to correction of the acid–base imbalance. However, there are situations that require specific treatment of the acid–base disorder to deliver optimal outcomes for the patient.

Bicarbonate Therapy

Bicarbonate therapy is commonly used in critically ill patients and is most often provided by the intravenous (IV) route. The primary indication for use of IV bicarbonate is severe acidemia (pH <7.15) that is not caused by a condition such as ketoacidosis.[5] Unnecessary bicarbonate use can easily result in a metabolic alkalosis, particularly in a disease state like ketoacidosis that corrects relatively quickly once the underlying disorder is remedied. Most often the use of bicarbonate is directed toward conditions such as renal tubular acidosis or metabolic acidosis caused by significant diarrhea fluid losses.[6,20] Some experts recommend against ever using bicarbonate to treat lactic acidosis and other metabolic acidoses because of lack of supportive data for the therapy and potential adverse effects.[20]

Sodium bicarbonate is available in 50 ml vials or ampules (amps) that contain 50 mEq of bicarbonate. Bicarbonate is given in bolus doses of 50 to 150 mEq or is commonly ordered as the number of amps desired added to a volume of IV diluent to run as a continuous IV infusion. Many institutions have disallowed the practice of ordering any medication by amps or volume because of patient safety concerns.

For continuous infusions of bicarbonate, 50 to 150 mEq (1 to 3 amps) of sodium bicarbonate is added to one liter of solution. The sodium content must be taken into account when adding bicarbonate to a solution so as not to create a hypertonic saline solution, unless that is the intended therapy. For example, 150 mls of $NaHCO_3$ added to 1 liter of D5W (after 150 mls of the D5W bag is removed and discarded) would create a saline concentration very close to that of normal saline. However, adding 150 mls of $NaHCO_3$ to a liter of normal saline would result in a solution that is approximately 1.8% sodium. It is possible for errors to occur when orders that involve adding bicarbonate to IV solutions are not clearly written and sodium content is not carefully considered.

When used for the treatment of severe acidemia, bicarbonate therapy should be monitored closely and only used until the underlying disorder is resolved, so as to avoid overcorrection resulting in a metabolic alkalosis. Bicarbonate therapy is typically discontinued prior to serum levels reaching 18 or 20 mEq/L to also avoid overcorrection.[6] In patients with ketoacidosis or lactic acidosis, if bicarbonate is used at all, the goal would only be to correct HCO_3 levels to 10 or 12 and a pH of about 7.2 since ketones and lactate will be metabolized to base as the condition resolves.

Acetazolamide

Acetazolamide is a carbonic anhydrase inhibitor that interferes with the reabsorption of HCO_3 at the renal tubule, thereby resulting in a decreased serum HCO_3 level. While this appears to be an easy option to treat metabolic alkalosis, therapy should be applied cautiously because overcorrection can result in acidosis quite easily. The best example to illustrate the possibility of overcorrection is in the patient with underlying chronic lung disease. These patients commonly have a chronic compensatory increase in serum HCO_3 to account for persistent elevations of CO_2. When this patient is intubated and admitted to an ICU, if mechanical ventilation decreases CO_2 levels to normal values, the compensatory increase in HCO_3 will now lead to a metabolic alkalosis because HCO_3 does not correct as quickly at CO_2. Aggressive use of acetazolamide may decrease HCO_3 to normal and therefore correct pH, but when the patient is liberated from the mechanical ventilator, CO_2 will most likely return to baseline levels because of the chronic lung disease; now the patient will experience a respiratory acidosis that is uncompensated. Therefore, only judicious, short-term use of acetazolamide in the treatment of acute metabolic alkalosis should be considered, particularly when chronic respiratory disease is present.

Acid Therapy

On very rare occasions, a patient with severe life-threatening metabolic alkalosis requires IV infusion of acid as hydrochloric acid (HCl).[6] Hydrochloric acid solution should only be given through a central line and at a rate of no more than 0.2 mmol/kg of body weight per hour. The specific calculation to determine the amount of HCl that needs to be given is based on the amount of HCO_3 reduction desired multiplied by the patient's weight in kilograms multiplied by 0.5. Therefore, in an 80 kg patient where HCO_3 is desired to be decreased from 65 to 55 mmol/L (mEq/L), the dose of HCl would be $(65-55) \times 80 \times 0.5$, which would equal 400 mmols. Since the maximum concentration of HCl is 0.2 N (200 mmols/L), this would require at least 2 liters of solution. It should be reiterated that this therapy is only indicated for life-threatening alkalosis that cannot be resolved via other means.

Diuresis and Dialysis

The kidneys play a key role in acid–base balance; therefore, it makes sense that diuretic agents will also affect acid–base equilibrium. Adjustment of diuretic doses, changes from one agent to another, and the adjustment of IV fluids will all have an effect on the patient's overall acid–base status. The previously described contraction alkalosis can be improved by adjusting the loop diuretic dose or by infusing appropriate fluids.

Dialysis and continuous renal replacement therapy is commonly used to manage metabolic acidosis and alkalosis. The dialysate bath is set to a desired bicarbonate concentration, and this will lead to a normalization of the bicarbonate level. The rapidity with which acid–base status changes will be dependent upon the dialysis prescription, the concentration of HCO_3 in the dialysate, and the degree of the acid–base disorder. Furthermore, if the underlying disorder is not resolved, dialysis will only temporarily correct the acidemia or alkalemia.

ACID–BASE ABNORMALITIES AND EFFECTS ON MEDICATIONS

Many medications are affected by alterations of pH within the body. Medications such as phenytoin experience altered protein binding in an acidic environment, which leads to increased free drug available for binding at the active site. Recombinant human activated factor VII (rFVIIa), as a clotting factor, is significantly less effective at a pH of less than 7.0, so pH should be corrected if at all possible prior to use. Potency of vasopressor agents may also be affected as the acidemia affects intracellular function of the smooth muscle cells.[21]

There are some instances where alterations of acid–base are used as a therapeutic treatment. Tricyclic antidepressant renal elimination can be increased by alkalinizing the urine, so therapy with intravenous bicarbonate therapy can be helpful in some cases of overdose. Furthermore, bicarbonate therapy has been commonly used as a renal protective strategy in multiple settings, including rhabdomyolysis and radiocontrast exposure.[22] While the utility of alkalinizing the patient as a renal protective strategy has not always proven beneficial, and clinician opinions vary, it remains a rather common practice and can be effective in select situations. Furthermore, changes in pH cause changes in the intracellular shift of several electrolytes and clinicians may therapeutically alter pH to help manage electrolyte abnormalities, particularly hyperkalemia.

SUMMARY

The evaluation and management of acid–base disorders is a common part of critical care practice. The pharmacist must understand the appropriate therapies involved in treatment of these disorders and provide appropriate recommendations regarding the initiation and discontinuation of medications used to correct acid–base disturbances.

KEY POINTS

- Differentiating between respiratory and metabolic causes is an important part of patient assessment for acid–base abnormalities.
- Bicarbonate therapy should only be used in severe acidemia and should be used judiciously to avoid overcorrection and a resultant metabolic acidosis.
- Acid therapy should only be used in severe life-threatening alkalosis settings unresolved by other therapies.
- Bicarbonate therapy may be a helpful prophylactic and treatment approach in certain settings.

SELECTED SUGGESTED READING

- Liamis G, Milionis HJ, Elisaf M. Pharmacologically-induced metabolic acidosis: a review. *Drug Saf.* 2010;33:371–391.
- Ayers P, Warrington L. Diagnosis and treatment of simple acid–base disorders. *Nutr Clin Pract.* 2008;23:122–127.
- Kellum JA. Disorders of acid–base balance. *Crit Care Med.* 2007;35:2630–2636.
- Kellum JA. Determinants of plasma acid–base balance. *Crit Care Clin.* 2005;21:329–346.
- Rastegar A. Clinical utility of Stewart's method in diagnosis and management of acid–base disorders. *Clin J Am Soc Nephrol.* 2009;4:1267–1274.

REFERENCES

1. Liamis G, Milionis HJ, Elisaf M. Pharmacologically-induced metabolic acidosis: a review. *Drug Saf.* 2010;33:371–391.
2. Ayers P, Warrington L. Diagnosis and treatment of simple acid–base disorders. *Nutr Clin Pract.* 2008;23:122–127.
3. Vanek VW. Assessment and management of acid–base abnormalities. In: Scott A. Shikora RGM, Schwaitzberg SD, eds. *Nutritional considerations in the intensive care unit.* Dubuque: Kendall/Hunt; 2002:101–109.

4. Gennari FJ, Weise WJ. Acid–base disturbances in gastrointestinal disease. *Clin J Am Soc Nephrol.* 2008;3:1861–1868.

5. Adrogue HJ, Madias NE. Management of life-threatening acid–base disorders. First of two parts. *N Engl J Med.* 1998;338:26–34.

6. Adrogue HJ, Madias NE. Management of life-threatening acid–base disorders. Second of two parts. *N Engl J Med.* 1998;338:107–111.

7. Morris CG, Low J. Metabolic acidosis in the critically ill: part 1. Classification and pathophysiology. *Anaesthesia.* 2008;63:294–301.

8. Kellum JA. Determinants of plasma acid–base balance. *Crit Care Clin.* 2005;21:329–346.

9. Kellum JA. Disorders of acid–base balance. *Crit Care Med.* 2007;35:2630–2636.

10. Gunnerson KJ, Kellum JA. Acid–base and electrolyte analysis in critically ill patients: are we ready for the new millennium? *Curr Opin Crit Care.* 2003;9:468–473.

11. Kaplan LJ, Kellum JA. Fluids, pH, ions and electrolytes. *Curr Opin Crit Care.* 2010;16:323–331.

12. Wooten EW. Science review: quantitative acid–base physiology using the Stewart model. *Crit Care.* 2004;8:448–452.

13. Kaplan LJ, Cheung NH, Maerz L, et al. A physicochemical approach to acid–base balance in critically ill trauma patients minimizes errors and reduces inappropriate plasma volume expansion. *J Trauma.* 2009;66:1045–1051.

14. Rastegar A. Clinical utility of Stewart's method in diagnosis and management of acid–base disorders. *Clin J Am Soc Nephrol.* 2009;4:1267–1274.

15. Kellum JA. Acid–base disorders and strong ion gap. *Contrib Nephrol.* 2007;156:158–166.

16. Kellum JA. Clinical review: reunification of acid–base physiology. *Crit Care.* 2005;9:500–507.

17. Herd AM. An approach to complex acid–base problems: keeping it simple. *Can Fam Physician.* 2005;51:226–232.

18. Taylor D, Durward A, Tibby SM, et al. The influence of hyperchloraemia on acid base interpretation in diabetic ketoacidosis. *Intensive Care Med.* 2006;32:295–301.

19. Mycyk MB, Aks SE. A visual schematic for clarifying the temporal relationship between the anion and osmol gaps in toxic alcohol poisoning. *Am J Emerg Med.* 2003;21:333–335.

20. Gehlbach BK, Schmidt GA. Bench-to-bedside review: treating acid–base abnormalities in the intensive care unit - the role of buffers. *Crit Care.* 2004;8:259–265.

21. Landry DW, Oliver JA. The pathogenesis of vasodilatory shock. *N Engl J Med.* 2001;345:588–595.

22. Massicotte A. Contrast medium-induced nephropathy: strategies for prevention. *Pharmacotherapy.* 2008;28:1140–1150.

Chapter 7

Fluid and Electrolyte Management

Billie Bartel and Elizabeth Gau

LEARNING OBJECTIVES

1. Identify and understand basic fluid and electrolyte abnormalities in critically ill patients.
2. Differentiate between the types of fluids used for fluid replacement in different disease states commonly seen in the intensive care unit.
3. Recognize the causes of electrolyte abnormalities in critically ill patients.
4. Understand when and how to replace or replete electrolytes in critically ill patients.

INTRODUCTION

Fluid and electrolyte abnormalities are common in critically ill patients and often represent complications from underlying disease states or medication therapies. Critically ill patients often experience alterations in absorption, distribution, and excretion of fluids and electrolytes. Changes in hormonal and homeostatic processes and fluid status are also common in intensive care unit patients.

Significant complications can result from fluid and electrolyte abnormalities, and the severity of these complications usually parallels the magnitude of the disorder. Fluid and electrolyte disorders occurring acutely and rapidly are often associated with increased symptoms and complications when compared to chronically occurring imbalances; these symptomatic abnormalities require more urgent treatment. Recognizing the cause of fluid and electrolyte abnormalities is important when making treatment decisions. Critically ill patients often require very frequent monitoring and evaluation of fluid status and serum electrolyte concentrations throughout their treatment course.

Pharmacists often assist in the management of fluid and electrolyte abnormalities in the intensive care unit. Working with physicians, pharmacists play an important role in the determination of underlying causes of these disorders, particularly when disorders are medication-related, and in providing knowledge of the potential implications of individual medications. Pharmacists also often evaluate and recommend treatment of fluid and electrolyte disturbances. This chapter will review body water composition and electrolyte regulation, focusing on the recognition, presentation, treatment, and monitoring of fluid and electrolyte disorders.

WATER AND FLUID IMBALANCES IN THE CRITICALLY ILL

Water comprises a high percentage of body fluid, with the exact percentage dependent on sex, age, and weight; the approximate percentages of body weight as water in men and women are 50% and 60%, respectively. Total body water is distributed into the intracellular and extracellular space, with the extracellular space broken down further into the intravascular and interstitial space. A complete breakdown of body water distribution is detailed in Figure 7–1.

The body maintains equilibrium between these spaces by maintaining osmolality in the extracellular space and intracellular space via allowing water permeation between cell membranes. Osmolality is the solute or particle content per liter of water (mOsm/L) with normal osmolality in the plasma between 285 and 295 mOsm/L.[1] Serum osmolality can be calculated based on serum levels of sodium, glucose, and BUN using the following equation:[2]

$$\text{Serum Osmolality} = 2(\text{Na}) + \text{Glucose}/18 + \text{BUN}/2.8$$

Fluid movement between the intravascular and interstitial spaces occurs across capillary walls by either filtration or diffusion and is determined by

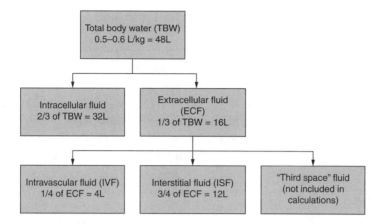

Figure 7–1 Body water distribution and example for 80kg male

Data from: Kaplan LJ, Kellum JA. Fluids, pH, ions, and electrolytes. *Cur Opin Crit Care.* 2010;16:323–331.

Starling forces. Normal distributions of fluid between compartments are commonly altered in critically ill patients before arriving in the intensive care unit (ICU) and will continue if not corrected. Causes of normal fluid loss are skin evaporation, urination, breathing, and through the gastrointestinal tract, but in critically ill patients, these normal losses are altered and increased through various mechanisms. It is important for pharmacists to evaluate patients in the ICU for fluid loss and accumulation and to note that each disease state has specific causes of and treatments for fluid imbalance.

Trauma and Surgery Patients

Trauma patients lose a significant amount of fluid through blood loss and third spacing,[3] which is a lack of equilibrium between the intracellular and extracellular fluid. The fluid remains extracellularly, but moves to areas that usually do not have fluid accumulation, like bowel lumen, subcutaneous tissues, retroperitoneal or peritoneal space, and the peritoneal cavity. Fluid accumulation in these areas exerts pressure on organs and removes fluid from the intravascular space, which requires sufficient volume to maintain cardiac output.

Surgical patients, either trauma or non-trauma, tend to begin surgery volume-depleted.[3] This is due to blood loss from trauma or because of dehydration caused by the long-term decreased fluid intake that occurs in disease states such as pancreatitis or cholecystitis. In contrast, post-operative patients tend to be fluid positive due to resuscitation during the procedure.[3]

Fluid is also lost through major burns. Intact skin will still lose fluid, but this occurs to a much greater extent with burns. Fluid resuscitation is extremely important in burn patients because they are at high risk for developing shock,[4] and so increased insensible fluid losses in these patients need to be replaced. The Consensus formula can be used to estimate fluid needs in burn patients. The resuscitation phase requires 4 ml/kg per percentage of body surface area burned. Fifty percent of needs should be given over the first 8 hours, then completed over the next 16 hours.[4] Ongoing maintenance fluid needs are then determined based upon patient condition.

Sepsis

Sepsis is another condition where systemic inflammation and vasodilation moves fluid from the intravascular space into the interstitial space. Patients with sepsis also experience fluid imbalances due to treatment strategies. Septic patients present with systemic vasodilation due to inflammatory cytokine release,[5] and fluids are used as treatment in sepsis to replace the lost volume in the intravascular space. Fluid resuscitation in sepsis adds many liters of fluid into a patient; however, after distribution, only a small portion of that fluid stays within the intravascular space, the amount of which is often determined by the osmolality of the fluid used in resuscitation.

In addition to disease states, fluid losses can also come from increased output from normal sites. Diarrhea and high ostomy output can affect fluid status, electrolytes, and acid–base balance. Increased urine output from diuretics can normalize fluid status, but can also affect electrolytes and cause dehydration.

FLUID REPLACEMENT

Fluid replacement is a large part of therapy in critically ill patients. Initial fluid replacement begins with the resuscitation phase. Rapid administration of large volumes of fluid replaces fluid lost from the intravascular space and prevents further decompensation due to low circulating volume. This strategy is important in treating many disease states, including shock, trauma, and burns. After the resuscitation period, fluid administration is adjusted to replace ongoing sensible and insensible losses.

Fluid replacement is provided in the form of either crystalloids or colloids. Each type of fluid has advantages and disadvantages in certain disease states. Crystalloids are fluids with a high volume of distribution. The main component of crystalloids is water, with additional electrolytes and/or dextrose.

Colloids are homogeneous non-crystalline substances also in a water base. Colloid particles are much larger than the electrolyte components in crystalloid solutions, so they tend to provide less free water and stay primarily in the intravascular space.

Examples of crystalloids are lactated Ringer's (LR) and normal saline (NS). These types of fluids may also contain dextrose to supply a glucose source and calories. Normal saline and LR distribute within the extracellular spaces. Lactated Ringer's solution contains electrolytes in amounts similar to serum levels and is used most often in trauma and surgery patients. Dextrose 5% in water (D5W) is also considered a crystalloid, but provides free water and distributes to both the intracellular and extracellular spaces. Since the goal of resuscitation is to replete intravascular volume, D5W is not typically used within this phase of treatment. Crystalloids are the primary fluid type for resuscitation and maintenance as they can be provided easily and at low cost.

Colloids contain large molecules such as proteins or starches to increase oncotic pressure in the intravascular space. Examples of colloids are hetastarch and dextran (starches), whole blood and packed red blood cells (PRBCs), and albumin (proteins). Blood is the only colloid that provides the advantage of intravascular volume expansion and increased oxygen-carrying capacity. The synthetic starches add to intravascular volume, but do not need blood typing and antigen matching as with blood products; similarly, albumin does not require typing and matching, but since it is derived from human sources, it still carries a very low risk of viral transmission. Each of these products has other advantages and disadvantages that will be discussed in individual disease states. Types of fluids are outlined in Table 7–1.[1]

Trauma and Surgery

Goals of fluid resuscitation in trauma are to replace intravascular volume loss due to blood loss, maintain blood pressure, and maintain oxygen delivery. Whole blood, or pRBCs, in addition to fluids are used to replace the functional capacity of oxygen delivery and clotting. Advance Trauma Life Support programs sponsored by the American College of Surgeons recommend crystalloids for resuscitation.[3] Most studies have found no difference in survival between crystalloids and colloids, except in specific subsets of trauma patients, but crystalloids allow faster, less expensive fluid replacement as compared to colloids.[6] Surgical patients are managed in a similar manner as they do have some loss of blood during surgery, but also compartmentalize fluid due to surgical manipulation. These patients may require blood and/or crystalloids depending on patient-specific factors.

Table 7–1 Types of Fluid Replacement[1]

Fluid	mOsm/L	Electrolytes/L	Distribution (1L)
Crystalloids			
Lactated Ringer's	273	130 mEq Na 109 mEq Cl 28 mEq lactate 4 mEq K 3 mEq Ca	1L ECF (250ml IVF)
0.9% NaCl	308	154 mEq Na 154 mEq Cl	1L ECF (250ml IVF)
0.45% NaCl	154	77 mEq Na 77 mEq Cl	333ml ICF/667ml ECF (166ml IVF)
D5%	252	50 g dextrose	667ml ICF/333ml ECF(83ml IVF)
D5% 0.9% NaCl	560	154 mEq Na 154 mEq Cl 50 g dextrose	1L ECF (250ml IVF)
Colloids			
Albumin 5%	300		1L ECF
Albumin 25%	1500		1L ECF
Hetastarch 6%	309		1L ECF

Traumatic Brain Injury

Large studies have examined the benefits of crystalloids vs. colloids in traumatic brain injury patients. The most well known study is the SAFE-TBI review of saline versus albumin for fluid resuscitation.[7] The theory behind the use of albumin is based on the physiological principle that if plasma oncotic pressure is maintained, less intravascular fluid will redistribute into the brain interstitium. However, this has not been proven in animal or human models. The SAFE-TBI trial found that fluid resuscitation in brain injury patients with albumin was associated with higher mortality rates than with saline. One of the mainstays for treatment of brain injury has become the use of hypertonic crystalloids, which is intended to increase plasma osmolality and decrease cerebral edema. Chapter 15 has a thorough discussion of fluid management in traumatic brain injury.

Sepsis

Fluid resuscitation is a first-line therapy in sepsis to improve tissue hypoperfusion. During the first 6 hours after presentation for sepsis, fluids are necessary to achieve and maintain goal central venous pressure, mean arterial pressure, urine output, and central venous oxygen saturation. Maximizing fluid resuscitation and other components of Early Goal Directed Therapy as recommended by the Surviving Sepsis Campaign has been shown to reduce 28-day mortality.[5] However, the type of fluid recommended by the Surviving Sepsis Campaign is nonspecific. Either crystalloids or colloids are recommended during the resuscitation phase; generally, normal saline is the crystalloid most commonly used. If adequate central venous oxygen saturation is not achieved, transfusion of PRBCs is recommended to maintain hematocrit ≥30%.[5] Chapter 10 provides additional details regarding sepsis resuscitation.

SODIUM HOMEOSTASIS

Sodium is the most abundant extracellular cation in the body and works to regulate extracellular and intravascular volume. Sodium is the major cation that determines serum osmolality, which regulates water flow, as water moves from one compartment to another of lower osmolality until homeostasis is achieved. Normal serum sodium levels are 133 to 145 mEq/L. The total amount of sodium in the body is a component of water balance, but the concentration of sodium in the serum does not determine water balance.

Serum sodium only determines the number of cations needed in the intravascular space to maintain hemostasis with the interstitial and intracellular spaces. Total body sodium may not be accurately reflected by serum sodium concentrations, thus inappropriate treatment of serum sodium alterations may result in further complications. Imbalances in sodium are best evaluated by first evaluating serum sodium, followed by serum osmolality, and then volume status.

Hyponatremia

Hyponatremia is defined as serum sodium <133 mEq/L. The signs and symptoms of hyponatremia are rather non-specific, and include headache, lethargy, disorientation, nausea, depressed reflexes, seizures, and coma.[8] Most of these reactions occur when serum sodium is <120 mEq/L and are due to changes in serum osmolality and fluid balance in the central nervous system. The treatment used to correct hyponatremia depends on the cause and duration of the imbalance, as well as the fluid status of the patient. Recent and acute onset hyponatremia is more likely to be symptomatic and can be more rapidly corrected compared to chronic hyponatremia, which is usually not associated with as severe of symptoms and should be corrected slowly. In the ICU, hyponatremia is one factor that leads to increased mortality, so appropriate correction should not be delayed.[8]

Isotonic Hyponatremia

Once a patient is identified as having hyponatremia, serum osmolality should be assessed. Patients with isotonic hyponatremia have a normal serum osmolality. Common causes of isotonic hyponatremia include hyperlipidemia and hyperproteinemia. This is a not a true state of hyponatremia, as sodium in the aqueous portion of the serum is normal. Isotonic hyponatremia is treated by correcting the underlying cause or discontinuing any protein-based fluids.

Hypertonic Hyponatremia

Patients with hypertonic hyponatremia have an elevated serum osmolality. Causes of hypertonic hyponatremia are hyperglycemia (e.g., diabetic ketoacidosis and hyperosmolar hyperglycemic syndrome) and administration of hypertonic sodium-free solutions such as mannitol. Hyperglycemia causes water to move into the extracellular space to decrease osmolality via sodium dilution. For every 100 mg/dL increase in glucose above 100 mg/dL, the measured serum sodium will decrease by 1.6 mEq/L.[8] Treatment for hypertonic hyponatremia is to correct the underlying cause or stop any IV hypertonic solutions.

Hypotonic Hyponatremia

Hypotonic hyponatremia occurs in patients with low serum osmolality and is typically the most common cause of severe hyponatremia. To further determine cause and treatment of hypotonic hyponatremia, volume status must be evaluated.

Hypovolemic hypotonic hyponatremia occurs with fluid losses, such as during excessive diuresis, hemorrhage, diarrhea, and burns. In these patients, volume and sodium are replaced with normal saline or lactated Ringer's solution.

Isovolemic hypotonic hyponatremia occurs during conditions of sodium wasting and water conservation, such as in syndrome of inappropriate antidiuretic hormone (SIADH), adrenal insufficiency, hypothyroidism, and as a side effect of some medications. In this condition, continued fluid administration will exacerbate the hyponatremia, and so water restriction is the preferred treatment. Diuresis with loop diuretics and administration of hypertonic saline can also be helpful. Possible medication-related types of isovolemic hypotonic hyponatremia are listed in Table 7–2.

Hypervolemic hypotonic hyponatremia occurs in cirrhosis, congestive heart failure, and renal failure, and is caused by the inability to maintain normal volume status. These patients demonstrate a dilutional effect on sodium and other solutes in the serum. Diuresis is the primary treatment in this type of hyponatremia.

Treatment

Treatment of hyponatremia depends on serum osmolality and volume status, but rate of correction is similar in all conditions. For patients requiring NS or hypertonic saline as part of their treatment regimen,

Table 7–2 Medications Causing Hyponatremia and Hypernatremia[9]

Hyponatremia	**Diuretics** (Loop, thiazide)
	Mannitol
	ACE Inhibitors
	Trimethoprim-sulfamethoxazole
	Proton pump inhibitors
	Carbamazepine
	NSAIDs
	Antipsychotics
	Antidepressants
Hypernatremia	Loop diuretics
	Mannitol
	Amphotericin B
	Demeclocycline
	Lithium
	Normal and hypertonic saline
	Hypertonic bicarbonate solution
	Lactulose

sodium deficit can be calculated to determine the amount of sodium needed to correct the hyponatremia:[1,8]

Sodium deficit (mEq) = Total body water x (140 – serum sodium)

It should be noted that clinicians often calculate a sodium deficit based upon a target level of 125 or 130 (instead of 140) mEq/L to avoid over-correction. This calculated sodium deficit can then be used to determine a sodium solution infusion rate with serum sodium corrected at a rate of 1 to 2 mEq/L/hr in acute, symptomatic hyponatremia and 0.5 mEq/L/hr in chronic hyponatremia, but not more than 12 mEq/L in 24 hours in either case. Fifty percent of the sodium deficit should be replaced within the first 24 hours (again not to exceed 12 mEq/L/24 hours), and be completed over 48 to 72 hours. Overly-rapid correction of sodium can lead to the serious complication of central pontine myelinolysis.[8] All patients should be monitored closely, but attention should be paid in particular to those receiving hypertonic saline at high infusion rates (e.g., 3% NS at >30ml/hr) due to this potential complication. Patients with severe symptomatic hyponatremia should have frequent serum sodium checks, sometimes as often as hourly, and this is especially important if hypertonic saline (3% or 5%) is used as part of the treatment regimen.

Hypernatremia

Similar to hyponatremia, signs and symptoms of hypernatremia are non-specific and include lethargy, irritability, thirst, hyperreflexia, seizures, and coma; most serious symptoms are due to osmolality changes in the central nervous system. Hypernatremia is a reflection of a volume deficit relative to serum sodium, or a concentrating effect. Volume loss in conditions such as burns, diarrhea, diabetes insipidus, and administration of hypertonic fluids leads to hypernatremia. Hypernatremia in the ICU is also associated with an increased mortality risk.[2] As with hyponatremia, serum sodium should be corrected at a rate of not more than 1 to 2 mEq/L/hr in order to prevent cerebral edema. A water deficit can be calculated based on serum sodium, and this can serve as a guide for fluid resuscitation and maintenance:

Water deficit (L) = TBW x [(serum sodium/140) – 1]

Fifty percent of the water deficit should be replaced over the first 24 hours, with the entire process completed within 48 to 72 hours. A 5% dextrose or 0.45% saline solution can be used to provide fluid and minimize sodium load; remember that sterile water should never be used alone as an IV infusion.

As with hyponatremia, hypernatremia can also occur in different volume states. Hypovolemic hypernatremia should be initially corrected with fluids such as NS or LR until any symptomatic hypovolemia is corrected, and then fluids can be changed to D5W or 0.45% saline. Isovolemic hypernatremia occurs from water loss or sodium excess, and this type of hypernatremia is usually seen in diabetes insipidus. Hypervolemic hypernatremia is usually the result of hypertonic saline administration. This type of hypernatremia is treated with loop diuretics and D5W or 0.45% saline.

POTASSIUM HOMEOSTASIS

Potassium is the most abundant intracellular cation in the body, with approximately 98% of the body's potassium found intracellularly and only 2% present extracellularly. The normal serum potassium concentration exists within the range of 3.5 to 5 mEq/L.[10,11]

The body utilizes potassium for many functions, including regulation of electrical action potential across cell membranes (especially in the heart), cellular metabolism, and glycogen and protein synthesis. The sodium–potassium–adenosine triphosphatase (Na–K–ATPase) pump is principally responsible for regulating potassium entry into cells. Potassium is primarily excreted by the kidneys.[2,12-13] Potassium homeostasis can be altered by many mechanisms that are often present in critically ill patients, including acid-base imbalances, organ dysfunction, trauma, and malnutrition. Alterations in potassium homeostasis can cause severe cardiac abnormalities requiring emergent treatment and close monitoring in the intensive care unit.

Hypokalemia

Hypokalemia is defined as a serum potassium concentration less than 3.5 mEq/L, and severe hypokalemia occurs when the serum potassium concentration is less than 2.5 mEq/L or any time symptoms are present. Hypokalemia can be caused by an intracellular shift of potassium ions, increased potassium losses, or reduced ingestion. Critically ill patients present with many of the underlying etiologies responsible for the development of hypokalemia, and the cause of hypokalemia is often multifactoral in these patients. [2,14-15] Intracellular shift of potassium ions is often caused by metabolic alkalosis. Malnourished patients are at risk for development of hypokalemia during refeeding. Several medications can also cause intracellular shift, including albuterol, insulin, theophylline, and caffeine. Increased potassium loss from the body may be due to gastrointestinal losses or renal replacement therapy. Several medications are often associated with potassium loss, including loop and thiazide diuretics, sodium polystyrene sulfonate, and amphotericin. Hypomagnesemia also can cause refractory hypokalemia by impairing the Na–K–ATPase pump in the kidneys, resulting in increased urinary potassium losses.[2,14-15]

The symptoms associated with hypokalemia are often associated with compromised muscular and cardiovascular function. Hypokalemia may result in membrane hyperpolarization with subsequent insufficient muscle contraction. Symptoms of hypokalemia include weakness, respiratory compromise, and paralysis. Electrocardiogram changes can occur, including T wave flattening, T wave inversion, ST segment depression, and presence of U waves. The most serious complications associated with hypokalemia are cardiac arrhythmias and sudden death.[2, 12-13]

The goals for treatment of hypokalemia include normalization of serum potassium concentration and avoidance or resolution of symptoms. Potassium replacement should be guided by serum levels. The patient's acid–base status has a significant effect on the cellular shift of potassium, so serum levels must be adjusted due to this redistribution secondary to pH. Serum potassium levels will fall by 0.6 mEq/L for every 0.1 increase in pH, and vice versa.[16-18] Careful attention to acid–base status is an important part of ongoing management of serum potassium. Magnesium should also be supplemented if serum magnesium concentrations are low.[19]

Enteral and intravenous potassium replacement are both effective options. Intravenous replacement should take precedence only with severe hypokalemia, presence of symptoms, or lack of an enteral route for administration. Empiric dosing recommendations are listed in Table 7–3. Patients with renal impairment should only receive approximately 50% of the recommended initial potassium dose. Intravenous potassium should be infused at a slow rate of 10 to 20 mEq per hour to avoid cardiac complications, and infusion rates greater than 10 mEq per hour require continuous cardiac monitoring. Potassium infusion rates as high as 40 mEq per hour may be used, but only in emergency situations. Potassium levels should be checked frequently during replacement therapy to avoid overcorrection and development of hyperkalemia.[2,16-18,20] Often, non-emergent replacement of potassium and other electrolytes is driven by institutional protocols (see Table 7–4).

Table 7–3 IV Potassium Replacement[10-12]

Serum Potassium Level (mEq/L)	IV Potassium Replacement Dosing
3–3.4	20–40 mEq
Less than 3	40–80 mEq

Table 7-4 Example IV Electrolyte Replacement Protocol[2,10-12,24,26-29,38-40]

Potassium Replacement:
  Normal:

Serum K+ Level	K+ Dose
3.6 or greater	None
3.3 to 3.5	20 mEq KCl
3 to 3.2	40 mEq KCl
Less than 3	40 mEq KCl AND call physician

  Aggressive:

Serum K+ Level	K+ Dose
4 or greater	None
3.5 to 3.9	20 mEq KCl
3.3 to 3.4	40 mEq KCl
3 to 3.2	60 mEq KCl
Less than 3	60 mEq KCl AND call physician

  Labs:
  __ Recheck serum K+ 1 hour after IV bolus
  __ Serum K+ level every _____ hours
  __ Serum magnesium with next blood draw
  __ Serum glucose with next blood draw
  __ Basic metabolic panel with next blood draw
  __ Arterial blood gas now

Magnesium Replacement:

Serum Mg Level	IV Magnesium Dose
1.5 to 1.9	Magnesium sulfate 2 g in 100 ml IV over 2 hours
1.1 to 1.4	Magnesium sulfate 4 g in 250 ml IV over 4 hours
Less than 1.1	Magnesium sulfate 6 g in 250 ml IV over 6 hours

  Fluid for IV admixture:
  __ 0.9% NaCl OR __ D5W
  Labs:
  __ Magnesium level 2 hours after end of infusion
  __ Magnesium level in AM

Phosphorus Replacement:

Serum Phos Level	IV Phosphorus Dose
1.8 to 2.4	10 mmol in 100 ml IV over 2 hours
1 to 1.7	20 mmol in __ 100 ml Or __ 250 ml IV over 4 hours
Less than 1	40 mmol in 250 ml IV over 6 hours

  Fluid for IV admixture:
  __ 0.9% NaCl OR __ D5W
  Labs:
  __ Phosphorus level 2 hours after end of infusion
  __ Phosphorus level in AM

(*continued*)

Table 7–4 Example IV Electrolyte Replacement Protocol[2,10-12,24,26-29,38-40]

Calcium Replacement:

Serum Ionized Calcium	IV Calcium Dose
1 to 1.11	Calcium gluconate 1 gram in 100 ml IV over 30 min
0.9 to 0.99	Calcium gluconate 2 grams in 100 ml IV over 1 hour
0.8 to 0.89	Calcium gluconate 3 grams in 100 ml IV over 1 hour
Less than 0.8	Calcium gluconate 4 grams in 100 ml IV over 2 hours

Fluid for IV admixture:

__ 0.9% NaCl OR __ D5W

Labs:

__ Ionized calcium 2 hours after end of infusion

__ Ionized calcium in AM

Hyperkalemia

Hyperkalemia is present when the serum potassium concentration exceeds 5 mEq/L, and it is potentially life threatening with serum concentrations above 6.5 mEq/L. Hyperkalemia can be caused by an extracellular shift in potassium ions, excessive potassium ingestion, or reduced potassium elimination. Extracellular shift of potassium ions often occurs in metabolic acidosis, trauma, or rhabdomyolysis; medications such as beta-blockers, succinylcholine, and digoxin can also cause extracellular shift of potassium. Impaired potassium excretion is most often problematic in patients with acute renal failure. There are also several medications that can reduce potassium elimination, including potassium-sparing diuretics, angiotensin-converting enzyme inhibitors, and nonsteroidal anti-inflammatory agents.[2,11]

Symptoms of hyperkalemia usually do not develop until serum potassium concentrations reach 5.5 mEq/L. Symptoms associated with hyperkalemia are caused by changes in neuromuscular and cardiac function and include muscle twitching, cramping, weakness, and paralysis. The most concerning symptoms are cardiac abnormalities, which are demonstrated by electrocardiogram changes including peaked T waves, widened QRS complexes, a prolonged PR interval, and a shortened QT interval; this can lead to potentially life-threatening cardiac arrhythmias.[2,11]

Goals of treatment of hyperkalemia include rapidly antagonizing the effects of potassium and facilitating potassium excretion. All exogenous potassium should be discontinued. Intravenous calcium (as chloride or gluconate salt) can be administered if symptoms or electrocardiogram changes are present, as calcium will antagonize the effects of potassium to rapidly stabilize cardiac muscle function. Insulin with dextrose, sodium bicarbonate, and albuterol will promote intracellular shift of potassium ions and are options for rapid correction of hyperkalemia; note that these methods will aid in normalization of serum potassium levels, but will not affect total body potassium stores, therefore therapies to promote potassium excretion are necessary. Potassium-wasting diuretics, specifically loop diuretics, will increase the renal excretion of potassium. Sodium polystyrene sulfonate acts as a cation exchange resin, binding to potassium in the gastrointestinal tract to facilitate elimination. Renal replacement therapy will permanently remove potassium from the body and is indicated in patients with renal impairment or after non-response to diuretics or sodium polystyrene sulfonate. Serum potassium levels must be frequently monitored to ensure effective therapy and avoid overcorrection.[2,11]

MAGNESIUM HOMEOSTASIS

Magnesium is an intracellular cation, found primarily in the bone, muscle, and soft tissue, with approximately 1% of total body stores present in extracellular fluid. The normal serum magnesium concentration is 1.5 to 2.4 mg/dL.[21,22]

Magnesium is utilized throughout the body as a cofactor for enzymes and is required in reactions involving adenosine triphosphatase (ATP). Magnesium is largely regulated by the kidneys; however, other factors, including gastrointestinal function, parathyroid hormone activity, and patient condition, affect magnesium homeostasis.[2,21-23] Magnesium homeostasis is important in critically ill patients due to its association with potassium and calcium homeostasis. Magnesium is also used in the treatment of life-threatening arrhythmias and preeclampsia.

Hypomagnesemia

Hypomagnesemia is defined as a serum magnesium concentration less than 1.5 mg/dL and is considered severe when the serum magnesium concentration is below 1 mg/dL. Hypomagnesemia can be caused by or associated with excessive gastrointestinal losses, renal losses, surgery, trauma, burns, sepsis, pancreatitis, malnutrition, and alcoholism.[2,21,24] Hypomagnesemia is very common among critically ill patients, and has been associated with increased mortality rates.[21,25-27] Medications associated with hypomagnesemia include thiazide and loop diuretics, amphotericin, cisplatin, cyclosporine, and digoxin.[21,24] Symptoms associated with hypomagnesemia include arrhythmias, torsades de pointes, seizures, coma, and death.

Hypomagnesemia can cause concomitant hypokalemia and hypocalcemia, which are often refractory to other treatments.[21]

Goals of treatment include normalizing serum magnesium concentrations and resolution of symptoms. Magnesium may be replaced by the intravenous or enteral route of administration, though intravenous is often preferred due to slow absorption and intolerances to magnesium-containing enteral products. Mild to moderate hypomagnesemia should be initially treated with 1 to 4 g of IV magnesium sulfate (8 to 32 mEq of magnesium), while severe hypomagnesemia will typically require 4 to 6 g (32 to 48 mEq). This dosing should be reduced in patients with renal dysfunction by approximately 50%.[2,24,28,29] In critically ill patients, magnesium is often replaced until serum concentrations reach 2 mg/dL due to the association between hypomagnesemia and other electrolyte abnormalities. Rapid renal elimination (50% of the IV dose is renally excreted) and slow distribution into tissues necessitate slow infusion of intravenous magnesium, with a suggested maximum rate of 1 g per hour. Patients often require multiple doses for complete repletion. An additional consideration is that magnesium levels drawn after infusion may be falsely elevated due to magnesium's slow distribution into body tissues.[2,21,29] Serum levels should be monitored at least daily during supplementation or replacement. Often, non-emergent replacement of magnesium and other electrolytes is driven by institutional protocols (see Table 7–4).

Hypermagnesemia

Hypermagnesemia is defined as a serum magnesium concentration greater than 2.4 mg/dL. Elevated serum magnesium concentrations are most often due to renal insufficiency or iatrogenic causes,[2,21,23] and most patients remain asymptomatic until serum magnesium concentrations exceed 4 mg/dL. Serum magnesium concentrations between 4 and 12.5 mg/dL are defined as moderate hypermagnesemia. Symptoms associated with moderate hypermagnesemia include nausea, vomiting, hypotension, bradycardia, and loss of deep tendon reflex. Severe hypermagnesemia is defined as serum magnesium concentration greater than 12.5 mg/dL; severe hypermagnesemia can cause respiratory paralysis, refractory hypotension, atrioventricular block, and cardiac arrest.[2,21,23,30]

Treatment of hypermagnesemia should focus on symptom reduction and normalization of serum magnesium concentrations. All magnesium-containing medications must be discontinued. In the presence of severe or symptomatic hypermagnesemia, intravenous calcium (chloride or gluconate) should be administered to stabilize cardiac and neuromuscular function.

Patients may be treated with loop diuretics or renal replacement therapy to promote magnesium elimination. Serum levels should be monitored at least daily during treatment.[2,21,30]

Magnesium as Treatment

Magnesium is the one electrolyte useful in the emergency treatment of medical conditions not specifically related to electrolyte abnormalities, such as preeclampsia, eclampsia, and torsades de pointes. In severe preeclampsia, magnesium is used to prevent seizure occurrence. While the exact mechanism of action is unknown, magnesium is thought to cause smooth muscle relaxation in cerebral blood vessels and to reduce calcium ion transport, which prevents nerve firing in the central nervous system. In severe preeclampsia, magnesium sulfate should be administered as a 4 to 6 g IV loading dose, followed by a continuous infusion of 1 to 3 g per hour. The same dosing regimen is recommended for treatment of eclamptic seizures.

Torsades de pointes is a polymorphic ventricular tachycardia characterized by a gradual twisting of the QRS complex on the electrocardiograph, and is associated with a prolonged QT interval. Magnesium sulfate is the drug of choice for terminating this arrhythmia. Magnesium acts to reduce calcium influx, slowing depolarization of the cardiac membrane. Magnesium sulfate 1 to 2 g IV infused over 30 to 60 seconds should be given at the onset of the arrhythmia, and a subsequent dose may be given after 5 to 15 minutes if needed, or a continuous infusion of 0.5 to 1 g per hour may be started. Magnesium treatment is effective even when serum magnesium concentrations are within normal limits.

Patients receiving IV magnesium sulfate for emergency treatment must be monitored for signs of magnesium toxicity. Respiratory rate, oxygen saturation, and patellar reflexes should be regularly assessed. Because magnesium is renally excreted, urine output should be monitored as well. Magnesium levels should be frequently monitored and must be checked when signs of toxicity are present. Critical care practitioners are often comfortable with serum levels as high as 6 to 9 mg/dL in patients receiving magnesium treatment, as long as the patient remains asymptomatic.

PHOSPHORUS HOMEOSTASIS

Phosphorus is the most abundant intracellular anion in the body. Phosphorus is found mostly in bone and soft tissue, with only 1% present in extracellular fluid. The normal serum phosphorus concentration is 2.7 to

4.5 mg/dL, with most existing as phosphate. Phosphorus is an essential component of bone and cell membranes, is necessary in all bodily functions requiring energy (as adenosine triphosphate), and is especially important in nerve and muscle function.[2,31,32] Critically ill patients often have imbalances in phosphorus homeostasis due to acute and chronic medical conditions. In addition, critically ill patients are often hypermetabolic, necessitating increased phosphorus requirements.

Hypophosphatemia

Hypophosphatemia occurs when serum phosphorus concentrations are less than 2.7 mg/dL and is considered severe with serum phosphorus concentrations less than 1.5 mg/dL. Many critically ill patients present with conditions that predispose to development of hypophosphatemia, including malnutrition, alcoholism, alkalosis, diabetic ketoacidosis, and significant gastrointestinal losses. Hypophosphatemia can also be caused by renal replacement therapy and by medications, including diuretics, antacids, and sucralfate. Patients receiving large carbohydrate loads, as with parenteral nutrition, may develop hypophosphatemia, especially in patients with malnutrition at risk for refeeding syndrome. The severity of illness in these patients results in increased energy expenditure, thus increasing phosphorus requirements.[2,32]

The symptoms associated with hypophosphatemia can be severe. Symptoms include impaired diaphragmatic contractility, acute respiratory failure, impaired myocardial contractility, weakness, paresthesias, and seizure.[31,32]

Goals of treatment include symptom reduction and normalization of serum phosphorus concentrations. Treatment is dependent on the severity of hypophosphatemia and the presence of symptoms. In patients with mild hypophosphatemia and without symptoms, phosphorus may be replaced by the enteral route, if available. A variety of enteral phosphate products are available, each with different phosphorus, sodium, and potassium concentrations. Product selection should be based on the needs of the individual patients. In patients with severe hypophosphatemia, or if symptomatic, phosphorus should be replaced intravenously. Empiric dosing recommendations for intravenous phosphorus replacement are listed in Table 7–5. Initial doses should be reduced by approximately 50% in patients with renal impairment.[2,33-36] Often, replacement of phosphorus is driven by institutional protocols (see Table 7–4).

Intravenous phosphorus is available as potassium phosphate and sodium phosphate salts. These intravenous products contain 4.4 mEq of potassium

Table 7–5 IV Phosphorus Replacement[26-29]

Serum Phosphorus Level (mg/dL)	IV Phosphorus Replacement Dosing
2–2.5	0.08–0.16 mmol/kg
1.5–2	0.16–0.24 mmol/kg
1–1.5	0.24–0.32 mmol/kg
Less than 1	0.32–0.64 mmol/kg

for each 3 mmol of phosphate, and 4 mEq of sodium for each 3 mmol of phosphate. Potassium phosphate may be used for replacement in patients with coexisting hypokalemia, and is generally safe to use with serum potassium concentrations less than 4 mEq/L. Phosphorus should be infused over several hours to reduce the risk of thrombophlebitis and calcium-phosphate precipitation in the body, with a maximum infusion rate of 7.5 mmols per hour. Serum phosphorus levels should be checked 2 to 4 hours after the IV infusion is complete. Phosphorus supplementation should continue until the serum phosphorus level is greater than 2 mg/dL and may be considered until serum levels reach the lower limit of normal.[32-36]

Hyperphosphatemia

Hyperphosphatemia occurs when serum phosphorus concentrations exceed 4.5 mg/dL. The most common cause of hyperphosphatemia is renal insufficiency, though other causes include excessive phosphorus administration, such as in enteral and parenteral nutrition therapies; acidosis; hemolysis; rhabdomyolysis; tumor lysis syndrome; and hypoparathyroidism.[2,32]

The clinical symptoms of hyperphosphatemia are caused by hypocalcemia associated with calcium-phosphorus precipitation, which can lead to tetany. Calcium-phosphate crystals can deposit into soft tissues, causing organ damage. The risk of calcium-phosphate precipitation increases when the product of the serum calcium and phosphorus concentrations exceeds 55 mg/dL.[2,32,37]

Treatment of hyperphosphatemia is focused on determination of the underlying etiology, with the primary goal of therapy to maintain the product of serum calcium and phosphorus concentrations less than 55 mg/dL.[32,37] In patients with renal insufficiency, daily phosphorus intake should be reduced. Patients who are eating a regular diet may be administered phosphate binders such as calcium carbonate, calcium acetate, and sevelamer orally with meals to reduce phosphorus absorption from the gastrointestinal tract. The effectiveness of these agents on lowering serum phosphate levels is delayed, and thus frequent monitoring of serum levels is unnecessary. In patients that are receiving nutrition through enteral or parenteral routes, the feeding formula should be adjusted to minimize phosphorus content. Phosphorus may also be minimally removed by renal replacement therapy, which requires more frequent monitoring of serum phosphorus concentrations.[2,32,37]

CALCIUM HOMEOSTASIS

Ninety-nine percent of total body calcium resides in bone, and calcium homeostasis is regulated by parathyroid hormone, calcitonin, and vitamin D. Calcium is essential to many bodily functions, including bone metabolism, neuromuscular activity, electrical conduction in the heart and smooth muscle, coagulation, and exocrine and endocrine functions.[2,38,39] Less than 1% of calcium exists in the extracellular fluid. The normal serum calcium concentration exists between 8.6 and 10.2 mg/dL. Nearly 50% of serum calcium is protein bound, primarily to albumin, and so hypoalbuminemia will result in a reduced serum calcium concentration. For every 1 g/dL decrease in serum albumin concentrations below 4 g/dL, serum calcium concentrations will decrease by 0.8 mg/dL, therefore serum calcium concentrations should be corrected in patients with hypoalbuminemia.[38,39]

$$\text{Corrected Calcium} = (0.8 * (4 - \text{albumin})) + \text{serum calcium}$$

The ionized serum calcium is the unbound and biologically active form. Normal serum ionized calcium concentrations are 1.12 to 1.3 mmol/L. Ionized calcium is a more reliable indicator of the functional status of serum calcium concentrations. Ionized calcium correlates poorly with total serum concentrations and is the recommended measure of serum calcium status, especially in critically ill patients, as these patients often present with hypoalbuminemia or acid–base imbalances, which will affect protein binding.[2,38,39] Calcium homeostasis is important in critically ill patients to prevent blood pressure and cardiac instabilities. It should also be noted that calcium is often used to stabilize cardiac function in critically ill patients with arrhythmias or severe hyperkalemia.

Hypocalcemia

Hypocalcemia is the more common disorder of calcium in critically ill patients and is defined as a serum calcium concentration less than 8.6 mg/dL, or an ionized calcium concentration less than 1.1 mmol/L. The primary cause of hypocalcemia is hypoalbuminemia, with other potential causes including hypomagnesemia, hyperphosphatemia, sepsis, pancreatitis, hypoparathyroidism, and renal insufficiency. Administration of citrated blood products can also cause hypocalcemia.[2,38,39]

Tetany is the characteristic symptom associated with acute hypocalcemia; other symptoms include neuromuscular, cardiovascular, and central nervous system dysfunction. Signs of chronic hypocalcemia included hair loss, dermatitis, eczema, and grooved nails.[2,38,39]

Goals of treatment of acute hypocalcemia primarily focus on symptom reduction. Asymptomatic hypocalcemia does not typically require treatment, but significantly reduced levels should generally be replaced to avoid symptom development. When symptoms are present, when serum calcium concentrations are less than 7.5 mg/dL, or ionized calcium is less than 0.9 mmol/L, intravenous calcium should be administered for rapid correction of serum levels.[2,38,40] Intravenous calcium is available as calcium chloride and calcium gluconate salts. Calcium chloride contains three times the amount of elemental calcium (13.6 mEq per gram) than an equivalent amount of calcium gluconate (4.56 mEq per gram), though calcium chloride use should be reserved for emergency situations primarily due to the risk of tissue necrosis with extravasation; this risk necessitates administration through a central IV line if at all possible. Initial supplementation of 1 to 3 g of calcium gluconate is appropriate for most patients, with repeated doses as necessary. Calcium gluconate undergoes hepatic metabolism, so calcium chloride should be considered for patients with liver failure. Some patients may require multiple doses and even continuous infusions of calcium to maintain adequate levels. Serum ionized calcium levels should be monitored at least daily, as well as 2 hours after a dose is finished infusing in symptomatic patients.[39,40] Often, non-emergent IV calcium is driven by institutional protocols (see Table 7-4). Evaluation for hypomagnesemia should also be completed and treated as necessary.[22] Oral calcium supplementation can be considered in patients with chronic hypocalcemia.

Hypercalcemia

Hypercalcemia is less commonly identified in the critically ill; it is defined as a serum calcium concentration exceeding 10.2 mg/dL, and is considered severe with serum concentrations of 13 mg/dL or greater. The most common causes of hypercalcemia are malignancy and primary hyperparathyroidism. Other potential causes include adrenal insufficiency, Paget's disease, milk-alkali syndrome, and rhabdomyolysis. Thiazide diuretics, lithium, vitamin D, and vitamin A can also be associated with hypercalcemia.[2,38,41]

Symptoms associated with acute hypercalcemia include fatigue, confusion, anorexia, bradycardia, and arrhythmias. Severe hypercalcemia can result in obtundation, acute renal failure, ventricular arrhythmias, and coma. Complications of chronic hypercalcemia include nephrolithiasis, metastatic calcifications, and renal failure.[2,38]

Severe hypercalcemia requires immediate treatment. Hydration should be initiated to reverse intravascular volume contraction, with NS at a rate of 200 to 300 milliliters per hour recommended. After hydration, loop diuretics may be used to increase renal elimination of calcium and avoid fluid overload. Renal replacement therapy may be needed in severe cases or in patients with renal failure. Goals of therapy include avoidance of symptoms, and treatment can be expected to reduce serum calcium concentrations by 2 to 3 mg/dL over the first 48 hours. Patients with mild or moderate hypercalcemia usually respond well to hydration therapy.[2,38,42]

Intravenous bisphosphonates are used for emergent treatment of severe hypercalcemia. These agents act on osteoblasts to inhibit bone resorption. Serum calcium levels will start to decrease approximately 2 days after bisphosphonate administration. Bisphosphonates are commonly used for hypercalcemia associated with malignancy, though glucocorticoids and calcitonin are other potential options for treatment of chronic hypercalcemia.[2,38,43]

SUMMARY

Fluid and electrolyte disorders are a common cause of in-hospital morbidity. Prompt recognition and treatment of severe fluid and electrolyte abnormalities is vital in critically ill patients to avoid significant and potentially fatal complications. Appropriate management of these disorders requires determination of the underlying cause. Pharmacists can greatly impact the assessment and treatment of fluid and electrolyte disturbance in intensive care unit patients, particularly as it relates to the patient's overall medication treatment plan.

KEY POINTS

- Total body water is divided into the extracellular and intracellular spaces. The extracellular space is further divided into the interstitial and intravascular space.

- Fluid resuscitation is an important initial therapy in critically ill patients with volume losses. After resuscitation is complete, fluid administration should be decreased to replace sensible and insensible losses and maintain appropriate fluid balance.
- Before treating hyponatremia, serum osmolarity and volume status should be determined to guide therapy.
- Hyponatremia treatment requires close monitoring to ensure a maximum correction rate of 12mEq/L/day.
- Potassium homeostasis can be altered by many mechanisms that are often present in critically ill patients. Alterations in potassium homeostasis can cause severe cardiac abnormalities, requiring emergent treatment and close monitoring in the intensive care unit.
- Magnesium homeostasis is important in critically ill patients due to its association with potassium and calcium homeostasis.
- Critically ill patients are often hypermetabolic, necessitating increased phosphorus requirements.
- Calcium homeostasis is important in critically ill patients to prevent blood pressure and cardiac instabilities.
- Calcium is often used to stabilize cardiac function in critically ill patients with arrhythmias or severe hyperkalemia.

Selected Suggested Reading

- Kaplan LJ, Kellum JA. Fluids, pH, ions, and electrolytes. *Cur Opin Crit Care*. 2010;16:323-331.
- Kraft MD, Btaiche IF, Sacks GS, et al. Treatment of electrolyte disorders in adult patients in the intensive care unit. *Am J Health-Syst Pharm*. 2005;62:1663-1682.
- The SAFE study investigators. A comparison of albumin and saline for fluid resuscitation in the intensive care unit. *New Engl J Med*. 2004;350:2247-2256.

References

1. Kaplan LJ, Kellum JA. Fluids, pH, ions, and electrolytes. *Cur Opin Crit Care*. 2010;16:323-331.
2. Kraft MD, Btaiche IF, Sacks GS, et al. Treatment of electrolyte disorders in adult patients in the intensive care unit. *Am J Health-Syst Pharm*. 2005;62:1663-1682.
3. Fouche Y, Sikorski R, Dutton RP. Changing paradigms in surgical resuscitation. *Crit Care Med*. 2010;38(9):s411-s420.
4. Latenser BA. Critical care of the burn patient: The first 48 hours. *Crit Care Med*. 2009;37(10):2819-2826.

5. Dellinger RP, Levy MM, Carlet JM, et al. Surviving Sepsis Campaign: International guidelines for management of severe sepsis and septic shock: 2008. *Crit Care Med.* 2008;36:296–327.

6. The SAFE study investigators. A comparison of albumin and saline for fluid resuscitation in the intensive care unit. *New Engl J Med.* 2004;350:2247–2256.

7. The SAFE study investigators. Saline or albumin for fluid resuscitation in patients with traumatic brain injury. *New Engl J Med.* 2007;357:874–884.

8. Adrogue HJ, Madias NE. Hyponatremia. *New Engl J Med.* 2000;342(21): 1581–1589.

9. Buckley MS, LeBlanc JM, Cawley MJ. Electrolyte disturbances associated with commonly prescribed medications in the intensive care unit. *Crit Care Med.* 2010;38(6):s253–s264.

10. Halperin ML, Kamel KS. Potassium. *Lancet.* 1998;352:135–140.

11. Williams ME. Hyperkalemia. *Crit Care Clin.* 1991;7:155–174.

12. Kunau RT, Stein JH. Disorders of hypo and hyperkalemia. *Clin Nephrol.* 1977;7:173–190.

13. Mandal AK. Hypokalemia and hyperkalemia. *Med Clin North Am.* 1997;81: 611–639.

14. Freedman BI, Burkart JM. Hypokalemia. *Crit Care Clin.* 1991;7:143–153.

15. Gennari FJ. Hypokalemia. *N Engl J Med.* 1998;339:451–458.

16. Hamill RJ, Robinson LM, Wexler HR, et al. Efficacy and safety of potassium infusion therapy in hypokalemic critically ill patients. *Crit Care Med.* 1991;9:694–699.

17. Kruse JA, Carlson RW. Rapid correction of hypokalemia using concentrated intravenous potassium chloride infusions. *Arch Intern Med.* 1990;150:613–617.

18. Kruse JA, Clark VL, Carlson RW, et al. Concentrated potassium chloride infusions in critically ill patients with hypokalemia. *J Clin Pharmacol.* 1994;34:1077–1082.

19. Ryan MP. Interrelationships of magnesium and potassium homeostasis. *Miner Electrolyte Metab.* 1993;19:290–295.

20. Agarwal A, Wingo CS. Treatment of hypokalemia. *N Engl J Med.* 1999;340: 154–155.

21. Reinhart RA. Magnesium metabolism: a review with special reference to the relationship between intracellular content and serum levels. *Arch Intern Med.* 1988;148:2415–2120.

22. Weisinger JR, Bellorin-Font E. Magnesium and phosphorous. *Lancet.*1998;352:391–396.

23. Wacker WE, Parisi AF. Magnesium metabolism. *N Engl J Med.* 1968;278: 658–663,712–717,772–776.

24. Salem M, Munoz R, Chernow B. Hypomagnesemia in critical illness: a common and clinically important problem. *Crit Care Clin.* 1991;7:225–252.

25. Reinhart RA, Desbiens NA. Hypomagnesemia in patients entering the ICU. *Crit Care Med.* 1985;13:506–507.

26. Ryzen E, Wagers PW, Singer FR, et al. Magnesium deficiency in a medical ICU population. *Crit Care Med.* 1985;13:19–21.

27. Rubeiz GJ, Thill-Baharozian M, Hardie D, et al. Association of hypomagnesemia and mortality in acutely ill medical patients. *Crit Care Med.* 1993;21:203–209.

28. Oster JR, Epstein M. Management of magnesium depletion. *Am J Nephrol.* 1988;8:349–354.

29. Hebert P, Mehta N, Wang J, et al. Functional magnesium deficiency in critically ill patients identified using a magnesium-loading test. *Crit Care Med.* 1997;25:749–755.

30. Van Hook JW. Hypermagnesemia. *Crit Care Clin.* 1991;7:215–223.

31. Knochel JP. The pathophysiology and clinical characteristics of severe hypophosphatemia. *Arch Intern Med.* 1977;137:203–220.

32. Peppers MP, Geheb M, Desai T. Hypophosphatemia and hyperphosphatemia. *Crit Care Clin.* 1991;7:201–214.

33. Vannatta JB, Whang R, Papper S. Efficacy of intravenous phosphorous therapy in the severely hypophosphatemic patient. *Arch Intern Med.* 1981;141:885–887.

34. Kingston M, Al-Siba'i MB. Treatment of severe hypophosphatemia. *Crit Care Med.* 1985;13:16–18.

35. Rosen GH, Boullata JI, O'Rangers EA, et al. Intravenous phosphate repletion regimen for critically ill patients with moderate hypophosphatemia. *Crit Care Med.* 1995;23:1204–1210.

36. Clark CL, Sacks GS, Dickerson RN, et al. Treatment of hypophosphatemia in patients receiving specialized nutrition support using a graduated dosing scheme: results from a prospective clinical trial. *Crit Care Med.* 1995;23:1504–1510.

37. Block GA, Port FK. Re-evaluation of risks associated with hyperphosphatemia and hyperparathyroidism in dialysis patients: recommendations for a change in management. *Am J Kidney Dis.* 2000;35:1226–1237.

38. Bushinsky DA, Monk RD. Calcium. *Lancet.* 1998;352:306–311.

39. Zaloga GP. Hypocalcemic crisis. *Crit Care Clin.* 1991;7:191–200.

40. Vincent JL, Bredas P, Jankowski S, et al. Correction of hypocalcaemia in the critically ill: what is the haemodynamic benefit? *Intensive Care Med.* 1995;21:838–841.

41. Mundy GR, Guise TA. Hypercalcemia of malignancy. *Am J Med.* 1997;103:134–145.

42. Chisholm MA, Mulloy AL, Taylor AT. Acute management of cancer-related hypercalcemia. *Ann Pharmacother.* 1996;30:507–513.

43. Davis KD, Attie MF. Management of severe hypercalcemia. *Crit Care Clin.* 1991;7:175–190.

Chapter 8

Pharmacologic Management of Blood Pressure

Thomas Johnson

LEARNING OBJECTIVES

1. Describe the alterations of blood pressure in critically ill patients.
2. Identify the common vasopressor agents used for treatment of hypotension and specify appropriate dosing strategies.
3. Define and classify hypertensive events commonly present in the critically ill.
4. List the antihypertensive agents commonly used in the intensive care unit.
5. Compare and contrast medications, and know how to select appropriate treatment for hypertension in the critically ill.

INTRODUCTION

Management of blood pressure is one of the most common pharmacologic interventions made in critically ill patients. Many patients develop alterations in blood pressure during their intensive care unit (ICU) stay, and some experience both hypotension and hypertension. Pharmacists can play a significant role in optimizing medication regimens to treat, as well as prevent, disorders of blood pressure. While the underlying causes of blood pressure disorders must be addressed and treated, pharmacologic management of blood pressure is a very important supportive measure. This chapter will primarily focus on the pharmacology and rationale for medication selection for the patient with blood pressure disorders; treatment of the specific underlying causative disorders is covered in other chapters and other texts.

HYPOTENSION

Hypotension is often simply defined as systolic blood pressure (SBP) of less than 90 millimeters of mercury (mmHg) or a mean arterial pressure (MAP) of less than 60 mmHg. Remember that MAP is equal to SBP plus 2 times diastolic blood pressure (DBP) divided by 3 (MAP = (SBP+2*DBP)/3). While this definition of hypotension does not take into account previous or baseline blood pressure readings, it does provide a common point of reference for clinicians to use. It should be noted that blood pressure alone does not provide information on oxygen delivery, which is ultimately the most important element in care of the critically ill patient.

Causes of hypotension are numerous and can include sepsis, cardiac failure, hypovolemia, medications, and allergic reactions. Definitive therapy for any underlying cause is important, as using medications to augment blood pressure is only a temporary solution.

Hypotension should almost always be first addressed with fluid resuscitation via administration of appropriate crystalloid or colloid solutions, which is described in Chapter 7 of this text. However, if the blood pressure response is inadequate to fluid resuscitation and other supportive measures, it often becomes necessary to provide blood pressure support with vasopressor medications.

Vasopressors

The vasopressors commonly used in the critically ill include dopamine, norepinephrine, epinephrine, and phenylephrine, and they are listed in Table 8–1 with a summary of their pharmacologic activity and typical doses. Vasopressin is also included in the table, although the mechanism and use of this agent for blood pressure support is rather unique as compared to the other agents. Dobutamine is not a vasopressor, but is listed in the table for comparison as it is commonly used alone or in combination with other adrenergic agents for hemodynamic support.

One of the best ways to remember the effects and side effects of these vasopressors is to have a clear understanding of the pharmacology of each agent. The agents used to increase blood pressure typically work on the alpha and beta receptors to varying degrees, and this is represented in Table 8–1 as a percentage designation.

While a full discussion of the complete pharmacology of the adrenergic receptors is best left to a pharmacology textbook, a brief, simplified review may be helpful.[1-3] Alpha-1 receptors are primarily present in the peripheral smooth muscles and, when stimulated, tend to cause vasoconstriction. Alpha-2 receptors are generally located pre-synaptically within the nervous system and alter the release and reuptake of norephinephrine. Beta-1 receptors are primarily located within the heart and affect heart rate and contractility, and beta-2 receptors are mostly located within smooth muscle and affect vasodilation and bronchial smooth muscle tone. Most of the catecholamine vasopressors will affect both alpha and beta receptors, and have varying effects on subtypes 1 or 2, but usually one of the overall effects will predominate.

A more detailed discussion of the literature surrounding each of the vasopressors and their specific effects on regional blood flow and oxygenation is beyond the scope of this introductory textbook. The critical care practitioner should be well versed in the literature that describes the variation in effect of the different vasopressors on regional blood flow and, ultimately, oxygen delivery. Selected suggested supplemental reading materials are listed within Table 8–2, and the reader is referred to this literature and other citations for a full understanding of the intricacies of vasopressor use.

Table 8–1 Continuous Infusion Vasopressor Medications Used for Hypotension[1-4]

Medication	Receptor effect*	Normal dose
Dopamine	Dose dependent:	1 to 20 mcg/kg/min
	Dopamine (low dose)	Low dose = <5 mcg/kg/min
	Beta (moderate dose)	Moderate dose = 5 to
	Alpha (high dose)	10 mcg/kg/min
Norepinephrine	90% alpha	High dose = >10 mcg/kg/min
	10% beta	2 to 20 mcg/min or
Phenylephrine	100% alpha	0.01 to 3 mcg/kg/min
Epinephrine	50% alpha	20 to 180 mcg/min
	50% beta	1 to 20 mcg/min or
Vasopressin	V1, V2, V3, OTR	0.05 to 0.5 mcg/kg/min
	V1 primarily in hypotension	Up to 0.04 units/min
Dobutamine	90% beta	0.03 units/min most common
	10% alpha	1 to 20 mcg/kg/min

*Note that this is a simplified way to remember primary effects, not absolute effects

Table 8-2 Selected Reference Readings for Vasopressor Differentiation

Medication	Citation
General Review	Dellinger RP, Levy MM, Carlet JM, et al. Surviving Sepsis Campaign: international guidelines for management of severe sepsis and septic shock: 2008. *Crit Care Med*. 2008;36:296-327.
	Dellinger RP. Cardiovascular management of septic shock. *Crit Care Med*. 2003;31:946-955.
	Landry DW, Oliver JA. The pathogenesis of vasodilatory shock. *N Engl J Med*. 2001;345:588-595.
	Beale RJ, Hollenberg SM, Vincent JL, Parrillo JE. Vasopressor and inotropic support in septic shock: an evidence-based review. *Crit Care Med*. 2004;32:S455-S465.
Dopamine	Povoa PR, Carneiro AI I, Ribeiro OS, Pereira AC. Influence of vasopressor agent in septic shock mortality. Results from the Portuguese Community-Acquired Sepsis Study (SACiUCI study). *Crit Care Med*. 2009;37:410-416.
	Patel GP, Grahe JS, Sperry M, et al. Efficacy and safety of dopamine versus norepinephrine in the management of septic shock. *Shock*. 2010;33:375-380.
Norepinephrine	Beloeil H, Mazoit JX, Benhamou D, Duranteau J. Norepinephrine kinetics and dynamics in septic shock and trauma patients. *Br J Anaesth*. 2005;95:782-788.
	Vasu TS CR, Hirani A, Kaplan G, Leiby B, Marik PE. Norephinephrine or dopamine for septic shock: a systematic review of randomized clinical trials. *J Intensive Care Med*. March 24, 2011. Epub ahead of print. DOI: 10.1177/0885066610396312.
Phenylephrine	Morelli A, Ertmer C, Rehberg S, et al. Phenylephrine versus norepinephrine for initial hemodynamic support of patients with septic shock: a randomized, controlled trial. *Crit Care*. 2008;12:R143.
Epinephrine	Myburgh JA, Higgins A, Jovanovska A, Lipman J, Ramakrishnan N, Santamaria J. A comparison of epinephrine and norepinephrine in critically ill patients. *Intensive Care Med*. 2008;34:2226-2234.
Vasopressin	Maybauer MO, Walley KR. Best vasopressor for advanced vasodilatory shock: should vasopressin be part of the mix? *Intensive Care Med*. 2010;36:1484-1487.
	Russell JA, Walley KR, Singer J, et al. Vasopressin versus norepinephrine infusion in patients with septic shock. *N Engl J Med*. 2008;358:877-887.
	Klinzing S, Simon M, Reinhart K, Bredle DL, Meier-Hellmann A. High-dose vasopressin is not superior to norepinephrine in septic shock. *Crit Care Med*. 2003;31:2646-2650.
Dobutamine	Annane D, Vignon P, Renault A, et al. Norepinephrine plus dobutamine versus epinephrine alone for management of septic shock: a randomised trial. *Lancet*. 2007;370:676-684.
Multiple Agents	De Backer D, Creteur J, Silva E, Vincent JL. Effects of dopamine, norepinephrine, and epinephrine on the splanchnic circulation in septic shock: which is best? *Crit Care Med*. 2003;31:1659-1667.

Dopamine

Dopamine is one of the more complex vasopressors to understand, simply because it is very difficult to discern the exact pharmacologic activity of the drug at any given dose in a specific patient. In general, dopamine given in low doses has the primary effect of being an agonist at dopamine receptor sites, which tends to cause vasodilation to the splanchnic and renal vasculature.[4] At moderate doses, dopamine tends to have the primary effect of beta-receptor stimulation, which leads to increased myocardial contractility and increased heart rate. At higher doses, dopamine has a primary effect of alpha agonist activity, which leads to peripheral vasoconstriction. Dopamine is actually a precursor of norepinephrine and also causes the release of norepinephrine from the nerve terminal, which is the primary means for dopamine to cause alpha agonist activity and therefore vasoconstrictor activity.[1]

While the dosing ranges provide a frame of reference and an increased ability to understand the action of dopamine, each patient will respond somewhat differently, and there is really no way to determine the exact effect dopamine will have at any given dosing range. Further, the effects listed are only the predominant effects, and effects at the other receptor sites will also be present at any dose. One of the main reasons that the use of low dose dopamine for prevention or treatment of renal dysfunction is discouraged is that while blood flow is increased to the kidneys, tachyarrhythmias and blood pressure alterations tend to offset any positive effects that may have been present.[5,6] Patients at higher doses (5 to 20 mcg/kg/min) also have variable effects, including increases in heart rate, blood pressure, and contractility, but the exact dose needed to reach the desired effect can be very difficult to ascertain. However, in certain patients, the variable effects of dopamine may be considered by some to be a positive. As initial therapy in a hypotensive patient where etiology has yet to be determined, dopamine can be titrated either until optimal hemodynamic effects are attained or adverse effects or lack of endpoint attainment necessitate the use of alternative agents.

Dopamine remains a first-line agent for the treatment of hypotension from a variety of causes, such as sepsis, or cardiogenic shock, despite some of the limiting factors.[4,5,7,8] The positive attributes of the medication include the ability for short-term administration through a peripheral line with relative safety as compared to norepinephrine or phenylephrine, as well as the common availability of dopamine as a premade product; this allows for easy storage and rapid availability through floor stock and in code carts. Furthermore, the mechanism of action on several receptor sites may allow for the ability to titrate the agent to achieve an optimal response. The negative aspects of the medication include the tachyarrhythmias, lack of definitive response, and unclear alterations in hemodynamic indices.

Norepinephrine

Norepinephrine (NE) is a naturally occurring catecholamine that is primarily an alpha agonist that causes peripheral vasoconstriction.[1] However, there is some beta activity present as well, which can lead to increased myocardial contractility or increases in heart rate. The cardiac effects from norepinephrine can range from minimal or none to significant, depending upon the patient. As a potent vasoconstrictor, NE can produce peripheral ischemia as well as alter blood flow to various vascular beds, although regional bloodflow alterations have proved to be variable and depend upon study design and measurement.[9-11] However, the need to maintain overall perfusion within the patient almost always supersedes the concerns of altered regional blood flow.

Norepinephrine can be dosed as either mcg/min or mcg/kg/min, and is typically chosen based upon institutional policy. Ultimately, the dosing scheme does not really matter, since the medication should be titrated as an IV infusion until the desired effect is obtained. If a non-weight-based dosing regimen is utilized, then the clinician should consider the overall size of the patient when determining initial and "maximum" doses. For example, a female patient who weighs 52 kg and a male patient who weighs 135 kg could be started on the same dose of NE if a mcg/min approach is used, but it would seem intuitive that the significantly larger patient would ultimately require a higher dose. Of course, the underlying condition and the relative sensitivity of the patient to norepinephrine will play a significant role as well, so it is quite possible that the same dose could be equally effective.[12] Nonetheless, some consideration should be given to patient differences even when using a standard mcg/min dosing approach.

Norepinephrine remains a first-line agent for the management of hypotension and is often considered the preferred vasopressor for the treatment of septic shock.[4,7] While there are no definitive studies that describe superiority of norepinephrine over other vasopressors, many head-to-head studies have been conducted over the years;[5,13-19] however, the varying patient types, dosing schemes, and underlying disease processes, as well the inherent difficulties in adjusting for co-morbidities and patient-specific factors, have made this line of literature difficult to interpret. Even so, the relative ease of use of norepinephrine, the potency at the alpha receptor site, and the minimal unwanted additional effects of the medication make it a very good choice for management of several types of hypotension in the critically ill, including sepsis- and medication-induced hypotension. Note that norepinephrine should only be infused through central IV access unless there is no way to quickly attain central access.

Phenylephrine

Phenylephrine is a pure alpha agonist that works solely to provide peripheral vasoconstriction.[1] While it only has effects on the alpha receptor, it is much less potent than norepinephrine at the receptor site, which necessitates the use of higher doses and therefore often higher fluid volumes for medication delivery. Similar to NE, phenylephrine is typically dosed on a mcg/min basis and titrated to effect via continuous IV infusion.

Phenylephrine is normally used in patients with significant tachycardia (>140 bpm) or in patients that cannot otherwise tolerate any beta stimulation. The Surviving Sepsis Campaign (SSC) guidelines list phenylephrine as a second-line agent primarily because of the expected negative cardiac stroke volume effects.[7] Occasionally, phenylephrine will be used when a pure alpha agonist medication is desired to help with diagnosis of a complex hemodynamic picture; when combined with a primarily beta medication like dobutamine, a complex patient can be managed by titration of each agent to allow the experienced clinician maximal control over the adrenergic system controlling vasoconstriction and myocardial contractility. Phenylephrine may also be used in patients that have hypotension due to significant vasodilation secondary to other medications. If at all possible, phenylephrine should be administered through a central venous catheter.

Epinephrine

Epinephrine (EPI) is a catecholamine that has significant effects on both beta and alpha receptors.[1] Epinephrine can be used in bolus doses during anaphylaxis or cardiac arrest situations, but for management of ongoing hypotension, it is typically given as a continuous IV infusion either as mcg/min or mcg/kg/min and titrated to the desired effect. Since EPI has significant effects on both beta and alpha receptors, patients will experience profound peripheral vasoconstriction, as well as tachycardia, increased myocardial contractility, and increased myocardial oxygen demand. Epinephrine is considered a second-line agent for the management of hypotension due to sepsis,[7] and may be considered first or second line for the treatment of cardiogenic hypotension. As with NE and phenylephrine, a central IV catheter should be used if at all possible.

Vasopressin

Vasopressin is a vasopressor that is typically utilized as an add-on therapy to one of the other primary vasopressors (NE, dopamine, phenylephrine, or EPI) in the treatment of septic shock.[7] Vasopressin can be utilized as a bolus dose during cardiac arrest (40 units IV X1 and may be repeated 20 minutes after the initial dose), but for hypotension due to sepsis, vasopressin is given as a continuous infusion. The typical dose is 0.03 units/min based upon the only randomized controlled trial to date,[20] but it is used in clinical practice within the range of 0.01 to 0.04 units/min. There is minimal, if any, literature support for doses greater than 0.04 units/min, and use of higher doses should be discouraged. Further, vasopressin should not be titrated to help manage blood pressure, but rather should be used as an add-on therapy; instead, the other vasopressors should be titrated to maintain blood pressure within the goal ranges.[21]

Vasopressin works on several receptors, including V1, V2, V3, and OTR, with the V1 receptor, the primary receptor for causing vasoconstriction.[22,23] In the setting of sepsis, patients tend to experience a relative vasopressin deficiency, and providing a continuous infusion of a set dose of vasopressin replaces this deficiency, improving smooth muscle responsiveness to other vasopressors or endogenous catecholamines.

Dobutamine

While dobutamine is not a vasopressor, it is used to augment cardiac output and can improve blood pressure and oxygen delivery, so it deserves discussion here. Dobutamine primarily acts as a beta-1 agonist and has minimal alpha effects.[1] It increases heart rate and contractility while causing peripheral vasodilation, which could cause or worsen hypotension in some patients, and this effect results in an increase in cardiac output, as well as reduced afterload from the peripheral vasodilation. This can be especially useful in patients with cardiac failure and in septic patients who may have a relative cardiac deficiency, and so are not able to provide adequate oxygen delivery to the tissues and organs. In septic patients, dobutamine is typically combined with a vasopressor agent such as norepinephrine to provide overall hemodynamic support.[24] Adverse effects associated with dobutamine include an increase in tachyarrhythmias and other arrhythmias. Dobutamine is typically dosed by mcg/kg/min via continuous IV infusion through a central line, when possible.

Other Agents

Hypotension is primarily managed with fluids and the vasopressors listed, but there are other agents that are used to assist with low blood pressure in certain situations. For example, steroids can be used to augment blood pressure. Hydrocortisone is recommended in septic shock patients who are not adequately responding to fluid resuscitation and vasopressors, and this will be discussed in more detail in Chapter 10.[7,25] Furthermore, patients who take chronic steroids often need steroid replacement to maintain blood pressure if they experience stressors such as critical illness or surgery because of hypothalamic pituitary axis (HPA) suppression. Acute use of steroids in this setting is typically called "stress-dose steroids" and the use of these agents in patients with HPA suppression is critical to ensure the patient has the best chance for recovery. Identifying patients who take chronic oral steroids should be a key point to address during medication reconciliation to ensure optimal patient outcomes.

HYPERTENSION

The causes of hypertension in critically ill patients are many. Pain, stress, sleep deprivation, underlying disease states, medications, and other influences all can cause alterations in blood pressure.[26] Therefore, it is important for the clinician to determine the underlying cause of hypertension prior to developing a treatment plan, as many times the patient does not need medication directed at altering blood pressure, but instead needs effective treatment of an underlying issue.

Selection of a treatment regimen for a patient whose primary issue of hypertension led to admission to the ICU may differ from patients that are hypertensive as a secondary problem during their ICU stay. Further, treatment goals will vary depending upon the patient and the scenario, and individual care plans are essential.

Hypertension treated in the ICU as the primary issue for admission is typically referred to as a hypertensive urgency or emergency. Urgency and emergency situations are defined as SBP of greater than 180 mmHg or a DBP of greater than 120 mmHg.[27,28] Emergency differs from urgency by the presence of target organ damage, which would include signs such as significant headache, kidney dysfunction, stroke, or myocardial damage.[29,30] The immediate treatment goals in this situation are to reduce MAP by approximately 20% to 25% using IV medications, followed by further reductions to a SBP of less than 160 and DBP to less than 100 if the patient is stable over the next several hours. Once initial control has been obtained, further reduction to goal levels should take place over the next few days and include either the initiation or resumption of oral medications.

While hypertensive urgency and emergency treatment is a fairly common occurrence in the ICU, hypertension is more often treated as a secondary issue in critically ill patients. Perioperative patients, patients with significant pain or anxiety, and patients with underlying hypertension who are unable to take their chronic medications because of their acute illness are common populations that require acute hypertension treatment in the ICU. Before IV antihypertensives are used, the cause of hypertension must be determined.

Patients with pain or anxiety are better treated with adequate analgesia and sedation rather than antihypertensive medications. If the underlying cause of hypertension is unable to be adequately identified or resolved, then antihypertensive medications should be considered.

Intravenous Antihypertensives

There are many choices of medication for intravenous use for the management of hypertension. They can be categorized by several methods, including pharmacologic mechanism, overall effect, or by intermittent vs. continuous IV infusion. For purposes of discussion in this text, they will be divided by intermittent vs. continuous IV infusion.

Intermittent IV Agents

Table 8-3 lists the common IV medications used for management of blood pressure that typically utilize intermittent dosing regimens. Each agent has a unique pharmacologic profile that helps with selection of the most appropriate medication based upon the individual patient.

Hydralazine   Hydralazine is a peripheral vasodilator that reduces blood pressure through arterial dilation.[29] The resultant drop in blood pressure due to afterload reduction typically results in a rebound tachycardia, so hydralazine is best used in patients with a heart rate of less than 100 beats per minute. Hydralazine is usually given as an intermittent IV bolus dose in response to acute increases in blood pressure. While hydralazine can be quite effective, it can also cause a precipitous drop in blood pressure that may

Table 8-3 Intermittent Intravenous Medications for Acute Hypertension[1,27,29,30]

Medication	Mechanism	Normal dose
Hydralazine	Peripheral vasodilator	5 to 10 mg every 4 or 6 hours, as needed
Labetalol	Non-selective beta blocker Alpha-1 blocker	20 to 80 mg every 2 to 6 hours
Metoprolol	Beta-1 selective blocker	2.5 to 5 mg every 4 to 6 hours
Enalaprilat	Angiotensin-converting enzyme inhibitor	0.625 to 1.25 mg every 6 hours
Phentolamine*	Peripheral alpha-1 and alpha-2 blocker	10 to 15 mg repeated as needed

*Use normally limited to catecholamine excess due to pheochromocytoma or overdose (cocaine, amphetamines, etc.).

require treatment with fluid or other medications. Further, the rebound tachycardia can limit the usefulness of the drug in certain patients.

Labetalol   Labetalol is a non-selective beta-blocker that also has alpha-blocking effects.[1,29] The beta-blockade provides a decrease in blood pressure through a decrease in cardiac output and via peripheral vasodilation caused by alpha blockade. The elimination half-life ranges up to 8 hours and it can take several doses of labetalol to achieve a blood level that actually leads to a decrease in blood pressure; this is most likely because of inter-patient variability in response and distribution.[1,29,31] Labetalol is available in both IV and oral form, which can allow for conversion from the IV to oral route if therapy is to continue beyond the acute illness. Labetalol can be dosed as either an intermittent IV bolus or as a continuous IV infusion, although the continuous infusion is most likely just serving as an extended "loading dose" by allowing the blood level of the drug to build up over time without the spikes in concentration that would be seen with IV bolus dosing. Labetalol is a reasonable choice for blood pressure control in patients that are tachycardic or at risk for tachycardia. Since labetalol is a non-specific beta-blocker, caution should be used in patients with a history of significant reactive airway disease. Overall, labetalol can be a very useful antihypertensive agent in patients with either primary or secondary hypertension in the ICU.

Metoprolol   Metoprolol is available in IV and oral forms and is typically used as a heart rate control medication, but it may be used to help facilitate blood pressure control as well; this can be particularly useful in patients who take oral metoprolol on a chronic basis. Oral to IV conversion is possible for patients on chronic metoprolol therapy, but exact conversions are not always reliable, primarily because of the differences between oral and IV doses in peak levels and overall elimination half-life. Therefore, a common strategy is to begin a standard IV dose of 2.5 to 5 mg every 6 hours and adjust the IV dose as needed to attain target heart rate or blood pressure. Metoprolol is also commonly used as a beta-blocker of choice within acute myocardial infarction protocols; it is given initially via the IV route every 5 minutes for up to three doses, as blood pressure tolerates, to improve outcomes in these patients.

Enalaprilat   Enalaprilat is the IV version of enalapril and is the only IV angiotensin-converting enzyme inhibitor (ACEi) available in the United States. The mechanism of action is to block conversion of angiotensin I to angiotensin II. The IV form tends to have a variable effect on blood pressure. While conversion doses exist to switch patients from an oral ACEi to enaprilat, the conversions are not clinically effective, and automatic PO to IV switches should generally be discouraged. Patients who are taking ACEi and are no longer able to take oral medication should be managed with other blood pressure medications or given standard doses of enalaprilat and monitored closely for response. Enalaprilat is also associated with significant abrupt decreases in blood pressure, particularly in patients with congestive heart failure, hypovolemia, or recent significant changes in volume status.[29]

Continuous Infusion Agents

Intermittent dosing of IV antihypertensive agents can be effective and is commonly used for management of patients with fluctuating blood pressure, patients needing blood pressure control perioperatively, or in patients that are unable to take oral medications. However, for patients that need tight blood pressure control with specific treatment targets, or in patients who have persistent hypertension that cannot be adequately controlled with intermittent agents, continuous IV medications are available. The commonly used continuous infusion antihypertensive agents are listed in Table 8-4.

Nitroglycerin Nitroglycerin (NTG) at lower doses reduces blood pressure primarily through preferential venous vasodilation, which decreases blood return to the heart and therefore reduces preload, which in turn leads to

Table 8–4 Continuous Infusion Intravenous Medications for Acute Hypertension[1,27,29,30]

Medication	Mechanism	Normal dose
Nitroglycerin	Venous vasodilation	5 to 20 mcg/min with a maximum rate of 200 mcg/min for refractory patients
Sodium nitroprusside	Venous and arterial vasodilation	0.1 to 3 mcg/kg/min Doses of 3 to 10 mcg/kg/min should only rarely be used and for very short time periods
Fenoldopam	Dopamine agonist; arterial vasodilation	0.1 to 1.6 mcg/kg/min
Nicardipine	Calcium channel blocker	Begin at 5 mg/hr Range: 2.5 to 30 mg/hr
Clevidipine	Calcium channel blocker	Begin at 1 or 2 mg/hr with rapid titration to goal blood pressure. Maximum rate: 32 mg/hr
Esmolol	Beta blocker	0.5 to 1 mg/kg bolus followed by 50 to 300 mcg/kg/min infusion
Diltiazem	Calcium channel blocker	0.25 mg/kg bolus followed by 5 to 25 mg/hr infusion

a decrease in blood pressure.[32] At higher doses, NTG will lead to arterial vasodilation, but side effects such as headache and flushing often limit the doses that can be given. Through several complex mechanisms, NTG decreases myocardial oxygen demand and improves coronary artery blood flow, making it an effective agent for the treatment of cardiac patients. Because nitroglycerin does not have a predominant effect on the arterial vasculature, it is typically only used for blood pressure management in the cardiac patient and results in the dual effect of blood pressure reduction and improved coronary circulation.

Sodium Nitroprusside   Sodium nitroprusside is the historical gold standard for continuous IV medications used to manage significant acute hypertension in critically ill patients. Dosed as mcg/kg/min, nitroprusside causes both venous and arterial vasodilation through a nitric oxide-mediated vasodilation similar to NTG, which leads to rapid blood pressure changes.[29,32] The medication is easily titratable, allowing blood pressure to be maintained within a specified goal range; however, significant potential toxicity exists with the medication as it is approximately 44% cyanide by weight.[33] When infused into the bloodstream, thiocyanate is released and then eliminated by the kidneys. Nitroprusside should be limited in dose (<3 mcg/kg/min) and duration (<48 hours) to minimize the chance of cyanide toxicity, and this is especially important in patients with kidney dysfunction. Some references advocate co-infusion of sodium thiosulfate as an antidote to the cyanide component during the nitroprusside infusion to minimize any toxicity associated with the medication.[34] Nitroprusside has also been associated with decreases in blood flow to selected vascular beds, including the brain, which may lead to detrimental outcomes in patients with brain injury,[32] so while sodium nitroprusside remains an effective treatment for significant hypertension, adverse events and regional effects on blood flow, as well as effective alternative medications, limit the use of this agent.

Fenoldopam   Fenoldopam is a dopamine-1 agonist that decreases blood pressure through arterial vasodilation.[1] Fenoldopam is unique in that it also has selective vasodilatory effects on the renal and splanchnic vascular beds, which increase blood flow to the kidneys and mesentery. This pharmacologic effect has been investigated on many different occasions to determine if fenoldopam may have renal protective effects, or if target organ damage to the kidneys may be minimized with the use of this agent. Despite success in small trials, and demonstrated increases in renal vascular blood flow, confirmatory studies have not been able to show any renal protective benefit in terms of targeted patient outcomes.[29,32] However, this does not detract from the effectiveness of fenoldopam as an antihypertensive agent that is easily titratable and consistently maintains blood pressures within the target ranges, even though lack of demonstrable significant patient outcomes and relative expense has historically limited the use of the agent. Fenoldopam is a reasonable choice for patients with significant kidney disease or damage who are either not responding to intermittent antihypertensives or where other continuous infusion agents are contraindicated.[27]

Nicardipine   Nicardipine is a dihydropyridine calcium channel blocker that provides rapid and effective blood pressure control.[35] The relatively short half-life of the medication allows for easy titration of the drug to attain target blood pressures. Nicardipine appears to have at least a neutral, if not a positive, effect on cerebral perfusion in patients with stroke or brain injury as compared to nitroprusside.[35-37] This property makes nicardipine one of the preferred agents for the management of hypertension related to stroke, intracranial hemorrhage, or head injury.[38-41]

Nicardipine must be diluted to a concentration of 0.1 mg/ml; therefore, at higher doses, fluid overload may become an issue.[42] The medication also has a risk of phlebitis, and so infusions should only be run through well-placed peripheral lines or, preferably, through a central line.

Clevidipine   Clevidipine is a recently introduced IV antihypertensive and is also a dihydropyridine calcium channel blocker. It is differentiated from nicardipine by its ultra-short half-life and highly lipophilic properties.[26,29,32] The ultra-short half-life allows for rapid and easy titration of the medication to attain target blood pressures; however, abrupt discontinuation can lead to rebound hypertension. Therefore, clinicians must be careful to start oral medications or other antihypertensive management strategies prior to discontinuation of clevidipine to avoid adverse events. Clinical trials with clevidipine have demonstrated its ability to maintain blood pressure within target ranges very effectively.[43] The agent has also demonstrated efficacy within specific patient populations with severe hypertension.[44,45]

The lipophilic properties of clevidipine actually require a formulation utilizing lipid emulsion to allow for stability. This creates some special handling properties for the drug that are similar to other IV lipid products. Specifically for clevidipine, once accessed, vials can only be hung for 4 hours, after which they should be discarded to minimize the risk of infection.[46] While there are advantages and unique properties of the medication, clear outcomes benefits are currently lacking compared to existing historical agents, and clevidipine has yet to become a first-line agent for the management of acute hypertension in many hospitals.[43]

Esmolol   Esmolol is a very short-acting beta-1 selective blocker that is used primarily for heart rate control, but can also be used for the acute management of blood pressure. With a half-life and onset of action of minutes, the medication is easy to titrate and effects dissipate quickly if adverse events are encountered.[1] Some clinicians suggest that esmolol frequently requires add-on therapy with another antihypertensive to attain effective blood pressure control.[27]

Diltiazem Diltiazem is a non-dihydropyridine (benzothiazepine) calcium channel blocker.[29] Like metoprolol and esmolol, diltiazem is commonly used as a rate control medication rather than a primary agent to manage blood pressure. Diltiazem is dosed as a continuous IV infusion and the IV product should typically not be given in doses of greater than 20 mg/hr to avoid precipitous changes in blood pressure and heart rate.

Other Agents

Clonidine

Clonidine is an alpha-2 agonist occasionally used to manage blood pressure in the critically ill patient. In the United States, it is available as both a transdermal patch and as an oral tablet. Because clonidine is available as a patch formulation, it is a possible option for patients unable to take oral medications and have a significant sympathetic component to their hypertension, such as patients who are withdrawing from narcotics or alcohol. Clonidine's activity on the alpha-2 receptor is helpful to both reduce blood pressure and overall anxiety associated with the withdrawal symptoms.[47] The oral tablets may also be given via an enteral tube if available.

Special Considerations in Pregnancy

Preeclampsia and eclampsia are hypertensive emergencies that require rapid treatment and resolution to prevent significant morbidity or mortality for both mother and baby. Medications of choice include hydralazine, labetalol, and calcium channel blockers such as nicardipine.[29,48] Magnesium sulfate infusion is also used for prevention and treatment of seizures, but not specifically for blood pressure reduction. For pregnant patients with hypertension without preeclampsia, hydralazine, labetalol, and nicardipine remain agents of choice. Remember that ACEi are contraindicated in pregnancy, so medications such as enalaprilat should not be used.

SUMMARY

Alteration of blood pressure is a common occurrence in the ICU and is often managed with medication therapy. The pharmacist plays a key role in optimizing regimens to both increase and decrease blood pressure.

By utilizing knowledge of pharmacology and potential adverse events associated with each therapy, individualized plans can be created to optimally manage patients with either hypo- or hypertension.

KEY POINTS

- Knowledge of receptor activity of the vasopressor agents is important in selecting appropriate regimens.
- Continuous infusions should be dosed based upon a protocol and titrated to the targeted blood pressure goals.
- Hypertension in the ICU is common and can be managed with a variety of medications.
- Selection between intermittent and continuous antihypertensive agents is based upon the underlying cause of hypertension, treatment goals, and potential side effects of the medication.

SELECTED SUGGESTED READINGS

- Dellinger RP, Levy MM, Carlet JM, et al. Surviving Sepsis Campaign: international guidelines for management of severe sepsis and septic shock: 2008. *Crit Care Med.* 2008;36:296–327.
- Landry DW, Oliver JA. The pathogenesis of vasodilatory shock. *N Engl J Med.* 2001;345:588–595.
- Rhoney D, Peacock WF. Intravenous therapy for hypertensive emergencies, part 1. *Am J Health-Syst Pharm.* 2009;66:1343–1352.
- Rhoney D, Peacock WF. Intravenous therapy for hypertensive emergencies, part 2. *Am J Health-Syst Pharm.* 2009;66:1448–1457.

REFERENCES

1. Thomas C, Westfall DPW. Adrenergic agonists and antagonists. In: Brunton LL, ed. *Goodman & Gilman's: The Pharmacologic Basis of Therapeutics. 11th ed.* New York: McGraw-Hill; 2006:237–295.
2. Dellinger RP. Cardiovascular management of septic shock. *Crit Care Med.* 2003;31:946–955.
3. Beale RJ, Hollenberg SM, Vincent JL, Parrillo JE. Vasopressor and inotropic support in septic shock: an evidence-based review. *Crit Care Med.* 2004;32: S455–S465.
4. Hollenberg SM, Ahrens TS, Annane D, et al. Practice parameters for hemodynamic support of sepsis in adult patients: 2004 update. *Crit Care Med.* 2004;32:1928–1948.

5. Patel GP, Grahe JS, Sperry M, et al. Efficacy and safety of dopamine versus norepinephrine in the management of septic shock. *Shock.* 2010;33:375–380.
6. Jo SK, Rosner MH, Okusa MD. Pharmacologic treatment of acute kidney injury: why drugs haven't worked and what is on the horizon. *Clin J Am Soc Nephrol.* 2007;2:356–365.
7. Dellinger RP, Levy MM, Carlet JM, et al. Surviving Sepsis Campaign: international guidelines for management of severe sepsis and septic shock: 2008. *Crit Care Med.* 2008;36:296–327.
8. Povoa PR, Carneiro AH, Ribeiro OS, Pereira AC. Influence of vasopressor agent in septic shock mortality. Results from the Portuguese Community-Acquired Sepsis Study (SACiUCI study). *Crit Care Med.* 2009;37:410–416.
9. Albanese J, Leone M, Garnier F, Bourgoin A, Antonini F, Martin C. Renal effects of norepinephrine in septic and nonseptic patients. *Chest.* 2004;126:534–539.
10. Nygren A, Thoren A, Ricksten SE. Norepinephrine and intestinal mucosal perfusion in vasodilatory shock after cardiac surgery. *Shock.* 2007;28:536–543.
11. De Backer D, Creteur J, Silva E, Vincent JL. Effects of dopamine, norepinephrine, and epinephrine on the splanchnic circulation in septic shock: which is best? *Crit Care Med.* 2003;31:1659–1667.
12. Beloeil H, Mazoit JX, Benhamou D, Duranteau J. Norepinephrine kinetics and dynamics in septic shock and trauma patients. *Br J Anaesth.* 2005;95:782–788.
13. Myburgh JA, Higgins A, Jovanovska A, Lipman J, Ramakrishnan N, Santamaria J. A comparison of epinephrine and norepinephrine in critically ill patients. *Intensive Care Med.* 2008;34:2226–2234.
14. Morelli A, Ertmer C, Rehberg S, et al. Phenylephrine versus norepinephrine for initial hemodynamic support of patients with septic shock: a randomized, controlled trial. *Crit Care.* 2008;12:R143.
15. Levy B, Perez P, Perny J, Thivilier C, Gerard A. Comparison of norepinephrine-dobutamine to epinephrine for hemodynamics, lactate metabolism, and organ function variables in cardiogenic shock. A prospective, randomized pilot study. *Crit Care Med.* 2011;39:450–455.
16. Havel C, Arrich J, Losert H, Gamper G, Mullner M, Herkner H. Vasopressors for hypotensive shock. *Cochrane Database Syst Rev.* 2011;5:CD003709.
17. Marik PE, Mohedin M. The contrasting effects of dopamine and norepinephrine on systemic and splanchnic oxygen utilization in hyperdynamic sepsis. *JAMA.* 1994;272:1354–1357.
18. Vasu TS CR, Hirani A, Kaplan G, Leiby B, Marik PE. Norephinephrine or dopamine for septic shock: a systematic review of randomized clinical trials. *J Intensive Care Med.* 2011.
19. Klinzing S, Simon M, Reinhart K, Bredle DL, Meier-Hellmann A. High-dose vasopressin is not superior to norepinephrine in septic shock. *Crit Care Med.* 2003;31:2646–2650.
20. Russell JA, Walley KR, Singer J, et al. Vasopressin versus norepinephrine infusion in patients with septic shock. *N Engl J Med.* 2008;358:877–887.
21. Maybauer MO, Walley KR. Best vasopressor for advanced vasodilatory shock: should vasopressin be part of the mix? *Intensive Care Med.* 2010;36:1484–1487.

22. Holmes CL, Patel BM, Russell JA, Walley KR. Physiology of vasopressin relevant to management of septic shock. *Chest.* 2001;120:989–1002.

23. Landry DW, Oliver JA. The pathogenesis of vasodilatory shock. *N Engl J Med.* 2001;345:588–595.

24. Annane D, Vignon P, Renault A, et al. Norepinephrine plus dobutamine versus epinephrine alone for management of septic shock: a randomised trial. *Lancet.* 2007;370:676–684.

25. Marik PE. Critical illness-related corticosteroid insufficiency. *Chest.* 2009;135:181–193.

26. Varon J, Marik PE. Perioperative hypertension management. *Vasc Health Risk Manag.* 2008;4:615–627.

27. Haas AR, Marik PE. Current diagnosis and management of hypertensive emergency. *Sem dialysis.* 2006;19:502–512.

28. Chobanian AV, Bakris GL, Black HR, et al. The Seventh Report of the Joint National Committee on Prevention, Detection, Evaluation, and Treatment of High Blood Pressure: the JNC 7 report. *JAMA.* 2003;289:2560–2572.

29. Rhoney D, Peacock WF. Intravenous therapy for hypertensive emergencies, part 1. *Am J Health-Syst Pharm.* 2009;66:1343–1352.

30. Cherney D, Straus S. Management of patients with hypertensive urgencies and emergencies: a systematic review of the literature. *J of Gen Intern Med.* 2002;17:937–945.

31. McNeil JJ, Louis WJ. Clinical pharmacokinetics of labetalol. *Clin Pharmacokinet.* 1984;9:157–167.

32. Varon J. Treatment of acute severe hypertension: current and newer agents. *Drugs.* 2008;68:283–297.

33. Schulz V. Clinical pharmacokinetics of nitroprusside, cyanide, thiosulphate and thiocyanate. *Clin Pharmacokinet.* 1984;9:239–251.

34. Hall VA, Guest JM. Sodium nitroprusside-induced cyanide intoxication and prevention with sodium thiosulfate prophylaxis. *Am J Crit Care.* 1992;1:19–25; quiz in the book, does the quiz appear before the info being covered? The quiz is on p. 6–7 and the info in on p. 19–25. Should the quiz page range be 26–27 instead? 6–7.

35. Reddy P, Yeh YC. Use of injectable nicardipine for neurovascular indications. *Pharmacotherapy.* 2009;29:398–409.

36. Qureshi AI. Acute hypertensive response in patients with stroke: pathophysiology and management. *Circulation.* 2008;118:176–187.

37. Rhoney D, Peacock WF. Intravenous therapy for hypertensive emergencies, part 2. *Am J Health-Syst Pharm.* 2009;66:1448–1457.

38. Summers D, Leonard A, Wentworth D, et al. Comprehensive overview of nursing and interdisciplinary care of the acute ischemic stroke patient: a scientific statement from the American Heart Association. *Stroke.* 2009;40:2911–2944.

39. Narotam PK, Puri V, Roberts JM, Taylon C, Vora Y, Nathoo N. Management of hypertensive emergencies in acute brain disease: evaluation of the treatment effects of intravenous nicardipine on cerebral oxygenation. *J Neurosurg.* 2008;109:1065–1074.

40. Morgenstern LB, Hemphill JC, 3rd, Anderson C, et al. Guidelines for the management of spontaneous intracerebral hemorrhage: a guideline for healthcare professionals from the American Heart Association/American Stroke Association. *Stroke.* 2010;41:2108-2129.
41. Rose JC, Mayer SA. Optimizing blood pressure in neurological emergencies. *Neurocrit Care.* 2004;1:287-299.
42. Cardene IV solution for IV infusion, nicardipine HCL solution for IV infusion [package insert]. Bedminster, NJ: EKR Therapeutics; 2010.
43. Ndefo UA, Erowele GI, Ebiasah R, Green W. Clevidipine: a new intravenous option for the management of acute hypertension. *Am J Health Syst Pharm.* 2010;67:351-360.
44. Peacock FWt, Varon J, Ebrahimi R, Dunbar L, Pollack CV Jr. Clevidipine for severe hypertension in patients with renal dysfunction: a VELOCITY trial analysis. *Blood Pressure.* 2011;20 (Suppl 1):20-25.
45. Peacock FWt, Varon J, Ebrahimi R, Dunbar L, Pollack CV Jr. Clevidipine for severe hypertension in acute heart failure: a VELOCITY trial analysis. *Congest Heart Fail.* 2010;16:55-59.
46. Cleviprex (clevidipine butyrate) injectable emulsion [package insert]. Parsippany, NJ: The Medicines Company; 2008.
47. Honey BL, Benefield RJ, Miller JL, Johnson PN. Alpha2-receptor agonists for treatment and prevention of iatrogenic opioid abstinence syndrome in critically ill patients. *Ann Pharmacother.* 2009;43:1506-1511.
48. Steegers EA, von Dadelszen P, Duvekot JJ, Pijnenborg R. Pre-eclampsia. *Lancet.* 2010;376:631-644.

Chapter 9

Management of Cardiac Issues in the Critically Ill Patient

James R. Clem

LEARNING OBJECTIVES

1. Provide an overview of the pharmacologic management of acute coronary syndromes.
2. Detail the use of anticoagulation for cardiac indications in the critically ill.
3. Summarize the management of post-cardiac artery bypass patients.
4. Describe the pharmacologic management of acute congestive heart failure.
5. Recognize the common arrhythmias and common arrhythmia management techniques.

INTRODUCTION

Management of cardiac conditions is common in almost every critical care setting. While cardiac disease is a common primary reason for admission to the intensive care unit (ICU), cardiac disease can also be a significant secondary issue within the ICU. Patients that are under stress from other conditions have a high risk of arrhythmias and cardiac ischemia, leading to acute coronary syndromes or acute myocardial infarction. Further, patients with underlying congestive heart failure (CHF) that may be well controlled in normal health are at high risk to experience exacerbations of the disease when stressed because of other critical illness. This chapter will provide an overview of the management of common medications and treatment algorithms used to treat cardiac disease and complications that are common to critically ill patients.

ACUTE CORONARY SYNDROME MANAGEMENT

Acute coronary syndromes (ACS) include unstable angina and non-ST segment elevation myocardial infarction (NSTEMI). Acute coronary syndromes are characterized by myocardial ischemia associated with partial occlusion of a coronary artery or a lack of blood flow due to hypoperfusion from another cause.

Management of ACS requires the appropriate use of medications that have proven benefit on improving outcomes from clinical trials. The medications that are recommended for use in acute coronary syndromes come from evidence-based consensus guidelines and their use is well-founded. These medications should be incorporated into treatment protocols to ensure that they are used when appropriate to achieve the best possible clinical outcomes.

Heparin and Low-Molecular Weight Heparin

Unfractionated heparin (UFH) has played a vital role in the treatment of acute coronary syndromes for quite some time. Due to the pathophysiology of coronary atherosclerosis and the subsequent thrombus formation on the atheroma that occurs in ACS, UFH use is critical because it interrupts the thrombotic process, stopping further growth of the thrombus and allowing other interventions to effectively open the area of coronary stenosis or occlusion and allow it to remain patent. The recommended dosing and monitoring parameters for UFH use in ACS are listed in Table 9–1.[1] One of the major drawbacks of UFH use is the unpredictable anticoagulation response that can occur, and the potential delay in achieving therapeutic levels of anticoagulation can lead to a greater chance for a poor outcome compared to those who achieve therapeutic anticoagulation quickly. However, in patients with ACS that occurs as a secondary complication of critical illness, many clinicians choose heparin because of the ability to easily monitor for anticoagulant effect and stop the infusion rapidly if an adverse bleeding event occurs or if an invasive procedure is necessary.

The low molecular weight heparins (LMWHs) are an alternative to heparin for use in acute coronary syndromes. Overall, the low molecular weight heparins have demonstrated equivalent efficacy when compared to UFH.[1] However, in a few clinical trials, enoxaparin demonstrated superiority over UFH in desired outcomes when used for acute coronary syndromes.[2-4] In those clinical trials, enoxaparin was more effective in achieving the cardiovascular outcomes of reducing death, myocardial infarction, or recurrent angina.[2-4] The major advantage of the LMWHs over UFH is that LMWHs generally have a more predictable absorption pattern and effect; however, in the critically ill patient, alterations in peripheral perfusion may affect absorption patterns, although this has not been proven consistently. Further, LMWHs have longer half-lives and therefore do not reverse as quickly as heparin should bleeding occur or if an invasive procedure is necessary. Due to the predictable response that is seen with LMWH therapy, routine monitoring with anti-Xa levels is not needed in most patients, resulting in lower lab monitoring costs compared to UFH therapy. However, monitoring of LMWH therapy may be necessary in those patients that are at extremes in weight (high and low) and those with renal insufficiency. The dosing and monitoring parameters for the LMWHs with an indication for ACS are also listed in Table 9–1.

Table 9–1 Heparin Dosing for Acute Coronary Syndromes[1]

Drug	Dosing	Monitoring Parameters
Unfractionated heparin (UFH)	LD = 60 units/kg (max dose: 4,000 units) MD = 12 units/kg/hour (max: 1,000 units per hour)	aPTT (target range 1.5 to 2 times control) or equivalent heparin level Hgb, Hct Platelets Signs and symptoms of bleeding
Enoxaparin	MD = 1 mg/kg subq every 12 hours (extend interval to every 24 hours if creatinine clearance is less than 30 ml per min)	Anti-Xa level if poor renal function or extremes in weight Hgb, Hct Platelets Signs and symptoms of bleeding
Dalteparin	120 units/kg subq every 12 hours (max dose: 10,000 units every 12 hours)	Hgb, Hct Platelets Signs and symptoms of bleeding

LD = Loading dose

MD = Maintenance dose

Subq = Subcutaneous

IIb/IIIa Inhibitors

The role of the glycoprotein IIb/IIIa receptor inhibitors in the setting of ACS has varied significantly over the years as more clinical evidence of their safety and efficacy in achieving outcomes has been identified. The glycoprotein IIb/IIIa receptor inhibitors possess antiplatelet activity by inhibiting the final pathway of platelet aggregation. The glycoprotein IIb/IIIa receptor inhibitors can be utilized in the medical management of ACS when percutaneous coronary intervention (PCI) is either not planned or not possible, or they can be used as adjunct therapy to improve the clinical outcomes of someone undergoing an intervention such as angioplasty or stent placement.[1] Although glycoprotein IIb/IIIa inhibitors block the final common pathway of platelet aggregation, aspirin and/or clopidogrel still need to be administered concomitantly along with heparin or another parenteral anticoagulant. The major risks associated with glycoprotein IIb/IIIa receptor inhibitors is increased risk of major bleeding and thrombocytopenia.

The glycoprotein IIb/IIIa inhibitors that are available in the United States are abciximab and the "small molecule" agents eptifibatide and tirofiban. While they all inhibit the IIb/IIIa receptor, they do so via different mechanisms. Abciximab, a relatively large molecule compared with other agents, irreversibly binds to the IIb/IIIa site; therefore, the only way to even partially reverse the effects of abciximab is to transfuse platelets. The small molecule agents also inhibit the IIb/IIIa receptor but do so by occupying the receptor site in a reversible manner, and so adequate serum levels of the agent are needed in order to ensure inhibition of platelet aggregation. This difference in mechanism may be one of the reasons that the agents seem to perform slightly differently in practice and explain the differences in labeled indications.

In patients managed without the use of PCI for acute coronary syndromes, only two of the three available glycoprotein IIb/IIIa receptor inhibitors should be utilized based on available clinical trials. Eptifibatide and tirofiban are the only glycoprotein IIb/IIIa receptor inhibitors that have demonstrated evidence of benefit when used for the medical management of acute coronary syndromes.[1]

When an interventional approach is used for the treatment of acute coronary syndromes, any of the three available glycoprotein IIb/IIIa receptor inhibitors can be used. Clinical trial evidence has demonstrated that the glycoprotein IIb/IIIa receptor inhibitors have beneficial effects that lead to improvements related to PCI outcomes.[1] The recommended dosing and monitoring parameters for the glycoprotein IIb/IIIa receptor inhibitors are listed in Table 9–2.

Table 9–2 Glycoprotein IIb/IIIa Receptor Inhibitors for Acute Coronary Syndromes[1]

Drug	Dose	Monitoring Parameters
Abciximab	For PCI use only:	Hgb, Hct
	LD = 0.25 mg/kg IV bolus	Platelets
	MD = 0.125 mcg/kg/minute	Signs and symptoms of
	(max: 10 mcg/minute)	bleeding
Eptifibatide	LD = 180 mcg/kg IV bolus	Hgb, Hct
	(Administer a second bolus of	Platelets
	180 mcg/kg IV after 30 minutes if	Signs and symptoms of
	for PCI use)	bleeding
	MD = 2 mcg/kg/min	
	(reduce infusion rate by 50% if creatinine clearance is less than 50 ml per minute)	
Tirofiban	LD = 0.4 mcg/kg/minute for 30 minutes	Hgb, Hct
	MD = 0.1 mcg/kg/minute	Platelets
	(reduce infusion rate by 50% if creatinine clearance is less than 30 ml per minute)	Signs and symptoms of bleeding

LD = Loading dose

MD = Maintenance dose

Treatment Protocol Medications for Acute Coronary Syndromes

In addition to anticoagulation with heparin or LMWH, several other medications should also be used in ACS patients, unless contraindications are present, to ensure optimal outcomes and compliance with quality protocols. Table 9–3 highlights the medications and dosing regimens for each of the common additional medications.

Aspirin, Clopidogrel, and Prasugrel

Numerous medications play a critical role in ACS treatment. For example, aspirin plays a fundamental role in treatment algorithms based on demonstrated efficacy data from clinical trials.[1,5,6] It is important that aspirin be administered as quickly as possible, as platelet aggregation has been shown to be one of the most important pathophysiologic processes that initiates and leads to an acute thrombus formation on an atheroma. Aspirin's antiplatelet effect prevents further platelet aggregation and halts continued thrombus formation. It is important to use a non-enteric coated aspirin product for the initial doses to avoid

Table 9-3 Protocol Medications for Acute Coronary Syndromes[1]

Drug	Dose	Monitoring Parameters
Aspirin	162 to 325 mg (non-enteric coated) po daily	Signs and symptoms of bleeding
Clopidogrel	LD = 300 to 600 mg orally MD = 75 mg po daily	Signs and symptoms of bleeding
Nitroglycerin	Starting dose: 5 to 10 mcg/min continuous infusion and titrate to desired effect	Blood pressure, heart rate Symptoms of ischemia
Morphine	2 to 5 mg IV bolus every 5 to 30 minutes as needed for ischemic symptoms	
Beta-adrenergic blockers	Metoprolol: 5 mg IV bolus (over 1 to 2 minutes) every 5 minutes for 3 doses, then 25 to 50 mg po every 6 hours Atenolol: 5 mg IV bolus then 50 to 100 mg po daily Propranolol: 0.5 to 1 mg IV bolus then 10 to 80 mg po every 6 to 8 hours	Blood pressure, heart rate, respiratory rate Signs and symptoms of adverse effects
Calcium channel blockers	Diltiazem: LD = 0.25 mg/kg IV bolus, a repeat bolus of 0.35 mg/kg may be given if the first bolus is not effective MD = 5 to 15 mg/hr continuous infusion	Blood pressure, heart rate Symptoms of ischemia

LD = Loading dose
MD = Maintenance dose

any delay in the onset of aspirin's antiplatelet activity and the first dose should be chewed and swallowed.[1] For patients that have a true aspirin allergy, clopidogrel is an appropriate alternative.[1,7] In addition, it is important to note that when a patient has a coronary stent placed, the concomitant combination use of aspirin and clopidogrel is required to prevent platelet aggregation and subsequent thrombus formation on the coronary stent.[1,8]

A second thienopyridone, prasugrel, has recently been approved by the U.S. Food and Drug Administration (FDA) for use in ACS treatment. Prasugrel was included in the most recent focused update of the unstable angina/non-ST elevation myocardial infarction treatment guidelines.[9] Based on the clinical trials that assessed prasugrel's efficacy and safety, the focused update lists prasugrel as an alternative to clopidogrel in patients undergoing PCI for ACS treatment.[9,10] Based on the clinical evidence that is currently available, prasugrel was associated with better efficacy compared to clopidogrel; however, bleeding rates were higher with prasugrel use compared to clopidogrel.[10] Prasugrel should not be used in patients 75 years of age or older due to an association to increased bleeding risk.[9] Additional clinical trials are needed to further determine prasugrel's place in ACS treatment.

Nitroglycerin

Nitroglycerin is routinely used to help relieve the symptoms associated with myocardial ischemia. Nitroglycerin is a vasodilator that acts on both the peripheral and coronary vasculature. It predominantly works as a venous vasodilator, which in turn results in a reduction in preload pressures in the heart. This reduction in preload then leads to decreased myocardial oxygen demand, because myocardial contraction is decreased. Additionally, nitroglycerin can cause vasodilation in the coronary vasculature and collateral blood vessels to increase oxygen delivery to ischemic myocardial tissues.[1] The combination of these effects is likely how nitroglycerin helps relieve ischemic symptoms in acute coronary syndromes and myocardial infarction.

Nitroglycerin is typically given by intravenous (IV) continuous infusion in the critical care setting, while sublingual administration of nitroglycerin is most often utilized outside of a hospitalized setting. The overall goal in using nitroglycerin in any situation is to relieve the symptoms of ischemic pain. In the acute setting, the goal with nitroglycerin use is to titrate the infusion to relieve the ischemia symptoms while still maintaining an adequate blood pressure.

Morphine

When nitroglycerin is not completely effective in relieving the ischemic pain associated with ACS, intravenous morphine can be utilized.[1] Morphine can be very beneficial in treating the ischemic symptoms associated with acute coronary syndromes by two different mechanisms. The first pharmacologic benefit with its use is fairly obvious: morphine's analgesic effect can help in reducing the pain a patient may be suffering due to cardiac ischemia. Secondly, when morphine is given by the IV route, it has a venous vasodilatation effect that can reduce preload pressures in the heart and thus decrease myocardial oxygen demand. Morphine should be given in low doses on a frequent basis as needed for ischemic pain symptoms to help alleviate those symptoms.

Beta-Adrenergic Antagonists

Beta-adrenergic antagonists (beta-blockers) can have a significant beneficial impact on improving outcomes associated with ACS. Beta-blockers decrease heart rate and reduce myocardial contractility resulting in decreased myocardial oxygen demand. By decreasing the myocardial oxygen demand, the area of myocardial ischemia can potentially be reduced, resulting in less immediate damage to the myocardial tissue. Additionally, beta-blockers have demonstrated an overall short-term and long-term mortality reduction in patients with acute coronary syndromes. It is important to note that only beta-blockers that do not have intrinsic sympathomimetic activity (non-ISA beta-blockers), specifically atenolol, metoprolol, and propranolol, have been shown to have a mortality reduction benefit in acute coronary syndromes. The routine use of beta-blockers, unless they are contraindicated, in the setting of ACS is crucial in obtaining positive outcomes.

The intravenous administration of beta-adrenergic antagonists in acute coronary syndromes has historically been recommended in the treatment guidelines. This was essentially based on the premise that by administering the beta-blocker via the IV route, the onset of its beneficial effects would be quicker. However, it has been determined that the overall risk of aggressive beta-blocker dosing in the setting of ACS carries more risks than benefits, especially in hemodynamically unstable patients.[1] Therefore, the most recent evidence-based consensus guidelines recommend that beta-adrenergic antagonists in this setting should routinely be given by the oral route.[1,9]

Unless contraindicated, all patients who are being treated for ACS should receive beta-blocker therapy. In addition, the use of beta-blocker therapy for secondary prevention of ACS is important as well.

Calcium Channel Blockers

In patients who have severe reactive airway disease, beta-blockers are often avoided, and an alternative in this situation are the calcium channel blockers, diltiazem, or verapamil. They can be used to help decrease heart rate and cardiac output, thus reducing myocardial oxygen demand.[1] However, the impact of diltiazem or verapamil on clinical outcomes is limited and they are second-line agents used only when beta-blockers are contraindicated.

ACUTE MYOCARDIAL INFARCTION (ST-ELEVATION) MANAGEMENT

The treatment approach for an acute myocardial infarction and acute coronary syndromes are very similar; however, a few subtle differences do exist. In the setting of an acute myocardial infarction, complete coronary occlusion has occurred, whereas in acute coronary syndrome, only partial, but significant, narrowing of the coronary artery in the area of the atheroma has occurred. Both of these conditions result in an inadequate supply of oxygen to the myocardial tissue, but in the setting of acute myocardial infarction, no oxygen is being supplied to the affected myocardial tissue. This complete lack of oxygen results in the eventual death of myocardial cells if oxygen supply does not return in a timely manner. Therefore, it is very important to treat patients with an acute myocardial infarction very quickly to prevent myocardial cell death.

The most significant difference in treating an acute coronary syndrome patient and an acute myocardial infarction patient is the potential treatment option of utilizing fibrinolytic therapy in an ST-elevation myocardial infarction (STEMI) patient. In the setting of an acute coronary syndrome, fibrinolytic therapy has no significant demonstrated benefit in clinical trials.[1,11] Therefore, based on evidence-based clinical trials, fibrinolytic therapy is only beneficial in the setting of an acute myocardial infarction when invasive reperfusion strategies are not available in a timely fashion.

If an acute myocardial infarction patient is able to get to a healthcare facility with the ability to perform PCI (e.g., angioplasty, stenting) in a timely manner, that is the treatment approach of choice and has demonstrated the best overall outcome.[1,12] However, if for any number of reasons the patient is not able to be rapidly transported to a facility with the ability to perform PCI, then fibrinolytic therapy is the next best alternative treatment approach, as long as the patient has no contraindications to fibrinolytic therapy.[13]

PERIOPERATIVE CARDIOVASCULAR MANAGEMENT

Coronary Artery Bypass Graft Surgery and Valve Replacement

Patients who have open heart surgery for either coronary artery bypass and/or valve replacement with minimal or no complications are routinely in the intensive care unit for 24 hours or less. Duration of stay beyond 24 hours is dependent upon not only the amount of cardiac damage that may be present, but also upon co-morbid conditions such as lung disease, obesity, diabetes, or other chronic diseases. Any of these conditions can lead to complications, including extended mechanical ventilation times, increased risk of infection, gastrointestinal ileus, or acute kidney injury. Therefore, developing pharmacy care plans for cardiac surgery patients will be very dependent upon complications and co-morbid disease states. It is beyond the scope of this chapter to discuss all possible complications in detail, and the supportive care for patients with mechanical ventilation, infection, acute bleeding, and acute kidney injury (AKI) are discussed in other chapters of this text. However, there are several complications that should be monitored very closely.

One major risk for cardiac surgery patients is surgical wound infection. Beyond appropriate use of antibiotics during the perioperative period, it is very important to maintain control of blood glucose levels. While the exact range for glucose control in ICU patients remains elusive, a target blood glucose level of 150 mg/dL or less is common.

Significant bleeding during the postoperative period is also a potential complication, and this is typically monitored by closely watching the volume of output through the chest tubes that are placed in surgery. Increased amounts of drainage, or changes in the drainage from serosanguinous to bloody, for example, may indicate the need for treatment. Often this treatment requires re-operation, but agents such as recombinant factor VIIa, tranexamic acid, or aminocaproic acid have been used. Chapter 14 provides a discussion on use of procoagulant agents for bleeding complications.

Postoperative cardiac patients often require vasopressor and inotropic support to maintain cardiac output. Dobutamine, dopamine, ephinephrine, and phenylephrine are common agents used as pharmacologic support and these agents are described in detail in Chapter 8 of this text.

Balloon Counterpulsation

As described in Chapter 3, the intra-aortic balloon pump, or balloon counterpulsation therapy, is a mechanical device utilized to help stabilize patients who have recently undergone either cardiovascular surgery or a cardiovascular procedure and have remained or become unstable because of reduced cardiac output. The balloon counterpulsation therapy is utilized with the intent to increase cardiac output, as well as increase coronary artery, organ, and tissue perfusion. To date, there is limited evidence for balloon counterpulsation on outcomes.[1]

Balloon counterpulsation therapy is administered by inserting the balloon catheter into the femoral artery and threading the balloon catheter into the descending aorta. The balloon is inflated and deflated in a synchronized manner with the patient's heartbeat. The balloon deflates during systole, when the ventricle is contracting, thereby reducing afterload. During diastole, the balloon inflates, displacing blood in the aorta, which results in increased cardiac output. This, in turn, leads to increased coronary artery perfusion and increased organ and tissue perfusion.

Abdominal Aortic Aneurysm

Abdominal aortic aneurysms (AAA) are bulges of the descending aortic wall that commonly lead to pulsatile masses within the abdomen. The major concern of AAAs is aneurysm rupture, which has a very high mortality rate. Treatment guidelines suggest that AAA repair should generally occur when the AAA reaches a size greater than 5.5 centimeters, although there are exceptions to this, and other factors come into play when determining when repair should occur.[14] When repair is required, AAAs are treated either by open repair (surgery) or endovascularly. The surgical repair of an AAA involves the placement of a synthetic graft within the aneurysm to strengthen the aorta. The second treatment option is a less invasive endovascular approach. It is now more common for AAAs to be repaired endovascularly, which is achieved through the use of stent materials that repair the aneurysm without the need for major abdominal surgery that would include cross-clamping of the aorta and interruption of blood supply to major organs, most notably the kidneys, liver, and spine. However, if an AAA is identified upon rupture of the aneurysm, emergent surgery is the best hope for survival. Patients with ruptured AAA have often had a significant ischemic insult as well as required many units of transfused blood products prior to and during surgery. In the postoperative period, they are at risk for multiple complications including significant acid–base imbalance, AKI, acute respiratory distress syndrome (ARDS), disseminated intravascular coagulopathy (DIC), and infection. Management of the multiple possible complications requires intense monitoring and appropriate use of many medications that are detailed throughout this text.

Preventative approaches also need to be utilized for AAAs that do not require repair. Since high blood pressure is one of the major factors that contribute to the formation of AAA, adequate control of blood pressure in a patient with an AAA is an important part of treatment.

ACUTE DECOMPENSATED HEART FAILURE

Acute decompensated heart failure can be a primary reason for admission to the ICU, but it is often a co-morbid condition in the critically ill patient population that makes overall care of the patient more challenging. Whether a primary or secondary cause, acute heart failure is treated similarly, but it should be noted that some concomitant disease states and complications can lead to alterations in treatment pathways.

Acute decompensated heart failure is typically caused by two primary mechanisms: low cardiac output or fluid overload. The combination of

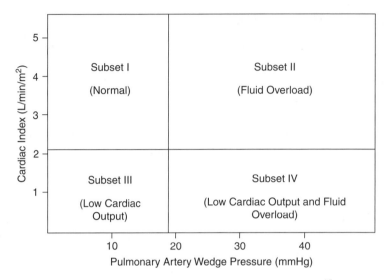

Figure 9-1 Subset Categories of Acute Decompensated Heart Failure[15]

both low cardiac output and fluid overload may also be present simultaneously. Invasive hemodynamic monitoring with a Swan–Ganz catheter or some type of non-invasive hemodynamic monitoring system is typically utilized to assist in determining the type of acute decompensated heart failure as well as to guide treatment. The classification system is then divided into four distinct subsets that are illustrated in Figure 9-1,[15] and the general treatment approach is guided by the patient's subset and overall response to therapies.

Loop Diuretics

The treatment approach in a patient with fluid overload (subsets II and IV) is generally with the use of aggressive diuresis; specifically, IV administration of a loop diuretic is the most common initial treatment, because loop diuretics cause a more vigorous diuresis compared to other diuretic classes, resulting in significant excretion of fluid from the body.[16] The dose of an IV diuretic depends significantly on a patient's chronic maintenance diuretic dose, as diuretic resistance is common in patients that have been taking loop diuretics for a significant amount of time. Furosemide or bumetanide are the most commonly used loop diuretics and are given by IV administration; however, torsemide is also available. Either intermittent bolus doses or continuous infusion may be utilized for diuresis.[16] Close monitoring of urine output and the patient's weight is critical to assist in determining the effectiveness of the diuresis and to prevent too rapid of a diuresis, as rapid diuresis or overdiuresis can lead to azotemia or even acute kidney injury, therefore, careful monitoring of fluid status and laboratory values including BUN and serum creatinine are necessary.

Dobutamine

For acutely decompensated heart failure patients that present with a reduced cardiac index, the use of positive inotropes is often adopted.[14] Dobutamine is a beta-adrenergic agonist that causes an increase in myocardial contraction and an increase in heart rate, both of which generally result in an increased cardiac index. If a patient is on a beta-adrenergic antagonist, then dobutamine may not be effective in increasing the cardiac index. Dobutamine should be titrated to increase the cardiac index but not cause more than a 20% increase in heart rate. Monitoring parameters for dobutamine are hemodynamic monitoring, specifically cardiac index, heart rate, blood pressure, and an electrocardiogram (ECG) for dysrhythmia monitoring. It should be noted that while short and long term use of dobutamine has demonstrated an improvement in symptoms, an overall increase in mortality is also observed, so the medication should only be used when absolutely necessary.[16]

Nesiritide

Nesiritide is recombinant human b-type naturetic peptide (BNP) indicated for use in acute decompensated heart failure. BNP is normally released by the ventricles when the ventricular wall is stretched more than normal. BNP has a naturetic and diuretic effect that reduces intravascular volume and vasodilating properties that reduce pulmonary capillary wedge pressure and preload.

Exogenous administration of BNP with nesiritide in acute decompensated heart failure is intended to improve symptoms and relieve acute decompensated heart failure. In clinical trials, nesiritide administration resulted in reductions in pulmonary capillary wedge pressure and dyspnea; however, no reduction in mortality or other endpoints has been demonstrated compared to other vasodilators.[17] The lack of confirmatory clinical evidence for outcome differences significantly limits use of the product.

Phosphodiesterase-3 Inhibitors

The phosphodiesterase-3 inhibitors (PDE) (e.g., milrinone) were developed for treatment of acute decompensated failure due to their positive inotropic effect in the myocardial tissue. The short-term use of milrinone in acute decompensated heart failure has been shown to improve hemodynamic parameters.[18] The monitoring of milrinone use includes hemodynamic monitoring of cardiac index and blood pressure. The phosphodiesterase-3 inhibitors have also been studied for use as long-term treatment for congestive heart failure; however, both short-term and long-term use have been associated with increased mortality, thus they should only be used short term in the critical care setting when indicated.[18]

Ultrafiltration Therapy

Ultrafiltration is a relatively new treatment approach for congestive heart failure. The therapeutic purpose of ultrafiltration is to remove excess fluid in heart failure patients, especially those patients that are demonstrating resistance to diuretic therapy.[18] Ultrafiltration works by forcing water through a semipermeable membrane and removing excess fluid from the body in an acutely decompensated heart failure patient who has fluid overload.[19] Ultrafiltration has been shown to effectively remove fluid from the body in a relatively short period of time with minimal problematic effects on blood pressure, heart rate, or other hemodynamic parameters.[19-21] In one early clinical trial,[19] up to nearly five liters of fluid was removed in a nine-hour period without any adverse effects or symptoms reported. Patients must have adequate blood pressure to be able to tolerate the significant fluid shifts associated with ultrafiltration therapy and patients typically need systemic anticoagulation with heparin to keep the system from clotting. Ultrafiltration may be a useful option in patients with significant diuretic resistance in the treatment of acute decompensated heart failure when fluid overload is a significant problem.

Ventricular Assist Devices

Left ventricular assist devices (LVADs) are mechanical pumps that are utilized to increase cardiac output and organ perfusion. LVADs are typically considered for use in the treatment of severe heart failure only when maximal medication therapy has been utilized but the patient still has inadequate cardiac output and organ perfusion.[22] The use of LVADS is primarily to maintain patients while awaiting transplantation, although technology in this area continues to advance.

ACUTE ARRHYTHMIA MANAGEMENT

Atrial Fibrillation

Acute atrial fibrillation and atrial flutter are common arrhythmias that occur in the general population as well as the critical care patient population.[23] In the critical care setting, atrial fibrillation is often a result of a secondary cause related to the severity of illness, such as recent cardiovascular surgery or severe pulmonary disease. Often, once the underlying illness improves, the atrial fibrillation will resolve spontaneously. However, the acute treatment of atrial fibrillation is very important in the critical care setting to avoid increased risk for potential complications, most commonly thromboembolic stroke. In addition, it is important to optimize cardiac function and reestablishing a regular cardiac rhythm will often benefit the patient by improving cardiac output.

The treatment approach to atrial fibrillation in the intensive care setting is very similar to the non-ICU setting. The first goal of therapy is to control the rapid ventricular rate with atrioventricular (AV) nodal blockade.[23] Often this will be with AV nodal blocking agents, most commonly beta-blockers and non-dihydropyridine calcium channel antagonists, given by the IV route.[23] The medications as well as appropriate dosages and monitoring parameters for the ICU setting are listed in Table 9–4. Digoxin may also be used to control ventricular rate, but is typically reserved for patients with heart failure or left ventricular dysfunction.[23]

Once the ventricular rate has been controlled at a goal of fewer than 100 beats per minute, the decision to attempt electrical or pharmacological cardioversion versus anticoagulation therapy needs to be determined. Many factors determine which approach is best for a given scenario. For example, any time a patient develops atrial fibrillation accompanied with life-threatening complications (ischemic chest pain, hemodynamic instability), direct current (DC) electrical cardioversion should be performed.[23] If the patient is relatively stable, then pharmacological cardioversion can be attempted. Drugs that are commonly used for pharmacologic cardioversion include amiodarone, dofetilide, and ibutilide; other options are available, but are less commonly used. The third option is to simply establish rate control, and then anticoagulate the patient to reduce the risk of thromboembolic complications of atrial fibrillation. Recent clinical trials demonstrated that rate control with anticoagulation was similar in safety and efficacy to rate control and pharmacologic cardioversion.[24] In the critical care setting, anticoagulation is typically done with either the low molecular weight heparins or unfractionated heparin.

Table 9–4 Atrioventricular Node Blocking Agents for Rate-control of Atrial Fibrillation/Flutter[18]

Drug	Dose	Monitoring Parameters
Diltiazem	LD = 0.25 mg/kg IV bolus; a repeat bolus of 0.35 mg/kg may be given if the first bolus is not effective. Max dose should not exceed 25 mg. MD = 5 to 15 mg per hour continuous infusion.	Blood pressure and heart rate
Beta-adrenergic antagonists	Esmolol: 500 mcg/kg IV bolus, then 60 to 200 mcg/kg/min IV continuous infusion. Metoprolol: 5 mg IV bolus (over 1 to 2 minutes) every 5 minutes for up to 3 doses for acute control. 2.5 to 5 mg IV every 6 hours for on-going control. Propranolol: 0.15 mg/kg IV bolus.	Blood pressure, heart rate, respiratory rate
Verapamil	LD = 2.5 to 5 mg IV bolus (slow push over 2 minutes).	Blood pressure and heart rate

LD = Loading dose

MD = Maintenance dose

A risk-to-benefit assessment should be made before using full anticoagulation if the patient is at significant risk for bleeding complications. The CHADS(2) score is a commonly-used method to determine overall risk of stroke as an embolic event caused by atrial fibrillation.[25] Use of this scoring system can help compare the risk of significant stroke to the immediate risk of severe bleeding.

Paroxysmal Supraventricular Tachycardia

Paroxysmal supraventricular tachycardia (PSVT) is another supraventricular arrhythmia that can occur in the critical care setting because of the stress of other underlying, severe diseases placing additional stress on the myocardial tissues. If the patient is having life-threatening symptoms associated with the arrhythmia, proper sedation and immediate DC electrical cardioversion should be administered. If the patient is relatively stable with PSVT, then vagal maneuvers or pharmacologic approaches should be pursued to resolve the arrhythmia. Based on practice guidelines, the drug of choice in treating PSVT is adenosine.[26] The initial dose of adenosine is

6 mg IV rapid push followed immediately by a saline flush to ensure all of the medication reaches the circulation, as adenosine has a very short half-life of just seconds. Clinicians should be aware that adenosine will often lead to a short period (seconds) of asystole followed by a resumption of electrical activity; therefore, only trained personnel should administer the medication. If the initial dose is ineffective, then a subsequent 12 mg dose should be administered, and an additional 12 mg IV bolus can be administered if this first 12 mg dose is ineffective. If the 6mg–12 mg–12 mg sequence of dosing is not effective, then either the rhythm is actually not PSVT or adenosine simply will not work and other approaches need to be attempted. Other AV nodal blocking agents such as beta-blockers or calcium channel blockers can be used and have demonstrated similar efficacy to adenosine.[26]

VENTRICULAR ARRHYTHMIAS

Tachycardia

The treatment of ventricular tachycardia in the critical care setting depends entirely on the specific ventricular rhythm and the symptoms or complications that result from the rhythm. Anytime a ventricular tachycardia rhythm causes a patient to become hemodynamically unstable or have life-threatening symptoms, proper sedation (if needed) and DC electrical cardioversion should be utilized. If the patient is otherwise relatively stable, pharmacological treatment may be used to treat the tachycardia as the initial approach. Medication administration should be by the IV route to ensure an immediate response to resolve the tachycardia.

Intravenous amiodarone is considered the initial antiarrhythmic agent of choice for most types of ventricular tachycardia.[26] Amiodarone is effective in suppressing ventricular tachycardia and is listed as the first choice for most arrhythmias based on the Advanced Cardiac Life Support guidelines.[26] Lidocaine is listed as a second choice agent in most ventricular tachycardias due to evidence in clinical trials that it may have a higher rate of adverse effects in the critical care setting.

Bradycardia

The treatment approach to bradycardia in the critical care setting is based on the severity of the symptoms associated with the low heart rate. Of note, asymptomatic bradycardia does not need any specific treatment intervention, but should be closely monitored in case it becomes symptomatic and requires treatment. A patient's medication profile should be reviewed for any medication that may cause bradycardia and any offending medication should be discontinued if possible.

The two main treatment approaches for bradycardia are either pharmacologic or pacing.[26] Atropine, in doses of 0.5 mg IV, can be effective at increasing a patient's heart rate; however, because of atropine's short half-life, the effect will be temporary. The electrical approach to treating bradycardia is with a pacemaker. Transcutaneous pacing can be used as a short-term solution until a temporary (transvenous) pacemaker can be inserted. If the bradycardia is resolved, then no further treatment is needed; however, if the bradycardia becomes permanent, then a permanent pacemaker needs to be placed.

ADVANCED CARDIAC LIFE SUPPORT OVERVIEW

Medications in the Code Tray

Medications play a vital role in most Advanced Cardiac Life Support (ACLS) situations. Proper utilization of medications in these life-threatening events improves the likelihood of a positive outcome. Over the years, the use of medications during acute cardiac resuscitation has become more streamlined and first-line agents have evolved as the amount of clinical trial data has increased. For example, IV amiodarone is now a primary agent for most ventricular arrhythmias and lidocaine is a second-line agent, even though lidocaine was a first-line agent in the past.

The medications used in these acute life-threatening situations serve many different purposes for a variety of medical conditions. Table 9–5 lists the common medications found in crash cart medication trays and their primary purpose, and Figure 9–2 illustrates a typical crash cart medication tray. Note that most medications come in a pre-filled syringe to facilitate the rapid use of the medications. A full review of the most up-to-date ACLS guidelines is an important part of understanding the appropriate use of medications in life-threatening emergencies, and those guidelines can be found through the American Heart Association.[26]

Mechanical Piston Devices for Aiding Cardiopulmonary Resuscitation

One of the most important elements in cardiopulmonary resuscitation is chest compressions. Unfortunately, chest compressions are frequently done incorrectly, resulting in minimal or no benefit to the patient. In addition, provider fatigue can become an issue, especially with prolonged

Table 9–5 Medications Typically Included in Crash Cart Trays

Drug	Indication
Adenosine	PSVT
Amiodarone	Atrial and ventricular arrhythmias
Atropine	Asystole or bradycardia
Calcium chloride	Cardioprotection in hyperkalemia and treatment of calcium channel blocker toxicity
Dextrose	Hypoglycemia
Diphenhydramine	Anaphylactic reactions
Epinephrine	To aid CPR effect and anaphylactic reactions
Furosemide	Acute pulmonary edema
Lidocaine	Ventricular arrhythmias
Magnesium	Torsdes de Pointes and refractory ventricular arrhythmias
Methylprednisolone	Anaphylactic reactions
Naloxone	Narcotic toxicity
Norepinephrine	Shock
Sodium Bicarbonate	Hyperkalemia and prolonged metabolic or respiratory acidosis
Vasopressin	To aid CPR effect and shock

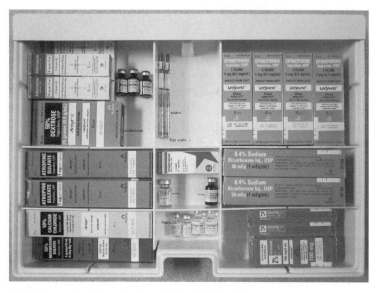

Figure 9–2 Example of Tray for Crash Cart Medication

chest compressions. However, a mechanical device called the LUCAS chest compression system provides continuous, hands-free chest compression via a plunger that pushes down on the chest and recoils back at a constant rate, providing more effective chest compressions compared to manual chest compressions.[27] The LUCAS device is powered by either compressed air, which requires no electricity, or by a battery. The device can be set up relatively easily, allowing for chest compressions to begin very quickly.

The most recent American Heart Association guidelines for cardiopulmonary resuscitation[28] state that mechanical piston devices may be used in appropriate settings, with specially trained personnel, in situations where manual cardiopulmonary resuscitation is difficult. However, there is not enough evidence to date to recommend for or against the routine use of a mechanical piston device during cardiopulmonary resuscitation.

SUMMARY

Cardiac disease and complications are common in the critical care setting. Whether the initiating event or a secondary complication, cardiac events require rapid evaluation and treatment to ensure positive patient outcomes. Medications play a significant role in the treatment of cardiac disease and use is often highly protocolized. Pharmacists must ensure that appropriate medication choices and monitoring are implemented to optimize patient outcomes and ensure adherence to quality measures.

KEY POINTS

- Acute coronary syndromes are common in the ICU as either primary or secondary events. Treatment pathways are similar for either presentation.
- Management of cardiac events in the ICU often requires anticoagulation, and appropriate dosing and careful monitoring are important to provide optimal outcomes.
- Acute heart failure can be a significant illness leading to ICU admission, or it can be a major co-morbid disease state that can make treatment of other conditions more difficult.
- Atrial fibrillation is a common disease encountered in the critically ill that can lead to tachyarrythmias, hypotension, and complications such as stroke.
- Ventricular arrhythmias are life-threatening events that must be treated rapidly and according to protocol.

SELECTED SUGGESTED READINGS

- Anderson JL, Adams CD, Antman EM, et al. ACC/AHA 2007 Guidelines for the management of patients with unstable angina/non–ST-elevation myocardial infarction—Executive summary. *JACC.* 2007;50(7):652–726.
- Wright RS, Anderson JL, Adams CD, et al. 2011 ACCF/AHA focused update of the guidelines for the management of patients with unstable angina/non–ST-elevation myocardial infarction (Updating the 2007 Guideline): A report of the American College of Cardiology Foundation/American Heart Association Task Force on Practice Guidelines *JACC.* 2011;57:1920-1959.
- Kushner FG, Hand M, Smith Jr SC, et al. 2009 Focused Updates: ACC/AHA guidelines for the management of patients with ST-elevation myocardial infarction (Updating the 2004 Guideline and 2007 Focused Update) and ACC/AHA/SCAI guidelines on percutaneous coronary intervention (Updating the 2005 Guideline and 2007 Focused Update). *JACC.* 2009:54(23):2205-2241.
- Brewster DC, Cronenwett JL, Hallett Jr JW, et al. Guidelines for the treatment of abdominal aortic aneurysms: Report of a subcommittee of the Joint Council of the American Association for Vascular Surgery and Society for Vascular Surgery. *J Vasc Surg.* 2003;37:1106-1117.

REFERENCES

1. Anderson JL, Adams CD, Antman EM, et al. ACC/AHA 2007 Guidelines for the management of patients with unstable angina/non–ST-elevation myocardial infarction—Executive summary. *JACC.* 2007;50(7):652–726.
2. Cohen M, Demers C, Gurfinkel EP, et al. A comparison of low-molecular-weight heparin with unfractionated heparin for unstable coronary artery disease. Efficacy and safety of subcutaneous enoxaparin in non–Q-wave coronary events study group. *N Engl J Med.* 1997;337:447–452.
3. Antman EM, McCabe CH, Gurfinkel EP, et al. Enoxaparin prevents death and cardiac ischemic events in unstable angina/non-Qwave myocardial infarction: results of the Thrombolysis In Myocardial Infarction (TIMI) 11B trial. *Circulation.* 1999;100:1593–1601.
4. Ferguson JJ, Califf RM, Antman EM, et al. Enoxaparin vs unfractionated heparin in high-risk patients with non–ST-segment elevation acute coronary syndromes managed with an intended early invasive strategy: primary results of the SYNERGY randomized trial. *JAMA.* 2004;292:45–54.

5. Lewis HDJ, Davis JW, Archibald DG, et al. Protective effects of aspirin against acute myocardial infarction and death in men with unstable angina: results of a Veterans Administration Cooperative Study. *N Engl J Med.* 1983;309:396–403.
6. Theroux P, Ouimet H, McCans J, et al. Aspirin, heparin, or both to treat acute unstable angina. *N Engl J Med.* 1988;319:1105–1111.
7. CAPRIE Steering Committee. A randomised, blinded, trial of clopidogrel versus aspirin in patients at risk of ischaemic events (CAPRIE). *Lancet.* 1996;348:1329–1339.
8. Mehta SR, Yusuf S, Peters RJ, et al. Effects of pretreatment with clopidogrel and aspirin followed by long-term therapy in patients undergoing percutaneous coronary intervention: the PCI-CURE study. *Lancet.* 2001;358:527–533.
9. Wright RS, Anderson JL, Adams CD, et al. 2011 ACCF/AHA focused update of the guidelines for the management of patients with unstable angina/non–ST-elevation myocardial infarction (Updating the 2007 Guideline): A Report of the American College of Cardiology Foundation/American Heart Association Task Force on Practice Guidelines *JACC.* 2011;57:1920–1959.
10. Wiviott SD, Braunwald E, McCabe CH, et al. Prasugrel versus clopidogrel in patients with acute coronary syndromes. *N Engl J Med.* 2007;357:2001–2015.
11. Fibrinolytic Therapy Trialists' (FTT) Collaborative Group. Indications for fibrinolytic therapy in suspected acute myocardial infarction: collaborative overview of early mortality and major morbidity results from all randomised trials of more than 1000 patients. *Lancet.* 1994;343:311–322.
12. Mehta SR, Cannon CP, Fox KA, et al. Routine vs selective invasive strategies in patients with acute coronary syndromes: a collaborative meta-analysis of randomized trials. *JAMA.* 2005;293:2908–2917.
13. Kushner FG, Hand M, Smith Jr SC, et al. 2009 Focused Updates: ACC/AHA guidelines for the management of patients with ST-elevation myocardial infarction (Updating the 2004 Guideline and 2007 Focused Update) and ACC/AHA/SCAI guidelines on percutaneous coronary intervention (Updating the 2005 Guideline and 2007 Focused Update). *JACC.* 2009;54(23):2205–2241.
14. Brewster DC, Cronenwett JL, Hallett Jr JW, et al. Guidelines for the treatment of abdominal aortic aneurysms: Report of a subcommittee of the Joint Council of the American Association for Vascular Surgery and Society for Vascular Surgery. *J Vasc Surg.* 2003;37:1106–1117.
15. Forrester JS, Diamond G, Chatterjee K, Swan HJC. Medical therapy of acute myocardial infarction by application of hemodynamic subsets. *N Engl J Med.* 1976;295:1356–1362.
16. Hunt SA, Abraham WT, Chin MH, et al. ACC/AHA 2005 guideline update for the diagnosis and management of chronic heart failure in the adult—summary article. *Circulation.* 2005;112;1825–1852.
17. O'Connor CM, Starling RC, Hernandez AF, et al. Effect of nesiritide in patients with acute decompensated heart failure. *N Engl J Med.* 2011;365:32–43.
18. Joseph SM, Cedars AM, Ewald GA, et al. Acute decompensated heart failure: Contemporary medical management. *Tex Heart Inst J.* 2009;36(6):510–520.
19. Kamath SA. The role of ultrafiltration in patients with decompensated heart failure. *Int J Nephrol.* 2011;190–230.

20. Marenzi G, Lauri G, Grazi E, et al. Circulatory response to fluid overload removal by extracorporeal ultrafiltration in refractory congestive heart failure. *JACC.* 2001;38:963–968.
21. Giglioli C, Landi D, Cecchi E, et al. Effects of ULTRAfiltration vs. DIureticS on clinical, biohumoral and haemodynamic variables in patients with deCOmpensated heart failure: the ULTRADISCO study. *Eur J Heart Fail.* 2011;13(3):337–346.
22. Ramani GV, Uber PA, and Mehra MR. Chronic heart failure: contemporary diagnosis and management. *Mayo Clin Proc.* 2010;85(2):180–195.
23. Fuster V, Rydén LE, Cannom DS, et al. ACC/AHA/ESC 2006 guidelines for the management of patients with atrial fibrillation—Executive summary. *Circulation.* 2006;114(7):700–752.
24. Wyse DG, Waldo AL, DiMarco JP, et al. A comparison of rate control and rhythm control in patients with atrial fibrillation. *N Engl J Med.* 2002;347:1825–1833.
25. Gage BF, Waterman AD, Shannon W, et al. Validation of clinical classification schemes for predicting stroke: results from the National Registry of Atrial Fibrillation. *JAMA.* 2001;285:2864–2870.
26. Neumar RW, Otto CW, Link MS, et al. Part 8: adult advanced cardiovascular life support 2010 American Heart Association guidelines for cardiopulmonary resuscitation and emergency cardiovascular care circulation. *Circulation.* 2010;122[Suppl 3]:S729–S767.
27. LUCAS Chest compression system. Physio-control, Inc. http://www.physio-control.com/ProductDetail.aspx?id=886&terms=lucas. Accessed January 8, 2011.
28. Cave DM, Gazmuri RJ, Otto CW, et al. Part 7: CPR techniques and devices 2010 American Heart Association guidelines for cardiopulmonary resuscitation and emergency cardiovascular care. *Circulation.* 2010;122[Suppl 3]:S720–S728.

Chapter 10

Severe Sepsis and Septic Shock Management

Garrett Schramm

LEARNING OBJECTIVES

1. Review the epidemiology and pathophysiology of severe sepsis and septic shock.
2. Determine the stage of sepsis and evaluate the initial resuscitation treatment goals and subsequent ongoing management.
3. Evaluate the pharmacotherapeutic goals related to the treatment of severe sepsis and septic shock.
4. Delineate a pharmacist's role in severe sepsis and septic shock quality improvement.

INTRODUCTION

Epidemiology and Pathophysiology

Severe sepsis and septic shock represent two severe manifestations on the continuum of acute, progressive organ dysfunction induced by infection. Each syndrome has a similar pathologic process, with septic shock representing the more severe manifestations of the two disorders. Both syndromes are characterized by the acute onset of systemic inflammatory response syndrome (SIRS) and evolve into a complex series of interacting pathways involving immune stimulation, immune suppression, hypercoagulation, and hypofibrinolysis.

Despite a decline in the associated mortality, the incidence of severe sepsis and septic shock continues to rise at a rate of 1.5% per year in the United States, and it is estimated that 934,000 cases of severe sepsis occurred in 2010 and 1,110,000 will occur in 2020.[1,2] The increasing incidence is likely due to a multitude of factors, including increased awareness for the diagnosis, advancement of invasive medical and technological treatments, increasing number of elderly and immunocompromised patients, and the number of multidrug-resistant pathogens. A 2001 publication estimated each case of severe sepsis to cost approximately $22,100, with an annual total cost in the United States of $16.7 billon.[1]

The urgency with which therapies should be initiated for severe sepsis and septic shock is a direct consequence of the rapid evolution of the disease course. Mortality rates of up to 50% have been reported for patients with complications secondary to severe sepsis, highlighting the need for aggressive diagnostic and effective management measures.[1] Even with such measures, the progression of sepsis to severe sepsis has been estimated to occur in 9% of hospitalized patients, and of those patients, 3% may progress to septic shock.[3]

The complex pathologic process involved with each stage of sepsis leads to the continuum of acute, progressive organ dysfunction. If this process is left unchecked, it may lead to multiple organ failure and death. As a result of such complex pathophysiology and the need for time-dependent interventions, it is recommended that the treatment of severe sepsis and septic shock be managed with a bundled treatment approach to improve patient survival.[4,5]

An all-encompassing single mechanism with regard to the immunopathophysiology of sepsis remains elusive. The host inflammatory response is theorized to lead to the SIRS and progression of sepsis that ultimately leads to immune dysregulation and tissue injury.[6] Cytokines, including tumor necrosis factor alpha (TNF-α) and interleukin-6 (IL-6), are low-molecular-weight glycoproteins that act as intracellular messengers in the host defense by attracting activated neutrophils to the site of infection. Entry of these cytokines into systemic circulation is associated with SIRS and the cascade of inflammatory and immune dysfunction commences. The activation of neutrophils and monocytes, along with platelet dysfunction, further increases cytokine production and a quadrad of dysfunction ensues, leading to increased coagulation, decreased fibrinolysis, apoptosis, and imbalances between inflammatory and anti-inflammatory mediators. Left unchecked, this process will progress to micro-thrombi formation and resultant endothelial damage, which subsequently leads to an increase in capillary permeability and edema formation that reduces the perfusion of body tissues with cellular hypoxia, eventually causing single or multi-site organ dysfunction and possibly death. Pharmacotherapy directed at the inflammatory cascade and/or the immune response have had both positive and negative results to date. Novel treatment therapies such as toll-like receptor 4 (TLR-4) antagonists for severe sepsis have recently completed Phase 2 trials and hopefully will add to a much-needed armamentarium of sepsis therapies.[7]

EVALUATION OF THE PATIENT AND TREATMENT GOALS

Determination of Sepsis Stage

The management of severe sepsis and septic shock typically requires the expertise of critical care clinicians who possess the ability to integrate evidence-based medicine into an individualized pharmacotherapeutic plan for patients who are rapidly progressing to or are already in multiple organ failure. It is imperative to objectively determine the stage of sepsis to aid in the determination of pharmacotherapy goals and treatment endpoints. Sepsis staging has previously been defined by the consensus criteria of the American College of Chest Physicians and the Society of Critical Care Medicine, which is outlined in Table 10-1.[8] Once sepsis has progressed to severe sepsis or septic shock, individual organ or organ system function begins to decline. Table 10-2 lists the most commonly affected organs and their respective diagnostic thresholds, including cardiovascular, pulmonary, renal, and the hematologic/coagulation system.[5] Concurrent to SIRS criteria identification and sepsis staging, the clinician should also determine the most likely known or suspected source of infection. The most common sources of infection in sepsis include the lung (40%), intra-abdominal (20%), primary bacteremia (15%), and genitourinary (10%).[9]

Table 10-1 American College of Chest Physicians and the Society of Critical Care Medicine Sepsis Stage Definitions[5]

Condition	Definition
Systemic inflammatory response syndrome (SIRS)	Temperature >38°C or <36°C; heart rate >90 beats/min; respiratory rate >20 breaths/min or partial pressure of carbon dioxide <32 mmHg; and white blood cell count >12 x 10^3/mm^3 or <4 x 10^3/mm^3, >10% immature (band) forms
Sepsis	Infection plus two or more SIRS criteria
Severe sepsis	Sepsis plus organ dysfunction, hypoperfusion, or hypotension
Septic shock	Sepsis-related hypotension despite adequate fluid resuscitation with presence of perfusion abnormalities

Table 10-2 2008 Surviving Sepsis Campaign Organ Dysfunction definitions[5]

Organ Dysfunction	Definition
Cardiovascular	SBP <90 mmHg or a decrease in SBP by at least 40 mmHg for more than 1 hour that is unresponsive to fluid resuscitation
Pulmonary	Need for mechanical ventilation and a PaO_2 to FiO_2 ratio of <300
Renal	Urine output <0.5 ml/kg/hour for more than 2 hours despite adequate fluid resuscitation
	Creatinine increase of >0.5 mg/dL
Hematologic/ Coagulation	Platelet count <100,000/mm^3 or a 50% reduction over 3-day period
	INR >1.5 or aPTT >60 seconds

SBP = systolic blood pressure; PaO_2 = partial pressure of arterial oxygen; FiO_2 = fraction of inspired oxygen; INR = international normalized ratio; aPTT = activated partial thromboplastin time

GOALS OF PHARMACOTHERAPY

Initial Care of the Patient

Similar to other critically ill patients, the initial priority in the management of a septic patient focuses on establishment of an airway, breathing, and circulation. At the time of diagnosis, patients with severe sepsis or septic shock usually demonstrate signs of hypoperfusion as evidenced by a low blood pressure (systolic blood pressure (SBP) less than 90 mmHg or mean arterial pressure (MAP) less than 60 mmHg in most patients) in combination with clinical manifestations that may include respiratory failure, tachycardia, and diminished urine output, among a constellation of other symptoms. In addition to monitoring for hypoperfusion via blood pressure monitoring, the Surviving Sepsis Guidelines (SSG)[5] recommend obtaining a serum lactate concentration at the onset of suspected severe sepsis or septic shock. Once other causes of an elevated serum lactate concentration are ruled out (e.g., reduced elimination in hepatic insufficiency or an increase in skeletal muscle activity), a serum concentration greater than 4 mmol/L may be utilized as an indicator of tissue hypoperfusion and suggest the need for early and aggressive fluid resuscitation to restore tissue perfusion. Upon documentation or suspicion of infection-induced hypoperfusion, the pharmacist must be familiar with the goals of initial resuscitation and hemodynamic stabilization that are based on the principles of early-goal-directed therapy (EGDT), including: (1) insertion of a central venous catheter, (2) achievement of a central venous pressure (CVP) of 8 to 12 mmHg in non-mechanically ventilated patients and up to 12 to 15 mmHg in mechanically ventilated patients to account for potential filling impediment associated with positive pressure ventilation, (3) MAP ≥65 mmHg, (4) urine output ≥0.5 ml/kg/hour, and (5) central venous or mixed venous oxygen saturation of ≥70% or ≥65%, respectively.[10] The time frame for achieving these endpoints should occur as soon as possible and always within the first 6 hours of the presentation of severe sepsis or septic shock.

Hemodynamic Stabilization

Severe sepsis is often complicated by hypotension resulting from the failure of vascular smooth muscle to constrict (vasodilatory shock) and/or a maldistribution of blood flow in the microcirculation (distributive shock). The importance of aggressive fluid administration as one of the critical initial resuscitative maneuvers to restore tissue homeostasis was established in the landmark EGDT trial.[10] With regards to which volume resuscitation agent is preferred for the resuscitation of critically ill patients, a study compared crystalloids (normal saline or lactated Ringer's solution) to colloids (albumin or pentastarch).[11] The primary end point of 28-day mortality did not differ between groups (pentastarch 26.7% vs. lactated Ringer's 24.1%, p = 0.48); however, the pentastarch group had a significantly higher rate of acute renal failure (34.9% vs. 22.8%, p = 0.002) and a greater percentage of days in which renal replacement therapy was required (18.3% vs. 9.2%). These findings led to early stoppage of the trial and may limit assessment of the safety of colloid solutions in recommended doses in patients with severe sepsis. Additional prospective trials have attempted to delineate the optimal fluid to resuscitate critically ill patients, including those with sepsis; however, cumulatively, a clear benefit of one form of fluid over the other with regard to patient survival has not been established, and certainly there is little guidance as to the fluid of choice during the initial 6 hours of care.

With the publication of numerous quality improvement studies describing efforts to translate the methodology of EGDT to the bedside, it has become clear that under-resuscitation is a theme that has plagued many institutions prior to implementation of a resuscitation protocol. In the majority of cases, the initial fluid challenge should be administered as a rapid bolus of 20 to 30 ml/kg of crystalloid (or colloid equivalent); cumulatively, within the first 6 hours of the onset of fluid administration, patients may receive on average 3.5 to 5 liters of total fluid volume.

Concurrent with intravascular volume resuscitation, vasopressor agents (see Chapter 8) often need to be initiated to restore adequate arterial pressure and organ perfusion. Norepinephrine and dopamine are recommended as the first-line agents for increasing blood pressure in patients with septic shock.[5] Titration of the selected vasopressor to a MAP goal of 60 to 65 mmHg should be set and adjusted to higher levels if endpoints of regional and global perfusion are not met. In patients that require escalating doses of vasopressors to maintain MAP goals, the clinician is often tempted to add additional vasopressors such as vasopressin. Septic patients may have depleted neurohypophyseal and plasma concentrations of vasopressin, and the addition of vasopressin has been shown in numerous studies to improve vasoconstriction. However, in a randomized controlled trial, adjunctive vasopressin administration in doses up to 0.03 units/min did not offer a survival advantage compared to norepinephrine alone and may have contributed to a worsened outcome in this situation.[12] At this time, the utility of vasopressin as a vasopressor, either alone or in combination with norepinephrine, remains a possible option, but lacks conclusive evidence of end outcome benefit. If infused, doses of vasopressin higher than 0.04 units/min should not be administered to minimize the likelihood of adverse effects including skin, gut, and myocardial ischemia.

Patients that have continued impairment in perfusion as indicated by a central venous oxygen saturation of ≤70%, despite appropriate volume resuscitation and institution of vasopressors, may benefit from inotrope therapy. Dobutamine, added to norepinephrine, is recommended as the first-line agent for augmenting cardiac output and improving oxygen delivery.[5] Alternatively, epinephrine at a starting dose of 0.2 mcg/kg/min appears to be an option that is as efficacious and has a similar safety profile to norepinephrine plus dobutamine.[13] Vasopressor/inotrope titration should be directed to a central venous oxygen saturation of ≥70%. Targeting therapy to endpoints such as an elevated cardiac index (>4.5 L/min/m^2) has not consistently improved mortality. Figure 10–1 outlines the common algorithm approach to the resuscitation bundle advocated by the Surviving Sepsis Campaign guidelines.[5]

Infection Management

Concurrent to hemodynamic perfusion restoration, a thorough workup for infection should take place. The most common site of infection in patients with severe sepsis or septic shock is the lung, followed by the intra-abdominal compartment and the urinary tract. Microbiologic confirmation is determined with a pair of positive blood cultures drawn from different sites, with at least one drawn percutaneously. Since blood cultures alone are only positive in approximately one-third of patients, it is recommended that expectorated sputum, induced sputum, tracheal secretions, or

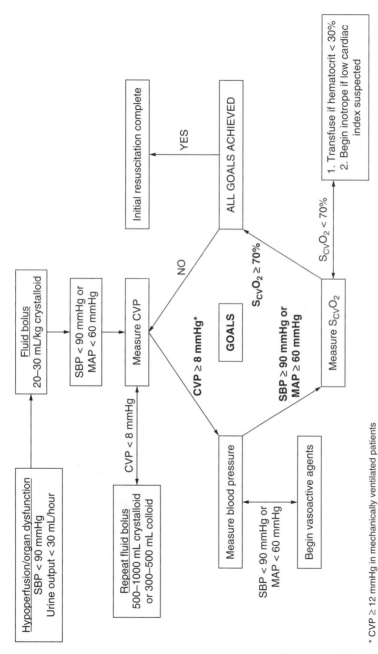

Figure 10–1 Resuscitation Bundle[10]

* CVP ≥ 12 mmHg in mechanically ventilated patients
SBP = systolic blood pressure; MAP = mean arterial pressure; CVP = central venous pressure; $S_{CV}O_2$ = central venous oxygen saturation

201

bronchoscopically obtained respiratory samples be obtained for culture if the lung is a suspected source of infection. Urine should also be obtained for culture and for determination of the presence of pyuria. Patients experiencing diarrhea should have a stool sample evaluated for *Clostridium difficile* toxin and other enteric pathogens if appropriate exposure or travel history exists. As part of a multidisciplinary team, the pharmacist may aid in the design of an appropriate empiric antimicrobial regimen for a patient with severe sepsis or septic shock and plays a key role with de-escalation practices.

Radiologic imaging studies should be performed to aid in the identification of the source of infection. Concurrently, emergent source control via drainage, debridement, or device removal should be considered for certain anatomical diagnoses of infection, including intra-abdominal abscess, septic arthritis, cholangitis, toxic megacolon, and necrotizing fasciitis. Although obtaining cultures, radiologic imaging, and source control are essential to confirm infection and facilitate de-escalation of antimicrobial regimens, they should not delay the prompt administration of appropriate antibiotics. Chapter 13 details an overall approach to antibiotic use in the critically ill.

The concrete diagnosis of sepsis is often complicated by the lack of both qualitative and quantitative infectious information at the bedside. Clinicians continue to rely upon the role of biomarkers such as C-reaction protein and white blood cell (WBC) count to aid in the diagnosis of sepsis; however, the sensitivity and specificity of these individual markers is variable. The role of the serum calcitonin-precursor procalcitonin has been the focus of research[14,15] in patients with sepsis, as procalcitonin levels have been shown to be elevated secondary to the release of bacterial cytokines and endotoxins, and then subsequently decline with the initiation of appropriate antimicrobial therapy. The utility of procalcitonin as a biomarker is compelling and would aid in the diagnosis of sepsis, individualize patient-specific antimicrobial therapy duration, and ideally promote judicious antimicrobial utilization. The effect of procalcitonin-guided treatment of patients with infections compared to standard treatment was evaluated in a meta-analysis that included seven randomized controlled trials and showed promising results with respect to decreasing exposure and shortening duration of antimicrobial therapy; however, no significant difference was found between the two groups with respect to mortality.[14]

The Procalcitonin to Reduce Antibiotic Treatments in Acutely Ill patients (PRORATA) is a prospective, open-label, multicenter trial that compared mortality rate and number of days without antimicrobials via non-inferiority and superiority analyses, respectively.[15] In the experimental arm, antimicrobials were started or stopped based on predefined cut-off ranges compared to the control arm, where therapy was guided by present guidelines.

The procalcitonin-guided algorithm resulted in a non-inferior 28 and 60-day mortality rate when compared to standard practice, with nearly 3 days less of antimicrobial therapy. Despite these positive findings, the results of PRORATA should be interpreted with caution given the open-label study design that may have introduced possible treatment bias and the fact that 53% of the patients did not receive algorithm-guided care.

Procalcitonin levels at baseline may be useful as an additional indicator of sepsis; however, the pharmacist must be aware that it may also be elevated in other inflammatory states, such as trauma and major surgery, and may decrease in the presence of existing appropriate antimicrobial therapy. Serial monitoring of procalcitonin may suggest when antimicrobial therapy for sepsis has succeeded, but until significant serum procalcitonin concentrations are more discretely defined, its role in the diagnosis and treatment of severe sepsis and septic shock remains controversial. At this time, procalcitonin levels greater than 0.25 mcg/L may be beneficial to help discern bacterial infections from viral or non-infectious inflammatory reactions and may help guide antimicrobial duration; however, the pharmacist must be aware that this information should be utilized in conjunction with other tools and within the context of the underlying disease.

ADJUNCTIVE THERAPIES

Corticosteroids

Throughout the history of sepsis research, the prevailing thought has been that the root of clinically observed morbidity and mortality is an uncontrolled inflammatory response to microbial invasion. Corticosteroids used to inhibit or limit the "cytokine storm" elicited by TNF-α and IL-6, amongst a host of other mediators, should result in a positive patient response. Dating back to the 1950s, steroids have been used as adjunctive therapy in bacterial infections;[16] however, these and other results were deemed to be non-beneficial in the majority of individual trials and also cumulatively when grouped together in a meta-analysis.[17] More recently, the focus of corticosteroids research has shifted to lower doses (300 mg/day or less of hydrocortisone or equivalent) for longer durations, of typically 5 days or more, with particular interest in patients lacking appropriate response to exogenously administered adrenocorticotropin.

The critical care community was re-invigorated with the potential benefit of corticosteroid administration after publication of a prospective trial that enrolled 300 patients with volume-refractory, vasopressor-dependent septic shock.[18] Patients were randomized to receive hydrocortisone 50 mg intravenously every 6 hours plus fludrocortisone 0.1 mg by mouth daily or placebo for 7 days. Relative adrenal insufficiency was tested for in patients with the administration of a corticotropin stimulation test. Non-responders, or patients having a response of 9 mcg/dL or less from time 0 to 60 minutes after administration of the 250 mcg adrenocorticotropin stimulation test, were the predefined subgroup of interest. Overall, there was no difference in 28-day mortality between hydrocortisone/fludrocortisone and placebo amongst the entire study population. However, a statistically significant reduction in the adjusted 28-day mortality was observed in the subgroup of 229 patients with adrenal insufficiency (non-responders), as well as a significantly shortened duration of vasopressor requirement. There were no differences between the groups with regard to the rate of adverse events. As a result of this trial, the 2004 SSG recommended the administration of the studied steroid regimen in patients with relative adrenal insufficiency and volume-refractory, vasopressor-dependent septic shock.[19]

Despite this recommendation, several important questions remained regarding the utilization of low dose, short duration corticosteroids for septic shock. First, debate ensued regarding the appropriate method to diagnose adrenal insufficiency in the setting of severe sepsis. The measurement of a baseline cortisol level in conjunction with a measured response as utilized in the previously mentioned trial versus a single or a random cortisol level with a concentration of less than 15 to 20 mcg/dL was debated as more compatible with a positive diagnosis. Arguments against the stimulation test held that patients with severe sepsis might have adequate cortisol concentrations at baseline, but fail to mount an appropriate response of 9 mcg/dL or greater, therefore falsely diagnosing patients with adrenal insufficiency. Other opponents disputed the use of the 250 mcg dose of adrenocorticotropin, claiming this approach could override normal adrenal resistance resulting in a false negative conclusion. To circumvent this possibility, a 1 mcg adrenocorticotropin stimulation test has been proposed to be more sensitive and specific for diagnosis in septic shock. The second issue of debate stemming from this trial surrounded the addition of fludrocortisone to hydrocortisone, since hydrocortisone provides both mineralocorticoid and glucocorticoid activity.

In an attempt to address the above concerns, a follow-up trial that enrolled 499 patients within 72 hours of severe sepsis or septic shock onset was conducted.[20] In contrast to the fixed regimen of the prior trial, patients were randomized to placebo or hydrocortisone 50 mg every 6 hours on days 1 through 5, with a tapered dose and frequency on days 6 through 11. Overall, the primary endpoint of 28-day mortality in non-responders did not differ between the hydrocortisone or placebo groups, though this finding is subject to type II error as the trial was significantly underpowered. Likewise, the duration of vasopressor administration was similar between hydrocortisone and placebo in both the adrenocorticotropin non-responders and responders. Despite the natural tendency to compare the follow-up trial to the original, several critical differences in methodology and patient demographics exist making such attempts problematic. However, the updated 2008 SSG no longer suggests routine testing for adrenal insufficiency with the adrenocorticotropin stimulation test, and concomitant fludrocortisone is only suggested if hydrocortisone is not available or the prescribed corticosteroid lacks mineralocorticoid activity. Intravenous corticosteroids are suggested in septic shock patients who are refractory to fluid resuscitation and are vasopressor dependent. Once vasopressors have been discontinued, weaning corticosteroids may be considered.

Drotrecogin Alfa (Activated)

Drotrecogin alfa (activated) (DAA), the recombinant formulation of human activated protein C, was the first biologic agent to be approved for the treatment of severe sepsis. Despite being withdrawn from the market in 2011, the research regarding DAA provides an interesting timeline in development, utilization, and safety for novel pharmacologic agent.

Drotrecogin alfa (activated), by way of inactivation of clotting factors Va and VIIIa and inhibition of fibrin-enhancing mediators such as plasminogen-activator inhibitor 1 (PAI-1), restored the imbalance of coagulation and fibrinolysis observed in patients with severe sepsis. Additionally, DAA may have offered anti-inflammatory and anti-apoptotic effects by limiting cytokine production, minimizing adhesion of leukocytes to capillary endothelium, and blunting B and CD4+ lymphocyte destruction in late sepsis. The Recombinant Human Activated Protein C Worldwide Evaluation in Severe Sepsis (PROWESS) study established the efficacy and safety of DAA.[21] This trial, which randomized 1,690 patients to a 96-hour continuous infusion of 24 mcg/kg/hour of DAA or placebo found the primary outcome of 28-day mortality from any cause to be significantly lower for patients treated with DAA after the second interim analysis, at which time the study was halted. Post hoc analysis indicated the mortality benefit was not consistent across different levels of severity of illness as measured by Acute Physiology and Chronic Health Evaluation II (APACHE II) score. The overall absolute 28-day mortality reduction was 6.1% in favor of DAA; however, upon subgroup analysis, the greatest benefit was seen in those patients with the highest predicted mortality (APACHE II score greater than or equal to 25).[22] Based on these findings, the U.S. Food and Drug Administration (FDA) gave an indication for DAA use only for the treatment of severe sepsis in patients with a high risk of death.

Given the apparent discrepancy in treatment effect for patients with a high vs. low risk of death, a follow-up trial deemed the Administration of Drotrecogin alfa (activated) Early Stage Severe Sepsis (ADDRESS) trial was conducted to evaluate the efficacy and safety of this agent compared to placebo in patients with a low risk of death, specifically as delineated by an APACHE II score less than 25 or single-organ dysfunction.[23] At the time enrollment was suspended due to futility of treatment with DAA, 2,640 patients were included. No significant difference in the primary outcome of 28-day mortality existed and a significantly increased rate of serious bleeding was observed among patients receiving DAA both during the infusion and at 28 days. Alarmingly, a subgroup analysis of 635 patients who had undergone recent surgery with single-organ dysfunction found patients treated with DAA to have a significantly greater 28-day mortality compared with the placebo group. This same trend was observed in 98 surgical patients from the PROWESS study and consequently a warning against use of DAA in low-risk surgical patients was issued in the package labeling.[24]

The Extended Evaluation of Recombinant Human Activated Protein C (ENHANCE) trial, a single-arm, open-label phase IIIb trial, evaluated DAA administration in 2,375 patients.[25] Similar to other sepsis therapies, those treated within 24 hours of sepsis onset had significantly lower 28-day mortality compared with those who began the infusion after 24 hours. Another significant finding from this trial was the higher rate of serious bleeding that occurred in patients during the infusion, after the infusion, and overall compared to those studied in PROWESS. Since the ENHANCE trial was open-label, this may suggest that the risk of bleeding in actual practice may have been greater than reported in PROWESS and ADDRESS.

Secondary analysis of the PROWESS trial revealed a slightly increased mortality rate in DAA patients who received prophylactic heparin as compared to those who did not and prompted the Xigris and Prophylactic HepaRin Evaluation in Severe Sepsis (XPRESS) trial.[26] All patients received DAA at 24 mcg/kg/hr for 96 hours and were randomly assigned to one of three groups: unfractionated heparin 5000 units subcutaneously twice per day, enoxaparin 40 mg subcutaneously once per day, or placebo (0.9% sodium chloride) in a 1:1:2 fashion. The primary outcome of 28-day mortality was non-significant lowering in the combined heparin group as compared to the placebo group, but did not satisfy the criteria to demonstrate equivalence. In a subgroup analysis, patients exposed to heparin at baseline and then randomized to the placebo group had a higher mortality than exposed patients subsequently randomized to the heparin group, and as a result, a warning was inserted into the package labeling to continue prophylactic heparin formulations when initiating DAA unless cessation is medically necessary.[24]

Based upon the findings of PROWESS, ADDRESS, ENHANCE, XPRESS and additional open label trials designed to determine the clinical effectiveness of DAA, the 2008 edition of the SSG segregated the use of DAA based on the patient's severity of illness. A strong recommendation against the use of DAA was given for patients with low severity of illness, while a weak recommendation was given for the use of this agent in patients at high risk of death.

With varied treatment response rates and multiple subgroups questioning the overall efficacy and safety of DAA, an additional prospective, randomized trial was completed in 2011. While the results of the confirmatory PROWESS-SHOCK trial have yet to be published at the time of writing this text, the manufacturer of DAA removed the product from the market due to lack of efficacy. Until the results of the PROWESS-SHOCK trial are fully available, many clinicians are left speculating about potential resons for DAA's lack of efficacy. Regardless, the development, utilization, and subsequent withdrawal of DAA from the market is an interesting case study in the evolution of a medication therapy over time. The history of DAA's role in the treatment of severe sepsis and septic shock is a good illustration of the need for a critical care pharmacist to be well-versed in the trial design and specific application of clinical data in order to provide optimal patient care.

RESUSCITATION BUNDLE AND QUALITY CARE

In the last decade, clinical studies have identified several strategies that reduce mortality in the critically ill, including EGDT[10], lung-protective measures,[27] and early appropriate antimicrobial therapy.[28,29] As a direct result of these evidence-based findings, professional organizations developed guidelines, facilitated through a core set of recommendations collectively known as sepsis bundles, to aid in the management of patients with severe sepsis and septic shock. The Institute for Healthcare Improvement (IHI) incorporated individual elements of evidence-based sepsis care into 6-hour resuscitation and 24-hour management bundles.

With the publication of numerous quality improvement studies describing efforts to translate the methodology of early-goal directed therapy to the bedside, it has become clear that inadequate initial resuscitation is common. The implementation of treatment pathways mimicking the interventions of well-scripted, carefully performed procedures in clinical trials is a challenging endeavor. For this reason, the SSC, in partnership with the Institute for

Healthcare Improvement, created the sepsis resuscitation bundle, which is described in Table 10–3, with a goal of a 25% reduction in worldwide, national, and local mortality. In essence, the bundle concept standardizes the care of patients with sepsis such that many of the complex interventions recommended in the SSG are at minimum considered in each patient, and instituted when appropriate. Numerous observational studies and quality improvement projects have been published documenting the positive effects of protocol-driven sepsis care.[30–36]

Various efforts, mainly focusing on education, have been used to implement evidence-based approaches for severe sepsis.[30,34,35] Although these approaches have led to improvement, the compliance rate with the standard processes of care and the mortality rate associated with severe sepsis remain alarmingly high.

Quality improvement initiatives, such as those dealing with severe sepsis and septic shock, commonly face several barriers to implementing changes. To circumvent some of the barriers, Sebat and colleagues[37] utilized a rapid

Table 10–3 Elements of the Surviving Sepsis Guidelines Sepsis Resuscitation Bundle[5]

Element	Definition
Lactate	Measured before or within 1-hour after blood culture
Blood culture	Drawn before antibiotics administered
Antibiotics	Administered within 1-hour of severe sepsis or septic shock onset
Fluid resuscitation	Given until one of the following: • CVP ≥8 mmHg (≥ 12 mmHg if mechanical ventilation) • MAP ≥65 mmHg without vasopressors and lactate <2.5 mmol/L and UOP >0.5 mL/kg/h
Vasopressor administration	Administered for one of the following: • MAP <65 mmHg despite fluid challenge 20 mL/kg of crystalloid • MAP <50 mmHg for ≥15 minutes
Red blood cell administration	Transfused if Hct <30% and $ScvO_2$ <70% or mixed venous O_2 saturation <65% despite fluid resuscitation
Inotrope utilization	Started if Hct ≥30% and $ScvO_2$ <70% or mixed venous O_2 saturation <65% despite fluid resuscitation

CVP = central venous pressure; MAP = mean arterial pressure; UOP = urine output; Hct = hematocrit; $ScvO_2$ = central venous oxygen saturation response system for the management of shock and were able to reduce the associated mortality rate; however, the study was not designed to focus exclusively on severe sepsis and septic shock. A similar multidisciplinary quality improvement approach dedicated to medical ICU patients with severe sepsis or septic shock improved the compliance with the process of care and decreased overall hospital mortality through weekly feedback and the activation of a multidisciplinary sepsis response team.[38] The sepsis response team phase, coupled with weekly feedback, was associated with 8.3% absolute mortality reduction.

Pharmacists continue to lead quality improvement projects related to improvement with sepsis resuscitation bundle implementation.[35,38,39] Given the complexity of severe sepsis and septic shock, a standardized systematic approach for this patient population appears to consistently improve the delivery of recommended therapies and may improve patient outcomes. A multidisciplinary approach may aid in the successful development of sepsis bundles by implementing quality improvement fundamentals. Pharmacists have a unique opportunity to lead or collaborate on sepsis protocols to further decrease patient mortality.

Despite the positive impact that the EGDT bundle has had on patient outcomes for over a decade,[40] debate still exists on whether or not individual components of the sepsis resuscitation bundle are necessary. Two multi-center clinical trials, the Australasian Resuscitation in Sepsis Evaluation Study (ARISE)[41] and the Protocolized Care for Early Septic Shock (ProCESS)[42] will aid in the determination of such issues.

SUMMARY

The diagnosis and management of severe sepsis and septic shock is a complex and dynamic process. New strategies to combat this syndrome are being developed, studied, and implemented with the purpose of improving morbidity and mortality. Investigations currently are being conducted in hospital environments to determine if educational initiatives and subsequent changes in clinician behaviors have the clinical impact delineated by the Surviving Sepsis Campaign. At the heart of the quality improvement initiatives are the prescription and timely administration of appropriate empiric antibiotics, restoration of tissue perfusion, and administration of adjunctive therapies in selected patients, all of which have been shown to improve patient survival. Pharmacists have a key role to fulfill in the management of septic patients by ensuring optimal medication regimens and monitoring plans are in place for these critically ill patients.

KEY POINTS

- An all-encompassing single mechanism of sepsis remains elusive; however, the host inflammatory response is theorized to lead to a SIRS with resultant increased coagulation, decreased fibrinolysis, apoptosis, and imbalances between inflammatory and anti-inflammatory mediators.
- It is imperative to objectively determine the stage of sepsis to aid in the determination of pharmacotherapy goals and treatment endpoints.
- Initial care and hemodynamic stabilization of septic patients is based upon the concept of EGDT.
- Adjunctive therapies such as corticosteroids should be considered, but remain controversial in the management of septic patients.
- Performance improvement projects highlighting a bundled care approach to the treatment of severe sepsis and septic shock have been shown to improve patient outcomes and represent an opportunity for critical care pharmacists to be patient advocates.

SELECTED SUGGESTED READINGS

- Severe sepsis bundles. Institute for Healthcare Improvement. Available from: http://www.ihi.org/IHI/Topics/CriticalCare/Sepsis/
- Dellinger RP, Levy MM, Carlet JM, et al. Surviving Sepsis Campaign: International guidelines for management of severe sepsis and septic shock: 2008. *Crit Care Med.* 2008;36:296–327.
- Rivers E, Nguyen B, Havstad S, et al. Early goal-directed therapy in the treatment of severe sepsis and septic shock. *N Engl J Med.* 2001;345:1368–1377.
- Annane D, Bellissant E, Bollaert PE, Briegel J, Keh D, Kupfer Y. Corticosteroids for severe sepsis and septic shock: a systematic review and meta-analysis. *BMJ.* 2004;329:480.

REFERENCES

1. Angus DC, Linde-Zwirble WT, Lidicker J, Clermont G, Carcillo J, Pinsky MR. Epidemiology of severe sepsis in the United States: analysis of incidence, outcome, and associated costs of care. *Crit Care Med.* 2001;29(7):1303–1310.
2. Martin GS, Mannino DM, Eaton S, Moss M. The epidemiology of sepsis in the United States from 1979 through 2000. *N Engl J Med.* 2003;348(16):1546–1554.
3. Rangel-Frausto MS, Pittet D, Hwang T, Woolson RF, Wenzel RP. The dynamics of disease progression in sepsis: Markov modeling describing the natu-

ral history and the likely impact of effective antisepsis agents. *Clin Infect Dis.* 1998;27:185–190.

4. Severe sepsis bundles. Institute for Healthcare Improvement. http://www.ihi.org/knowledge/Pages/Tools/SevereSepsisBundle.aspx. Accessed Oct 10, 2011.

5. Dellinger RP, Levy MM, Carlet JM, et al. Surviving Sepsis Campaign: International guidelines for management of severe sepsis and septic shock: 2008. *Crit Care Med.* 2008;36:296–327.

6. Cinel I, Opal SM. Molecular biology of inflammation and sepsis: A primer. *Crit Care Med.* 2009;37:291–304.

7. Tidswell M, Tillis W, Larosa SP, Lynn M, Wittek AE, Kao R, et al. Phase 2 trial of eritoran tetrasodium (E5564), a toll-like receptor 4 antagonist, in patients with severe sepsis. *Crit Care Med.* 2010;38:72–83.

8. Bone RC, Balk RA, Cerra FB, Dellinger RP, Fein AM, Knaus WA, Schein RM, Sibbald WJ. Definitions for sepsis and organ failure and guidelines for the use of innovative therapies in sepsis. The ACCP/SCCM Consensus Conference Committee. American College of Chest Physicians/Society of Critical Care Medicine. *Chest.* 1992;101:1644–1655.

9. Vincent JL, Abraham E. The last 100 years of sepsis. *Am J Respir Crit Care Med.* 2006;173:256–263.

10. Rivers E, Nguyen B, Havstad S, et al. Early goal-directed therapy in the treatment of severe sepsis and septic shock. *N Engl J Med.* 2001;345:1368–1377.

11. Brunkhorst FM, Engel C, Bloos F, Meier-Hellmann A, Ragaller M, Weiler N, et al. Intensive insulin therapy and pentastarch resuscitation in severe sepsis. *N Engl J Med.* 2008;358:125–139.

12. Russell JA, Walley KR, Singer J, Gordon AC, Hebert PC, Cooper DJ, et al. Vasopressin versus norepinephrine infusion in patients with septic shock. *N Engl J Med.* 2008;358:877–887.

13. Annane D, Vignon P, Renault A, Bollaert PE, Charpentier C, Martin C, et al. Norepinephrine plus dobutamine versus epinephrine alone for management of septic shock: a randomised trial. *Lancet.* 2007;370:676–684.

14. Tang H, Huang T, Jing J, Cui W. Effect of procalcitonin-guided treatment in patients with infections: a systematic review and meta-analysis. *Infection.* 2009;37:497–507.

15. Bouadma L, Luyt CE, Tubach F, Cracco C, Alvarez A, Schwebel C, et al. Use of procalcitonin to reduce patients' exposure to antibiotics in the intensive care units (PRORATA trial): a multicentre randomized controlled trial. *Lancet.* 2010;375:463–474.

16. Hahn EO, Houser HB, Rammelkamp CH Jr, Denny FW, Wannamaker LW. Effect of cortisone on acute streptococcal infections and poststreptococcal complications. *J Clin Invest.* 1951;30:274–281.

17. Annane D, Bellissant E, Bollaert PE, Briegel J, Keh D, Kupfer Y. Corticosteroids for severe sepsis and septic shock: a systematic review and meta-analysis. *BMJ.* 2004;329:480.

18. Annane D, Sebille V, Charpentier C, Bollaert PE, Francois B, Korach JM, et al. Effect of treatment with low doses of hydrocortisone and fludrocortisone on mortality in patients with septic shock. *JAMA.* 2002;288:862–871.

19. Dellinger RP, Carlet JM, Masur H, Gerlach H, Calandra T, Cohen J, et al. Surviving Sepsis Campaign guidelines for management of severe sepsis and septic shock. *Crit Care Med.* 2004;32:858–873.

20. Sprung CL, Annane D, Keh D, Moreno R, Singer M, Freivogel K, et al. Hydrocortisone therapy for patients with septic shock. *N Engl J Med.* 2008;358:111–124.

21. Bernard GR, Vincent JL, Laterre PF et al. Efficacy and safety of recombinant human activated protein C for severe sepsis. *N Engl J Med.* 2001;344:699–709.

22. Ely EW, Laterre PF, Angus DC, Helterbrand JD, Levy H, Dhainaut JF, et al. Drotrecogin alfa (activated) administration across clinically important subgroups of patients with severe sepsis. *Crit Care Med.* 2003;31:12–19.

23. Abraham E, Laterre PF, Garg R, Levy H, Talwar D, Trzaskoma BL, et al. Drotrecogin alfa (activated) for adults with severe sepsis and a low risk of death. *N Engl J Med.* 2005;353:1332–1341.

24. Xigris [package insert]. Indianapolis, IN: Eli Lilly and Co.; 2008.

25. Bernard GR, Margolis BD, Shanies HM, Ely EW, Wheeler AP, Levy H, et al. Extended evaluation of recombinant human activated protein C United States Trial (ENHANCE US): a single-arm, phase 3B, multicenter study of drotrecogin alfa (activated) in severe sepsis. *Chest.* 2004;125:2206–2216.

26. Levi M, Levy M, Williams MD, Douglas I, Artigas A, Antonelli M, et al. Prophylactic heparin in patients with severe sepsis treated with drotrecogin alfa (activated). *Am J Respir Crit Care Med.* 2007;176:483–490.

27. Ventilation with lower tidal volumes as compared with traditional tidal volumes for acute lung injury and the acute respiratory distress syndrome. The Acute Respiratory Distress Syndrome Network. *N Engl J Med.* 2000;342:1301–1308.

28. Kumar A, Roberts D, Wood KE, et al. Duration of hypotension before initiation of effective antimicrobial therapy is the critical determinant of survival in human septic shock. *Crit Care Med.* 2006;34:1589–1596.

29. Kumar A, Ellis P, Arabi Y, et al. Initiation of inappropriate antimicrobial therapy results in a fivefold reduction of survival in human septic shock. *Chest.* 2009;136:1237–1248.

30. Ferrer R, Artigas A, Levy MM, Blanco J, Gonzalez-Diaz G, Garnacho-Montero J, Ibanez J, Palencia E, Quintana M, de la Torre-Prados MV. Improvement in process of care and outcome after a multicenter severe sepsis educational program in Spain. *JAMA.* 2008;299:2294–2303.

31. Gao F, Melody T, Daniels DF, Giles S, Fox S. The impact of compliance with 6-hour and 24-hour sepsis bundles on hospital mortality in patients with severe sepsis: a prospective observational study. *Crit Care.* 2005;9:R764–R770.

32. Jones AE, Focht A, Horton JM, Kline JA. Prospective external validation of the clinical effectiveness of an emergency department-based early goal-directed therapy protocol for severe sepsis and septic shock. *Chest.* 2007;132:425–432.

33. Kortgen A, Niederprum P, Bauer M. Implementation of an evidence-based "standard operating procedure" and outcome in septic shock. *Crit Care Med.* 2006;34:943–949.

34. Levy MM, Dellinger RP, Townsend S, Linde-Zwirble W, Marshall JC, Bion J, et al. The Surviving Sepsis Campaign: Results of an international guideline-based performance improvement program targeting severe sepsis. *Crit Care Med.* 2010;38:367–374.

35. Micek ST, Roubinian N, Heuring T, Bode M, Williams J, Harrison C, Murphy T, Prentice D, Ruoff BE, Kollef MH. Before-after study of a standardized hospital order set for the management of septic shock. *Crit Care Med.* 2006;34:2707–2713.

36. Nguyen HB, Corbett SW, Steele R, Banta J, Clark RT, Hayes SR, Edwards J, Cho TW, Wittlake WA. Implementation of a bundle of quality indicators for the early management of severe sepsis and septic shock is associated with decreased mortality. *Crit Care Med.* 2007;35:1105–1112.

37. Sebat F, Musthafa AA, Johnson D, Kramer AA, Shoffner D, Eliason M, Henry K, Spurlock B. Effect of a rapid response system for patients in shock on time to treatment and mortality during 5 years*. *Crit Care Med.* 2007;35:2568–2575.

38. Schramm GE, Kashyap R, Mullon JJ, Gajic O, Afessa B. Septic shock: A multidisciplinary response team and weekly feedback to clinicians improve the process of care and mortality. *Crit Care Med.* 2011;39:252–258.

39. Patel GW, Roderman N, Gehring H, Saad J, Bartek W. Assessing the effect of the Surviving Sepsis Campaign treatment guidelines on clinical outcomes in a community hospital. *Ann Pharmacother.* 2010;44:1733–1738.

40. Rivers EP. Point: adherence to early goal-directed therapy: does it really matter? Yes. After a decade, the scientific proof speaks for itself. *Chest.* 2010;138:476–480.

41. Australasian Resuscitation In Sepsis Evaluation Randomised Controlled Trial (ARISE). http://clinicaltrials.gov/ct2/show/NCT00975793. Accessed June 20, 2011.

42. Protocolized Care for Early Septic Shock (ProCESS). http://clinicaltrials.gov/ct2/show/NCT00510835. Accessed June 20, 2011.

Chapter 11

Acute Kidney Injury, Renal Replacement Therapies, and Medication Dose Adjustment

Gregory J. Peitz and Keith M. Olsen

LEARNING OBJECTIVES

1. Describe the causes, pathophysiology, and complications of acute kidney injury.
2. Identify available therapy options and methods for the management of a critically ill patient with acute kidney injury.
3. Compare the different modalities of renal replacement therapy and understand each method's basic principles and issues associated with its delivery of dialysis.
4. Recognize the variability in pharmacokinetic and pharmacodynamic parameters that are experienced by critically ill patients when being treated pharmacologically.
5. Review available literature regarding appropriate antimicrobial dosing in critically ill patients receiving various modes of renal replacement therapy.

INTRODUCTION

Acute kidney injury (AKI), formerly known as acute renal failure (ARF), is characterized by a rapid reduction in kidney function resulting in a failure to maintain fluid, electrolyte, and acid–base homoeostasis. Acute kidney injury, which may occur in up to 30% of critically ill patients, is associated with a prolonged intensive care unit (ICU) stay, increased morbidity, and greater mortality.[1-5] Despite the understanding that AKI is caused by prerenal, intrinsic, or postrenal obstruction etiologies, there is little that practitioners can do to minimize kidney injury risk. However, following an AKI event, clinicians must manage subsequent consequences, such as uremia, fluid overload, and metabolic and electrolyte disturbances, and eliminate unnecessary exposure to nephrotoxic agents. Unlike patients with chronic renal insufficiency, critically ill patients who experience AKI often present with other acute medical problems such as life-threatening infections, organ failures, and systemic maldistributive states, making the management of these patients more complex.

The management of AKI is primarily accomplished by supportive measures and renal replacement therapy (RRT). Traditional RRT methods such as intermittent hemodialysis (IHD) have been used for patients with renal insufficiency for decades, but newer RRT options have been developed that may be better suited for the care of critically ill patients with AKI.[6] These modalities, such as continuous arteriovenous hemofiltration (CAVH), continuous venovenous hemofiltration (CVVH), continuous arteriovenous hemodialysis (CAVHD), continuous venovenous hemodialysis (CVVHD), continuous venovenous hemodiafiltration (CVVHDF), and sustained low efficiency dialysis (SLED), have been shown to have fewer hemodynamic effects on patients than IHD and provide equivalent solute removal.[7,8] These alternative dialysis methods have become increasingly utilized in the critically ill population, with no clear demonstration of mortality benefit along with the introduction of additional risks to patients.[4] Clinicians must be cognizant of the supportive measures and adjustments necessary when implementing these modalities. Given that each RRT method alters drug clearance and the critically ill patient has physiologic changes that may alter pharmacokinetic and pharmacodynamic parameters, appropriate changes in medical therapy and medication adjustments to patients receiving RRT are necessary.[6] This chapter will address the complications and challenges of managing AKI in the critically ill patient. The various modalities of RRT therapy will be reviewed, as well as supportive measures and monitoring that should be undertaken when utilizing these therapies. In addition, antimicrobial dosing recommendations will be made for the most commonly used

RRT modalities to provide this patient population with appropriate drug dosing regimens that optimize pharmacologic response to the ICU patient.

ACUTE KIDNEY INJURY: DEFINITIONS/TYPES/IDENTIFICATION

Acute kidney injury is generally described as a significant reduction in renal function over a short duration of time. Although no universal definition is available, AKI is often characterized as an increase in serum creatinine (Scr) of more than 0.5 mg/dL or more than 50% increase from baseline.[3,9] The Acute Kidney Injury Network (AKIN) definition of AKI is more inclusive, lowering the Scr requirement to a greater than 0.3 mg/dL increase over 48 hours or a demonstration of urine output less than 0.5 ml/kg/hr for 6 hours or more.[10] However, regardless of definition, the utility of using Scr as a marker and indicator for AKI remains in question by experts, as the Scr may lag behind real-time glomerular filtration rate (GFR). Furthermore, Scr values are affected by factors other than its urinary clearance, such as a patient's volume of distribution and overall production of creatinine.[11] A non-laboratory method that has been used to indicate AKI is the measurement of daily urine output; although not as specific as using other laboratory measurements, urine output can signify GFR decline. Measuring volume output classifies patients with AKI into the following categories: anuric (urine output <50 ml/d), oliguric (urine output 50 ml/d to 450 ml/d), or nonoliguric (urine output >450 ml/d).[12] Along with these methods for identifying and classifying AKI, there have been at least 35 other definitions used for AKI.[13,14] A relatively new classification system for determining the stage of AKI is the Risk, Injury, Failure, Loss, and End stage kidney disease (RIFLE) classification, which is described in detail in Chapter 2. Developed by the Acute Dialysis Quality Initiative (ADQI), the RIFLE classification uses both Scr and urine output data to classify and prognosticate patients following AKI. Validated in cardiac surgery, intensive care, and general hospital patients, the RIFLE classification helps delineate critically ill patients with severe AKI and suggests renal protection strategies for improving overall survival.[11,15]

CATEGORIES AND MECHANISMS OF ACUTE KIDNEY INJURY

Acute kidney injury results from any of the different pathophysiology mechanisms labeled as prerenal, intrinsic, or postrenal. The various causes are listed in Table 11–1. Each general etiology presents with separate risk

Table 11-1 Etiologies of Acute Kidney Injury[13]

Acute Kidney Injury Etiologies

Prerenal Causes	Hypoperfusion
	-Congestive heart failure
	-Liver insufficiency
	-Elevated intra-abdominal pressure
	Volume depletion
	-Blood loss
	-Septic shock
	Vascular issues
	-Renal artery stenosis
	Autoregulatory disturbances in glomerular perfusion pressure
	-Non-steroidal anti-inflammatory drugs
	-Angiotensin converting inhibitors
	-Angiotensin II receptor antagonists
	-Cyclosporine
Acute Intrinsic Causes	Acute Tubular Necrosis
	-Ischemic
	Exogenous toxins
	-Aminoglycosides
	-Amphotericin B
	-Intravenous contrast dye
	-Heavy metals
	Endogenous toxins
	-Myoglobin
	-Hemoglobin
	Acute interstitial nephritis
	-Penicillins
	-Sulfonamides
	Acute glomerulonephritis
	-Vascular
Obstructive Causes	Bladder obstruction
	Prostate hypertrophy
	Catheter obstruction
	Crystal deposition
	-Acyclovir
	-Sulfonamides
	-Indinavir

factors, prognostic indicators, and treatment strategies.[13] Evaluation of patient symptoms and relevant timing of events may provide a differential list of causes of AKI. Additionally, urinalysis and urine chemistry may aid in determining the etiology of AKI. When used in combination, these two measures can determine the kidney's ability to concentrate urine, evident by the fractional excretion of sodium (FeNa), which can help distinguish mechanisms of renal failure. In the event that the underlying mechanism of AKI cannot be determined, a renal biopsy could be performed, which has been described as a reliable method for confirming causes of AKI.[16]

Prerenal Kidney Injury

Prerenal failure, or prerenal azotemia, is caused by hypoperfusion to the glomerulus, which leads to reduced glomerular perfusion pressure.[13,17] An inadequate glomerular perfusion pressure for extended periods of time can precipitate renal injury to the parenchymal tissue. Damage to the parenchyma coincides with ischemia, which activates the renin-angiotensin-aldosterone system (RAAS) and subsequently causes the retention of sodium and water, evident in urine chemistry. In the presence of prerenal AKI, the fractional excretion of sodium is usually below 1%.[17,18] Several causes may be responsible for hypoperfusion episodes resulting in prerenal AKI. Comorbid disease states indirectly causing hypoperfusion to the kidneys, such as congestive heart failure (CHF), renal artery stenosis, decompensated liver failure, and intra-abdominal hypertension, as well as dehydration and volume loss, can all be risk factors.[13,14,17,18] Alterations in the glomerular perfusion pressure by hemodynamic modifying medications such as nonsteroidal anti-inflammatory drugs (NSAIDS), angiotensin-converting enzyme inhibitors (ACEI), angiotensin receptor blockers (ARBs), or cyclosporine can also lead to prerenal AKI.[13] This alteration in glomerular pressure is also referred to as functional AKI. Although prerenal AKI is often reversible and transient, failure to provide adequate glomerular perfusion either by fluid administration or balance of the autoregulatory compensation mechanisms can lead to further kidney injury, resulting in intrinsic AKI.[19]

Acute Intrinsic Kidney Injury

The majority of AKI events in the critically ill population are secondary to intrinsic renal failure.[17] Although the classification of acute intrinsic renal failure can be defined as damage to the kidney and its structures, it can be stratified according to location and nature of injury into the following categories: acute tubular necrosis (ATN), acute interstitial nephritis (AIN), acute glomerulonephritis, or vascular renal disease.

Acute tubular necrosis can follow ischemia, nephrotoxic agents, or a combination of the two insults. The ensuing death and destruction of tubular cells causes a reduction in GFR via increased tubular pressures resulting from the formation of intratubular casts. Subsequently, the nephron loses its ability to concentrate urine and regulate sodium reabsorption.[20,21] Ischemic ATN can be a complication of sepsis, blood loss, or any prolonged prerenal failure event. Patients with a history of chronic kidney disease, diabetes, atherosclerosis, low serum albumin, or impaired auto-regulation are at an increased risk for experiencing ischemic ATN.[22,23] Medications often responsible for causing nephrotoxic ATN include aminoglycosides, amphotericin B, cisplatin, and intravenous contrast.[13,24] Failure to dose these nephrotoxic medications according to a patient's renal function or foregoing pre-contrast fluid administration increases the risk of ATN.[24,25]

Acute kidney injury secondary to acute interstitial nephritis is the result of an inflammatory response within the kidney's interstitium, leading to lymphocyte and neutrophil-induced tubular epithelial cell necrosis.[26,27] The majority of AIN cases are caused by hypersensitivity reactions from medications, most notably antibiotics such as penicillins, cephalosporins, sulfonamides, and NSAIDs. Patients experiencing AIN may present with symptoms of rash, fever, and the presence of blood or urinary eosinophils, but these findings are not definitive for diagnosis. Renal biopsy remains the confirmatory test in AIN.[24]

Acute glomerulonephritis is a rapidly progressing insult to the glomerulus that precipitates an AKI event. Glomerulonephritis occurs via humoral and cell-mediated immune reactions, resulting in antigen-antibody complexes that produce glomerular and parenchymal damage.[28] Acute glomerulonephritis often manifests as a complication of a systemic disease such as Goodpasture's syndrome, lupus nephritis, poststreptococcal glomerulonephritis, membranoproliferative glomerulonephritis, IgA nephropathy, polyarteritis nodosa, Wegener's granulomatosis, or idiopathic crescentic glomerulonephritis.[29]

Large vessel or small vessel vascular disease can also lead to renal failure. Events such as a renal artery stenosis or either renal artery or vein thrombosis can lead to renal infarction and may progress to acute renal insufficiency if both functional kidneys are affected. The disease will also manifest if affecting a solitary kidney. Small vessel vascular disease arises from atherosclerosis and affects the kidneys when atheroembolisms or cholesterol emboli cause an inflammatory response in the vascular lumen, eventually causing obstruction and renal failure.[24]

Urinalysis and urine chemistry may determine the presence of red blood cells (RBC) and RBC casts that indicate kidney damage. Also, the fractional excretion of sodium will generally be >1%, unlike AKI events occurring from prerenal causes.

Postrenal Acute Kidney Injury

Defined as obstructive renal failure, this type of renal insult occurs anywhere within the renal system from the tubule to the urethra. However, renal function will only decline if both kidneys are simultaneously affected, or in the event of a patient presenting with only one active kidney.[30] Offending factors in obstructive AKI cases can include comorbid factors such as benign prostatic hyperplasia (BPH), active malignancies, prostate cancer, or neurogenic bladder.[24] Patients with urinary catheters may also experience obstructive AKI through occlusion of the catheter. Medications can contribute to obstructive AKI via the formation and deposition of crystals in the tubules.[31] Acyclovir, sulfonamides, methotrexate, and indanavir can all cause crystallization, especially with inadequate fluid administration. Urine output during postrenal AKI varies from anuria to polyuria. The treatment of postrenal AKI requires the alleviation of the obstruction. Patients with post renal AKI typically show cellular debris on urinalysis, but the urine chemistry can be variable due to concurrent factors that may be contributing to the event. Obstructive AKI is best diagnosed by imaging studies.

ACUTE KIDNEY INJURY CONSEQUENCES AND TREATMENT

With an incidence of 3% to 30% and a mortality rate up to 90% in the presence of multiple organ dysfunction syndromes (MODS), AKI in the critically ill patient is a common and detrimental occurrence.[4,32] Septic shock is the leading cause of AKI in the critically ill patient and may lead to ischemic prerenal and intrinsic kidney injury due to release of cytokine and inflammatory mediators.[2,4,24] Despite advances in the care of critically ill patients, including improved survival of sepsis, the overall mortality rate for patients with AKI remains elevated.[33] The initial treatment strategy for AKI is attentive management of fluid and electrolytes to avoid undesired complications of volume overload or electrolyte induced disturbances such as arrhythmias or neurologic sequelae. It is also important to initiate early enteral nutrition in the critically ill patient with AKI, as the intervention has been shown to improve patient outcomes.[32] Early initiation of RRT in appropriate patients leads to better outcomes, although determining the ideal patient, correct timing, and most beneficial mode of RRT can be difficult. Factors that may contribute to the decision regarding RRT initiation can be based on complications that arise following renal dysfunction.

The most urgent factor requiring RRT in AKI is the development of metabolic abnormalities. The failure of the nonfunctioning kidney to remove uremic toxins, manage the acid–base equilibrium, or maintain appropriate electrolyte balance may result in further unwarranted consequences.[4,13,32] Patients with acidemia are more likely to experience a decrease in myocardial contractility. The shift towards an acidemic state causes a diminished response to inotropic catecholamines as calcium transfer is slowed via the sodium calcium exchange during cardiac contraction and also results in the down regulation of beta-2 receptors.[34] Furthermore, vasodilation and a reduction in blood pressure may result from nitric oxide (NO) and inducible nitric oxide synthase (iNOS) displayed in hyperchloremic acidemic states.[17] Lung inflammation and injury have also been described with elevations in NO secondary to acidosis in animal models.[35]

In addition, the failure of fluid removal and development of volume overload poses separate risks for complications. Due to increases in intra- and extravascular fluid volume, critically ill patients with AKI are at risk for reduced pulmonary gas exchange from pleural effusions and congestion. In the event of impaired gas exchange leading to mechanical ventilation, the risk for nosocomial pneumonia increases, particularly in the presence of this patient population's altered immune status.[13] The greatest source of mortality in AKI comes from infectious etiologies. Acute kidney injury can profoundly affect critically ill patients' immune status, as they lose the ability to adequately remove free radical species from the body. This shifts the antioxidant equilibrium and predisposes these patients for infectious complications.[36] Anemic episodes, coagulopathic abnormalities, increases in muscle catabolism, and neuropathies have also been documented during an AKI event.[37] A consensus agreement on the timing and type of RRT is absent for AKI in the critically ill.[13,24,38,39] When RRT is under consideration, the chosen modality's hypotensive and coagulopathic risks should be considered. RRT methods can also cause imbalances in an individual's antioxidant equilibrium, thus further compromising a patient's immune function.[1,40] Special considerations should be made with each method of RRT to ensure that the risks of these extracorporeal modalities are minimized. Understanding the mechanisms, functions, limitations, and risks of each RRT method is important in the management of AKI in the critically ill patient.

COMPARING RENAL REPLACEMENT THERAPIES

Renal replacement therapy is a mechanism of purifying the blood via an extracorporeal circuit. Different forms of RRT exist, with each modality causing variations in water and solute transport via filtration, diffusion, convection, or a combination of mechanisms to remove fluid and waste products in AKI patients. Solute removal is also influenced by non-diffusion determinants. Variables such as the type of vascular access, filter size, and blood and dialysate flow rates can impact overall solute clearance.[39,41] Each RRT method poses risks of hypotension, thrombosis, and infectious complications. Understanding the functionality of each dialysis modality and awareness of the respective limitations and complications is essential in the choice of appropriate renal replacement therapy.

Mechanisms and Contributing Factors in RRT

Diffusion is defined as the movement of solute from a higher to lower concentration across a semipermeable membrane. This passive process of solute exchange is the primary mechanism responsible for solute removal in IHD.[42] When diffusion is utilized as a dialysis method, the process of solute exchange is influenced by both the size of the solute and speed of the dialysate flow rate. Higher flow rates result in greater solute clearance, and solutes with lower molecular weights and smaller size (<1500 Daltons) are removed more readily than larger molecules.[41,43]

Ultrafiltration is a method of volume removal that utilizes a pressure gradient to move fluid across a membrane. Defined as the difference between the oncotic pressure and hydrostatic pressure in the plasma, this is referred to as the "transmembrane pressure gradient." Ultrafiltration can be influenced by the membrane's surface area, pore size, and permeability. Unlike diffusion methods, ultrafiltration is not utilized for solute removal from the body.[41]

Convection is a process that relies on ultrafiltration to bring both water and solute across a semipermeable membrane and is referred to as hemofiltration.[39] As water is pulled across the membrane, the transfer of solute is made possible by utilizing a desired filter based on the specific solute of interest. Solute removal is possible if the molecule size is less than the sieving coefficient of the membrane.[4] The sieving coefficient describes the ratio of ultrafiltrate to plasma drug concentration as it enters the dialyzer.[6] Also, as the transmembrane pressure gradient increases, an increasing amount of solute and fluid can be moved across the semipermeable membrane.[41]

In any RRT mode, the type of filter is a major factor in the overall extent of solute exchange and removal. Filters for any given RRT method are selected based on membrane composition, surface area, electrostatic charge, permeability, cost, and biocompatibility.[39,44] Depending on the desired degree of extracorporeal solute removal, filters exhibiting more or less clearance capacities will be preferred.

Dialysis and CRRT Techniques

Intermittent hemodialysis is the primary mode for RRT in patients with renal insufficiency and continues to be the standard of care for patients with chronic renal failure. Exhibiting its mechanism of solute removal primarily through diffusion principles and fast dialysate rates, a rapid correction of plasma electrolytes and toxins occurs.[41] However, despite IHD's extended history of use and ability to remove toxins rapidly, the method is not always tolerated, especially in the critically ill population as hypotension and hypoperfusion can occur in up to 30% of patients treated with IHD.[41,45] Although prophylactic measures such as the cooling and alteration of the dialysate prescription may alleviate hypotensive episodes during IHD, the risk of hypotension still exists and can be detrimental to patient management. Hypotensive episodes can propagate further intestinal and renal ischemia, which may slow renal recovery and place the patient at increased risk for intestinal bacterial translocation.[46]

Continuous Renal Replacement Therapy Methods

Continuous renal replacement therapies (CRRT) offer a different approach to solute and volume management in patients with AKI. Utilizing highly permeable membranes and slower dialysate rates run continuously, CRRT methods provide AKI patients with an alternative method of renal replacement with less hemodynamic instability than IHD.[4,39,42] There are several types of CRRT, each one varying by the available access route and solute removal mechanism as summarized in Table 11–2. Initially, arteriovenous (AV) access was utilized for CRRT methods, but venovenous (VV) circuits provide better solute removal with fewer access line complications.[39]

Slow continuous ultrafiltration (SCUF) is used in patients experiencing volume overload in the absence of metabolic or electrolyte irregularities. SCUF does not require the coadministration of dialysate or replacement fluids and does not remove substantial amounts of solute.[39,41]

Continuous venovenous hemofiltration (CVVH) removes solute primarily through convection, which is directly dependent on ultrafiltration.[39,43]

Table 11–2 A Comparison of Renal Replacement Modalities[39]

RRT Modality	Mechanism of Solute Transport		Vascular Access	Fluid Replacement	Time of Therapy (hours)
	Convection	Diffusion			
IHD[a]	+	++++	Fistula	+	3–4
SLED[b]	+	++++	Fistula	+	6–12
CAVHD[c]	+	++++	AV[d]	+/0	24
CV VHD[e]	+	++++	V V[f]	+/0	24
CV VHFD[g]	++	++++	V V	+/0	24
CAVHFD[h]	++	++++	AV	+/0	24
CAVH[i]	++++	–	AV	+++	24
CV VH[j]	++++	–	V V	+++	24
CAVHDF[k]	+++	+++	AV	++	24
CV VHDF[l]	+++	+++	V V	++	24
SCUF[m]	+	–	Large vein	0	24

[a]intermittent hemodialysis
[b]sustained low efficiency dialysis
[c]continuous artiovenous hemodialysis
[d]artiovenous
[e]continuous venovenous hemodialysis
[f]venovenous
[g]continuous venovenous high-flux hemodialysis
[h]continuous arteriovenous high-flux hemodialysis
[i]continuous artiovenous hemofiltration
[j]continuous venovenous hemofiltration
[k]continuous artiovenous hemodialfiltration
[l]continuous venovenous hemodialfiltration
[m]slow continuous ultrafiltration

As the ultrafiltration rate increases, solute removal is enhanced. Unlike traditional IHD, dialysate is not required for CVVH, but replacement fluids need to be administered to the patient due to the volume loss that occurs with this modality. Patients may experience up to 1 to 2 L/hr volume loss from the ultrafiltration.[41]

Unlike CVVH, continuous venovenous hemodialysis (CVVHD) and continuous venovenous hemodiafiltration (CVVHDF) utilize a dialysate component to complement these modes' convection capability with simultaneous diffusion. Fluid replacement is not typically required in CVVHD due to its primary mechanism of diffusion, but for CVVHDF, replacement fluids would be appropriate as the concurrent ultrafiltration can cause volume losses up to 1.5 L/hr. The replacement fluids may be administered pre-filter or post-filter and should be compounded on an individual patient basis to maintain acid–base and electrolyte balances with respect to the clinical situation.[47]

Sustained Low-Efficiency Dialysis

Sustained low-efficiency dialysis (SLED) is the newest RRT for treating AKI with electrolyte and metabolic disturbances. The modality has been classified as a hybrid RRT secondary to the properties it exhibits from both IHD and CRRT methods. Acting similarly to IHD's mechanism of solute removal, SLED requires the use of a dialysate infusion to run counter current to blood flow. However, unlike IHD, which has dialysate fluid rates of 500 to 800 ml/min, SLED dialysate and blood flow rates typically run between 100 to 300 ml/min, and for longer periods of time, resembling CRRT methods. By utilizing the diffusion concept from IHD and slowing the rate (thus prolonging the dialysis time), a reduction in the incidence of hemodynamic alterations is observed. Since ultrafiltration does not occur with SLED, replacement fluids are not needed. Additionally, SLED is a less expensive method of RRT as conventional dialysate solutions and equipment can be utilized.[4,6,8,41]

Continuous Renal Replacement Therapy Complications and Considerations

Aside from the hypotensive effects associated with RRT modalities, several other complications may occur. Problems encountered with extracorporeal blood filtration techniques include bleeding events, line infections, air emboli, vascular access complications, and issues of circuit and filter clotting.[39] Renal replacement therapy methods with slower rates of ultrafiltration and solute removal are more prone to clotting complications than RRTs utilizing faster removal rates.[48] Through the use of several anticoagulation agents used both systemically and within the RRT dialysis circuit, practitioners face the task of providing an anticoagulation balance as they try to maintain filter patency while minimizing bleeding risks. Heparin is the anticoagulant of choice in patients undergoing CRRT.[48] If heparin is used systemically, maintaining an activated partial thromboplastin time (aPTT) of 35 to 45 seconds is desired, as this range has been shown to both reduce the risk of filter clotting while minimizing bleeding risk.[49] Heparin may also be administered within the extracorporeal circuit; however, this regional method of anticoagulation can be complicated, as it requires a simultaneous infusion of protamine sulfate postfilter for heparin neutralization prior to re-entry into systemic circulation.

The utilization of regional sodium citrate is an alternative method to provide anticoagulation within the extracorporeal circuit. Sodium citrate solution chelates ionized calcium, which is an essential component of the clotting cascade. When the sodium citrate is administered prefilter in RRT, it acts as a regional anticoagulant. After running through the extracorporeal circuit, the citrate enters the systemic circulation postfilter and is subsequently converted to bicarbonate by the liver, causing no systemic anticoagulation. Although this method of preserving filter life may provide fewer bleeding complications and forego the risk of heparin-induced thrombocytopenia (HIT), frequent monitoring of serum ionized calcium and other electrolytes are necessary. As the citrate binds the ionized calcium, the majority of the calcium-citrate complex is filtered from the circuit and the remaining citrate becomes metabolized to bicarbonate in the body. This removal of serum calcium creates a need for exogenous replacement of calcium, thereby mandating that a continuous calcium infusion be used in conjunction with citrate anticoagulation. Additionally, patients are at an increased risk for metabolic alkalosis as the residual citrate is converted to bicarbonate.[48,49] It should be noted that citrate anticoagulation should not be used with SCUF because there is only ultrafiltration and the risk of alkalosis is significant.

In addition to recognizing and managing the complications associated with RRT in the AKI patient, it is equally important to understand the alterations in medication clearance and removal for each given modality. Determining optimal medication regimens in the critically ill is crucial, as inappropriate selection and dosing of antimicrobial therapy has shown increases in mortality.[50] All clinicians involved in the care of the critically ill patient must evaluate the medication regimens during RRT and make therapeutic adjustments as needed to provide optimal treatment.

DRUG DOSING DURING DIALYSIS

Acute kidney injury and the use of dialysis present significant obstacles to dosing drugs.[6,7,51] These same obstacles are further enhanced in the critically ill patient, as the underlying disease and accompanying hemodynamic changes have a significant impacts on the pharmacokinetics of most medications, especially antimicrobials.[6,7,51] Many factors must be considered to assure effective dosing that maximizes the drug's pharmacodynamic effect while minimizing adverse events. The clinician must be aware of factors that impact the initial dose and maintenance doses; among the factors that affect a drug's dialyzability include the molecular size, protein binding, volume of distribution, water solubility, and plasma clearance.[6,7,51-57] Initial and maintenance doses of antibiotics are generally administered after an IHD dialysis session. The impact of critical illness on these factors and the influence on drug dosing will be discussed in greater detail. While many medications are affected by RRT, antibiotics are commonly affected and will be the focus of the remainder of the chapter.

Initial Doses

The initial or loading dose of a drug is influenced by the extent of distribution in the body.[6,55,56] Critically ill patients with multiple medical problems often have larger volumes of distribution (Vd) than observed in non-ICU patients, which may require larger initial doses. A large Vd may also result in a reduced drug clearance during dialysis. Some drugs have inherently large volumes of distribution because of wide tissue distribution, so dialysis may effectively remove drug in the plasma but have minimal impact on the total amount of drug in the body. Diseases that often result in higher Vds include AKI, sepsis, cirrhosis, uremia, and severe burns.[6,55,56] Sepsis is a complicated process that results in inflammatory cytokine release and disruption in endothelial cell function, which in turn produces capillary leakage of fluid from the vascular space to the extravascular space. The result is an increased Vd for many antibiotics. The aminoglycosides gentamicin and tobramycin have a Vd of 0.2 to 0.25 L/kg in non-ICU patients, but this figure may rise to 0.4 to 0.6 L/kg in the ICU patient with sepsis.[7,51,58] The resultant initial dose would change from a typical 2 mg/kg for these two antibiotics all the way up to 5 to 7 mg/kg for the ICU patient with significant volume expansion. However, not all antibiotics are affected in critically ill patients, as the Vd of ciprofloxacin and meropenem demonstrates no change. Understanding these potential changes in Vd allows the clinician to choose appropriate initial doses to achieve therapeutic goals in the ICU patient. When appropriate, serum drug concentrations should be measured to aid individual patient dosing.

Maintenance Doses

Following the initial drug dose, maintenance doses are determined by clearance.[54-56] Both renal and non-renal clearance can impact the amount of drug cleared in AKI and in patients receiving dialysis. During AKI, the GFR estimated by the determination of the creatinine clearance (Cl_{cr}) is the most common method used for dose adjustment. However, dialysis becomes more complicated as the membrane type, blood flow rate, and dialysate flow rate all alter drug clearance. The remaining intrinsic renal function in patients with AKI must be accounted for prior to and during dialysis episodes. Drugs dependent on renal elimination as their primary clearance mechanism will require extended dosing intervals in AKI as a patient's GFR decreases. Drugs that are predominantly eliminated by hepatic mechanisms generally do not require dosing adjustment during AKI, but may have increased clearance during dialysis.[6,7,55,56]

The dialysis membrane is an important determinant of drug removal and may subsequently impact the maintenance dose.[6-8,51-56] The dialytic membrane is a fixed pore synthetic material that allows the movement of drugs and solutes. Many studies of drug removal during dialysis were performed using standard intermittent hemodialysis equipment and membranes. However, newer techniques employ high permeability or high-flux dialysis. These dialysis membranes achieve an *in vitro* ultrafiltration coefficient of >8 mL/hr/mmHg. It is important that the clinician be aware of the membrane type and dialysis techniques used when applying dosing recommendations to their patients.

The molecular weight is the primary determinate of a drug's dialyzability in conventional hemodialysis equipment, although this becomes less important in CRRT. Generally, dialysis membranes allow the passage of molecules up to 5000 Daltons (Da).[51-56] If a drug is less than 5000 Da, it must have low protein binding to cross the dialysis membrane. Drug-binding proteins albumin and alpha-1-acid glycoprotein are large molecules that do not cross the dialysis membrane very well; therefore, drugs exhibiting high protein binding will only cross the membrane as the free or free fraction of the drug. However, critically ill patients are often hypercatabolic, resulting in a significant reduction of drug binding proteins, which leads to a higher free drug fraction. Critically ill patients also may receive drugs that displace highly bound drugs from proteins and increase the free fraction (e.g., aspirin). In contrast to conventional dialysis membranes, high-flux membranes used in CRRT have larger pore size ranging from 20,000 to 30,000 Da. These membranes present no significant barrier to large molecular-sized or protein bound drugs.[55,56] Vancomycin follows this pattern with minimal removal by IHD using conventional membranes, but significant removal when high-flux membranes are employed.[55,56,59]

ANTIMICROBIAL DOSING

Table 11–3 is a summary of selected antimicrobial agents and the recommended doses in critically ill patients receiving IHD, CRRT, and SLED. Minimal dosing recommendations are available for patients on SLED and

Table 11-3 Selected Intravenous Antimicrobial Agents and Recommended Doses in Critically Ill Patients with Acute Kidney Injury and Undergoing Hemodialysis or Continuous Renal Replacement Therapy.[6-8,51,54-59,61,63-66,68,69]

Antimicrobial	%[a] Excreted Unchanged	Usual Dose	Dose CL_{CR} 10-50[b]	Dose CL_{CR} <10	Dose for IHD[c,n]	Dose for CRRT[d] (CVVH[e])	Dosing for SLED[f]
Penicillins							
Ampicillin	75-85	1 g[g] q 6 h[h]	Same dose	Same dose q 12 h	Dose as CL_{CR} <10; dose after dialysis on dialysis days	1-2 g every 6-12 h	No data
		2 g q[i] 4 h	Same dose q 6 h	Same dose q 12 h			
Ampicillin-sulbactam	75-85	1.5-3 g q 6 h	Same dose q 8-12 h	Same dose q 24 h	Dose as CL_{CR} <10; dose after dialysis on dialysis days	1.5-3 g q 8-12 h	No data
Nafcillin	10-30	2-4 g q 4-6 h	No change	No change	No change	No change	No data
Oxacillin	42-50	1-2 g q 4-6 h	No change	No change	No change	No change	No data
Penicillin G	58-85	0.5-4 MU[j] q 4 h	75% of dose q 4 h	50% of dose q 4 h	50% of dose q 4 h; dose after dialysis	2 MU q 4-6h	No data
Piperacillin-tazobactam	Pip[k] 74-89 Taz[l] 74	3.375-4.5 g q 6-8 h	2.25-3.375 g q 6-8 h	2.25g q 6-8 h	2.25 g q 12 h and 0.75 g after dialysis	2.25-3.75 g q 6-8h	No data
Cephalosporins							
Cefazolin	60-80	1-2g q 8 h	Same dose q 12 h	Same dose q 24 h	0.5-1g q 24 h; dose after dialysis	1-2 g q 12 h	No data

Cefepime	70–85	1–2 g q 8–12 h	Same dose q 12 h	Same dose q 24 h (8 h) or 48 h (12 h)	Dose as CL_{CR} <10; dose after dialysis on dialysis days	1–2 g q 12 h	No data
Cefoxitin	50–85	1–2 g q 8 h	Same dose q 12 h	Same dose q 24 h	Dose as CL_{CR} <10; dose after dialysis on dialysis days	1–2 g q 12 h	No data
Ceftazidime	80–90	1–2 g q 8–12 h	Same dose q 12 h	Same dose q 24 h	Dose as CL_{CR} <10; dose after dialysis on dialysis days	1–2 g q 12 h	No data
Ceftriaxone	33–67	1–2 g q 12–24 h	No adjustment	No adjustment	1–2 g q 24 h	1–2 g q 12–24 h	No data
Carbapenems							
Ertapenem	38	1 g q 24 h	500 mg[m] q 24 h (CL_{CR} <30)	500 mg q 24 h (CL_{CR} <30)	500 mg q 24 h	*In vitro* data suggest increased clearance	No dose adjustment needed
Doripenem	70	500 mg q 8 h	250 mg q 8 h	250 mg q 12 h	No data	No data	No data, but likely similar to imipenem/meropenem
Imipenem	70	500 mg q 6 h or 1 g q 8 h	250–500 mg q 8 h	250 mg q 12 h	Dose as CL_{CR} <10; dose after dialysis on dialysis days	500 mg q 12 h	Imipenem 500 mg IV q 6 h while on SLED (if >70 kg)
Meropenem	62–70	0.5–1 g q 8 h	250–500 mg q 12 h	250–500 mg q 24 h	500 mg q 24 h	0.5–1 g q 12 h	Meropenem 500–1000 mg q 8 h while on SLED

(continued)

Table 11-3 Selected Intravenous Antimicrobial Agents and Recommended Doses in Critically Ill Patients with Acute Kidney Injury and Undergoing Hemodialysis or Continuous Renal Replacement Therapy.[6-8,51,54-59,61,63-66,68,69] (continued)

Antimicrobial	%[a] Excreted Unchanged	Usual Dose	Dose CL_{CR} 10-50[b]	Dose CL_{CR} <10	Dose for IHD[c,n]	Dose for CRRT[d] (CVVH[e])	Dosing for SLED[f]
Monobactam							
Aztreonam	60-75	1-2 g q 8-12 h	0.5-1 g q 8-12 h	250-500 mg q 8-12 h	Dose as CL_{CR} <10; dose after dialysis on dialysis days	1-2 g q 12 h	No data
Quinolones							
Ciprofloxacin	30-57	400 mg q 8-12 h	Same dose q 24 h (CL_{CR} <30)	Same dose q 24 h (CL_{CR} <30)	Dose as CL_{CR} <30; dose after dialysis on dialysis days	200-400 q 12-24 h	No data
Levofloxacin	87	500-750 mg q 24 h	250 mg q 24 h	250 mg q 24-48 h	250-500 mg q 48 h	250 mg q 24 h	No data
Moxifloxacin	20	400 mg q 24 h	No adjustment	No adjustment	No adjustment; dose after dialysis	400 mg q 24 h	No adjustment
Glycopeptides and Lipoglycopeptides							
Vancomycin	>80-90	10-15 mg/kg q 12 h	7.5 mg/kg q 24-48 h; Dose by levels	7.5 mg/kg q 48-96 h; Dose by levels	Dose as CL_{CR} <10; dose after dialysis on dialysis days; Dose by levels	10-15 mg/kg q 24-48 h; Dose by levels	Dose every 12-18 h while on SLED
Telavancin	72	10 mg/kg q 24 h	7.5 mg/kg q 24 h (CL_{CR} 30-50); 7.5 mg/kg q 48 h (CL_{CR} 10-30)	No data	No data	No data; in vitro study suggests sufficient clearance to alter dose	No data

Aminoglycosides						
Amikacin	84–94	10–20 mg/kg q 8–12 h	Adjust dose and interval by levels	Adjust dose and interval by levels	5–7.5 mg/kg q 48–72 h; Adjust dose and interval by levels	7.5 mg/kg q 48–72 h	No data. Expected to follow gentamicin recommendations with dose of 15–20 mg/kg
Gentamicin	70	1.5–3 mg/kg q 8–12 h	Adjust dose and interval by levels	Adjust dose and interval by levels	1.5–2 mg/kg q 48–72 h	1.5–2.5 mg/kg q 24–48 h (severe infection); redose when peak <3–5 mg/L	Initial loading dose 6 mg/kg lean body weight every 48 h as a 30 min infusion. Give 1 h prior to SLED. Doses should be adjusted according to serum concentrations observed during and after the SLED session
Tobramycin	70	1.5–3 mg/kg q 8–12 h	Adjust dose and interval by levels	Adjust dose and interval by levels		1.5–2.5 mg/kg q 24–48 h (severe infection); redose when peak <3–5 mg/L	Initial loading dose 6 mg/kg lean body weight every 48 h as a 30 min infusion. Give 1 hour prior to SLED. Doses should be adjusted according to serum concentrations observed during and after the SLED session
Miscellaneous Antibiotics						
Clindamycin	<1	300–900 mg q 6–8 h	No adjustment	No adjustment	No adjustment	No adjustment	No data

(continued)

Table 11–3 Selected Intravenous Antimicrobial Agents and Recommended Doses in Critically Ill Patients with Acute Kidney Injury and Undergoing Hemodialysis or Continuous Renal Replacement Therapy.[6–8,51,54–59,61,63–66,68,69] (continued)

Antimicrobial	%[a] Excreted Unchanged	Usual Dose	Dose CL_{CR} 10–50[b]	Dose CL_{CR} <10	Dose for IHD[c,n]	Dose for CRRT[d] (CVVH[e])	Dosing for SLED[f]
Daptomycin	78	4–8 mg/kg q 24 h	4–6 mg/kg q 48 h (CL_{CR} <30)	4–6 mg/kg q 48 h (CL_{CR} <30)	4–6 mg/kg q 48 h after dialysis on dialysis days	8 mg/kg q 48 h	Dose every 24 hours on SLED
Linezolid	30	600 mg q 12h	No adjustment	No adjustment	No adjustment	No adjustment	No adjustment; supplemental dose may be necessary for continuous SLED
Tigecycline	22	100 mg initial dose, 50 mg q 12 h	No adjustment	No adjustment	No adjustment	No adjustment	No data
Antifungals **Azoles**							
Fluconazole	80	400–800 mg q 24 h	50% of usual dose	50% of usual dose	100% of dose after dialysis session	200–400 mg q 24 h	No data
Echinocandins Anidulafungin	<1	200 mg initial dose, then 100 mg q 24 h	No adjustment	No adjustment	No adjustment	No adjustment	No adjustment

| Caspofungin | 1.4 | 70 mg initial dose, then 50 mg q 24 h | No adjustment | No adjustment | No adjustment | No adjustment | No data, but unlikely to require adjustment |
| Micafungin | <15 | 100–150 mg q 24 h | No adjustment | No adjustment | No adjustment | No adjustment | No data, but unlikely to require adjustment |

[a]percent
[b]creatinine clearance in milliliters per minute
[c]intermittent hemodialysis
[d]continuous renal replacement therapy
[e]continuous venovenous hemofiltration
[f]sustained low efficiency dialysis
[g]grams
[h]hours
[i]every
[j]million units
[k]piperacillin
[l]tazobactam
[m]milligrams
[n]doses are usually administered after the dialysis session

a review discusses dosing in greater detail.[51] In addition to renal function and dialysis method, individual antibiotic pharmacodynamic targets must be considered to determine the dosing regimen.

Beta-Lactam Antibiotics (Penicillins, Cephalosporins, Carbapenems)

The beta-lactam antibiotics are a structurally similar group of antibiotics, but possess widely varying pharmacokinetic parameters and antimicrobial activity. Most beta-lactam antibiotics have small, water-soluble molecular structures with low protein binding, and are eliminated primarily by renal mechanisms.[6,7] Therefore, most beta-lactam antibiotics require some dosage adjustment in AKI as GFR decreases. There are exceptions, as nafcillin and ceftriaxone have extra-renal routes of elimination and do not require dosage adjustments in patients with low GFRs;[6,7,57] because of these differences, the pharmacokinetics of each individual agent should be determined prior to dosing.

Most beta-lactam antibiotics are readily cleared by hemodialysis and CRRT. Again, nafcillin and ceftriaxone are notable exceptions as they are highly protein bound with only minimal removal by hemodialysis and only slightly greater clearance during CRRT modalities. The carbapenems differ in their clearance, with variations in protein binding being the most significant factor. Doripenem and imipenem have similar pharmacokinetic profiles with low protein binding and are therefore extensively removed by hemodialysis and CRRT, so supplemental dosages are required at the end of dialysis and normal or slightly modified regimens are required during CRRT.[60,61] Although meropenem has different pharmacokinetics than doripenem and imipenem, it follows a similar pattern of clearance. Ertapenem is 90% to 95% protein bound with only 30% of the drug cleared following hemodialysis, which may prompt a supplemental dose following dialysis. Continuous RRT increases ertapenem clearance and one study has recommended normal doses and intervals.[61]

Glycopeptides

Vancomycin and the lipoglycopeptide antimicrobial telavancin are large molecules, but distribute well to most tissues except into the cerebral spinal fluid.[62] Telavancin is 93% protein bound, while vancomycin binding ranges from 10 to 50%, with lower protein adherence in ICU patients.[62,63] Both drugs are primarily excreted renally through glomerular filtration resulting in prolonged half-lives during AKI. Due to the drug's predominant dependence on renal elimination, vancomycin requires close serum concentration monitoring in patients with AKI. Little data is available on telavancin clearance during dialysis.[63] Negligible amounts of vancomycin are removed by standard IHD; however, the use of high-flux membranes or CRRT may remove up to 40% of the drug, although this will vary depending the duration of dialysis.[6-8] It is important for the clinician to verify the membrane type being used in the dialysis equipment prior to making any dosing recommendation. Vancomycin loading dose regimens should not change in AKI or dialysis, though the frequency of maintenance doses to be administered post-dialysis should be guided by serum concentration determination.[6-8]

Aminoglycosides

Aminoglycosides are small, water-soluble molecules with low protein binding that display elimination rates closely following glomerular filtration rates.[51] These factors lead to significant pharmacokinetic changes in AKI and removal by IHD and CRRT. Loading doses in critically ill patients should be guided by an estimated Vd up to 0.4 to 0.6 L/kg that will result in loading doses up to 5 to 7 mg/kg for gentamicin and tobramycin and 15 to 20 mg/kg for amikacin.[51] It is important to make accurate estimates of the Vd to prevent giving too low or high doses, and an accurate assessment of overall fluid status is essential. Aminoglycosides are associated with nephrotoxicity, so their use may further worsen or prolong recovery from AKI. Therefore, all aminoglycoside dosing during hemodialysis should be cautiously guided by pre- and/or post-dialysis serum levels, with doses generally given after the dialysis session.

Daptomycin

Daptomycin, a lipopeptide antibiotic, is eliminated 50% unchanged in the urine and possesses a relatively long half-life of 8 to 9 hours.[64-67] It has a small Vd (0.1 L/kg) and is highly protein bound at 92%. Daptomycin is unique with a low Vd and high protein binding, thus predicting the impact dialysis on clearance is difficult. At minimum, clearance will be delayed in the patient with AKI without dialysis.[67] One study evaluated the impact of hemodialysis on daptomycin removal.[65] Over a 4-hour session of dialysis in patients with end-stage renal disease, only 15% of the drug was removed. Limited data describing the impact of CRRT on daptomycin clearance is available. In one *in vitro* dialysis simulation model using CVVH,[64] the clearances exceed the physiologic clearance described in patients with normal renal function. Daptomycin pharmacokinetics following CVVH was evaluated in eight adult ICU patients. The drug demonstrated significant clearance and a dose of 8 mg/kg every 48 hours was recommended. It would appear that conventional hemodialysis would have minimal impact on daptomycin clearance, while CRRT would remove significant amounts.[64–68]

Antifungals

Antifungal agents are structurally very different from class to class and substantial pharmacokinetic differences are observed in drugs from the same class. Amphotericin B has a large molecular structure and Vd, and therefore does not require dosage adjustment in AKI or patients receiving hemodialysis or CRRT.[6-8] The azole antifungal most often used in the ICU is fluconazole. Fluconazole has low protein binding and 60 to 80% is eliminated renally as unchanged drug, which necessitates dosage adjustment in patients with reduced GFR.[6-8] Supplemental fluconazole doses are necessary following IHD, while the dose in CRRT is similar to patients with normal renal function.[6-8] The echinocandins anidulafungin, caspofungin, and micafungin are highly protein bound (84 to 99%), have small volumes of distribution, and relatively long half-lives.[69,70] No dosage adjustment is generally required with dialysis due to their high protein binding; unfortunately, no studies have been published evaluating the echinocandins clearance during CRRT.[69] However, several review papers of antimicrobial dosing concepts in renal replacement therapy recommend no dosage adjustments with CRRT.[6,7]

Due to a paucity of guidelines, and given that the available recommendations for medication adjustments are largely based on small studies in a only a few drug classes, clinicians will need a thorough understanding of antimicrobial pharmacokinetics and pharmacodynamics when making dosing changes for RRT. Specific evidence may not be available for each medication a critically ill patient may be exposed to, but the use of clinical judgment in conjunction with a particular drug's pharmacokinetic profile must be utilized to provide appropriate therapy during RRT. In general, drugs that have a large molecular structure, high protein binding properties, and a large Vd are not going to be removed as extensively during RRT as medications exhibiting a smaller molecular size or Vd. Although the adjustment of medications in patients receiving RRT can be challenging, the use of available dosing resources and application of pharmacologic principles may result in the most efficacious dose while minimizing toxicity.

SUMMARY

Acute kidney injury and the resultant need for renal replacement therapy create unique challenges for the management of medications in the critically ill. An understanding of the different types of RRT is very helpful when designing individual patient care plans. It is important to evaluate patients with AKI on a daily basis and reassess dosing regimens based upon the type of RRT prescribed, as well as the progression or improvement of the underlying AKI to optimize medication use.

KEY POINTS

- Medication levels, if available, should be monitored in patients receiving RRT.
- CRRT modalities may have significant differences in clearance of medications.
- AKI is commonly described by the RIFLE classification.
- Protein binding, molecular size, water solubility, volume of distribution, and plasma clearance impact removal of drugs during IHD and CRRT.
- Volume of distribution significantly impacts initial doses of antibiotics in critically ill patients.
- Antibiotic maintenance doses are determined by renal and non-renal clearance.

SELECTED SUGGESTED READINGS

- John S, Eckardt K. Renal replacement strategies in the ICU. *Chest.* 2007;132:1379–1388.
- Heintz BH, Matzke GR, Dager WE. Antimicrobial dosing concepts and recommendations for critically ill adult patients receiving continuous renal replacement therapy or intermittent hemodialysis. *Pharmacotherapy.* 2009;29:562–577.
- Kellum JA, Bellomo R, Ronco C. Definition and classification of acute kidney injury. *Nephron Clin Pract.* 2008;109:182–187.
- Solomon R, Deray G. How to prevent contrast-induced nephropathy and manage risk patients: practical recommendations. *Kidney Int.* 2006;69(Suppl S100):S51–S53.
- Bogard KN, Peterson NT, Plumb TJ, Erwin MW, Fuller PD, Olsen KM. Antibiotic dosing during sustained low-efficiency dialysis: special considerations in adult critically ill patients. *Crit Care Med.* 2011;39:560–570.

REFERENCES

1. Metnitz GH, Fischer M, Bartens C, et al. Impact of acute renal failure on antioxidant status in multiple organ failure. *Acta Anaesthesiol Scand.* 2000;44:236–240.

2. Uchino S, Kellum JA, Bellomo R, et al. Acute renal failure in critically ill patients: a multinational, multicenter study. *JAMA.* 2005;294:813–818.
3. Clermont G, Acker CG, Angus DC, et al. Renal failure in the ICU: comparison of the impact of acute renal failure and end-stage renal disease on ICU outcomes. *Kidney Int.* 2002;62:986–996.
4. John S, Eckardt K. Renal replacement strategies in the ICU. *Chest.* 2007;132:1379–1388.
5. Levy EM, Viscoli CM, Horwitz RI. The effect of acute renal failure on mortality. A cohort analysis. *JAMA.* 1996;275:1489–1494.
6. Heintz BH, Matzke GR, Dager WE. Antimicrobial dosing concepts and recommendations for critically ill adult patients receiving continuous renal replacement therapy or intermittent hemodialysis. *Pharmacotherapy.* 2009;29:562–577.
7. Trotman RL, Williamson JC, Shoemaker DM, Salzer WL. Antibiotic dosing in critically ill adult patients receiving continuous renal replacement therapy. *Clin Infect Dis.* 2005;41:1159–1166.
8. Mushatt DM, Mihm LB, Dreisbach AW, Simon EE. Antibiotic dosing in slow extended daily dialysis. *Clin Infect Dis.* 2009;49:433–437.
9. Pruchnicki MC, Dasta JF. Acute renal failure in hospitalized patients: part I. *Ann Pharmacother.* 2002;36:1261–1267.
10. Mehta RL, Kellum JA, Shah SV, Molitoris BA, Ronco C, Warnock DG, Levin A, Acute Kidney Injury Network. Acute Kidney Injury Network: report of an initiative to improve outcomes in acute kidney injury. *Crit Care.* 2007;11(2):R31.
11. Abosaif NY, Tolba YA, Heap M, et al. The outcome of acute renal failure in the intensive care unit according to RIFLE: model application, sensitivity, and predictability. *Am J Kidney Dis.* 2005;46:1038–1048.
12. Sural S, Sharma RK, Singhal M, et al. Etiology, prognosis, and outcome of postoperative acute renal failure. *Ren Fail.* 2000;22:87–97.
13. Hoste AJ, Kellum JA. Acute kidney dysfunction and the critically ill. *Minerva Anestesiol.* 2006;72:133–143.
14. Kellum JA, Bellomo R, Ronco C. Definition and classification of acute kidney injury. *Nephron Clin Pract.* 2008;109:182–187.
15. Bellomo R, Kellum JA, Ronco C, et al. Defining and classifying acute renal failure: from advocacy to consensus and validation of the RIFLE criteria. *Intensive Care Med.* 2007;33:409–413.
16. Haas M, Spargo BH, Wit EJ, Meehan SM. Etiologies and outcome of acute renal insufficiency in older adults: a renal biopsy study of 259 cases. *Am J Kidney Dis.* 2000;35:433–447.
17. Kellum JA, Song M, Venkataraman R. Effects of hyperchloremic acidosis on arterial pressure and circulating inflammatory molecules in experimental sepsis. *Chest.* 2004;125:243–248.
18. Carvounis CP, Nisar S, Guro-Razuman S. Significance of the fractional excretion of urea in the differential diagnosis of acute renal failure. *Kidney Int.* 2002;62:2223–2229.
19. Macias-Nunez JF, Lopez-Novoa JM, Martinez-Maldonado M. Acute renal failure in the aged. *Semin Nephrol.* 1996;16:330–338.

20. Kelly KJ, Molitoris BA. Acute renal failure in the new millennium: time to consider combination therapy. *Semin Nephrol.* 2000:20:4–19.

21. Sutton TA, Fisher CJ, Molitoris BA. Microvascular endothelial injury and dysfunction during ischemic acute renal failure. *Kidney Int.* 2002;62:1539–1549.

22. Chawla LS, Abell L, Mazhari R, et al. Identifying critically ill patients at high risk for developing acute renal failure: a pilot study. *Kidney Int.* 2005;68:2274–2280.

23. Abuelo JG. Normotensive ischemic acute renal failure. *N Engl J Med.* 2007;357:797–805.

24. Abdel-Kader K, Palevsky P. Acute kidney injury in the elderly. *Clin Geriatri Med.* 2009;25:331–358.

25. Solomon R, Deray G. How to prevent contrast-induced nephropathy and manage risk patients: practical recommendations. *Kidney Int.* 2006;69(Suppl S100):S51–S53.

26. Rossert J. Drug-induced acute interstitial nephritis. *Kidney Int.* 2001;60:804–817.

27. Michel DM, Kelly CJ. Acute interstitial nephritis. *J Am Soc Nephrol.* 1998;9:506–515.

28. Schena FP, Gesualdo L, Grandaliano G, Montinaro V. Progression of renal damage in human glomerulonephritides: is there sleight of hand in winning the game? *Kidney Int.* 1997;52:1439–1457.

29. Couser WG. Rapidly progressive glomerulonephritis: classification, pathogenetic mechanisms, and therapy. *Am J Kidney Dis.* 1988;11:449–464.

30. Pascual J, Liaño F. Causes and prognosis of acute renal failure in the very old. Madrid Acute Renal Failure Study Group. *J Am Geriatr Soc.* 1998;46:721–725.

31. Perazella MA. Crystal-induced acute renal failure. *Am J Med.* 1999;106:459–465.

32. Metnitz PGH, Krenn CG, Steltzer H, et al. Effect of acute renal failure requiring renal replacement therapy on outcome in critically ill patients. *Crit Care Med.* 2002;30:2051–2058.

33. Kramer AA, Postler G, Salhab KF, Mendez C, Carey LC, Rabb H. Renal ischemia/reperfusion leads to macrophage-mediated increase in pulmonary vascular permeability. *Kidney Int.* 1999;55:2361–2367.

34. Marsh JD, Margolis TI, Kim D. Mechanism of diminished contractile response to catecholamines during acidosis. *Am J Physiol.* 1988;254:20–27.

35. Pedoto A, Caruso JE, Nandi J, et al. Acidosis stimulates nitric oxide production and lung damage in rats. *Am J Respir Crit Care Med.* 1999;159:397–402.

36. Metnitz PG, Bartens C, Fischer M, Fridrich P, Steltzer H, Druml W. Antioxidant status in patients with acute respiratory distress syndrome. *Intensive Care Med.* 1999;25:180–185.

37. Mitch WE. Mechanisms causing loss of muscle in acute uremia. *Ren Fail.* 1996;18:389–394.

38. Gibney RT, Bagshaw SM, Kutsogiannis DJ, Johnston C. When should renal replacement therapy for acute kidney injury be initiated and discontinued? *Blood Purif.* 2008;26:473–484.

39. Joy MS, Matzke GR, Armstrong DK, Marx MA, Zarowitz BJ. A primer on continuous renal replacement therapy for critically ill patients. *Ann Pharmacother.* 1998;32:362–375.

40. Druml W. Metabolic aspects of continuous renal replacement therapies. *Kidney Int.* Suppl 1999;72:S56–S61.

41. O'Reilly P, Tolwani A. Renal replacement therapy III: IHD, CRRT, SLED. *Crit Care Clin.* 2005;21:367–378.

42. Ronco C, Bellomo R, Ricci Z. Continuous renal replacement therapy in critically ill patients. *Nephrol Dial Transplant.* 2001;16:67–72.

43. Pea F, Viale P, Pavan F, Furlanut M. Pharmacokinetic considerations for antimicrobial therapy in patients receiving renal replacement therapy. *Clin Pharmacokinet.* 2007;46:997–1038.

44. Bressolle F, Kinowski JM, de la Coussaye JE, et al. Clinical pharmacokinetics during continuous haemofiltration. *Clin Pharmacokinet.* 1994;26:457–471.

45. Schortgen F, Soubrier N, Delclaux C, et al. Hemodynamic tolerance of intermittent hemodialysis in critically ill patients: usefulness of practice guidelines. *Am J Respir Crit Care Med.* 2000;162:197–202.

46. Manns M, Sigler MH, Teehan BP. Intradialytic renal haemodynamics—potential consequences for the management of the patient with acute renal failure. *Nephrol Dial Transplant.* 1995;10:1018.

47. Palevsky P. Continuous renal replacement therapy component selection: replacement fluid and dialysate solutions. *Semin Dial.* 1996;9:107–111.

48. Abramson S, Niles J. Anticoagulation in continuous renal replacement therapy. *Curr Opin Nephrol Hypertens.* 1999;8:701–707.

49. Tolwani AJ, Wille KM. Anticoagulation for continuous renal replacement therapy. *Seminars in Dialysis.* 2009;22:141–145.

50. Garnacho-Montero J, Garcia-Garmendia JL, Barrero-Almodovar A, Jimenez-Jimenez FJ, Perez-Paredes C, Ortiz-Leyba C. Impact of adequate empirical antibiotic therapy on the outcome of patients admitted to the intensive care unit with sepsis. *Crit Care Med.* 2003;31:2742–2751.

51. Bogard KN, Peterson NT, Plumb TJ, Erwin MW, Fuller PD, Olsen KM. Antibiotic dosing during sustained low-efficiency dialysis: special considerations in adult critically ill patients. *Crit Care Med.* 2011;39:560–570.

52. Pinder M, Bellomo R, Lipman J. Pharmacological principles of antibiotic prescription in the critically ill. *Anaesth Intensive Care.* 2002;30:134–144.

53. Choi G, Gomersall CD, Tian Q, et al. Principles of antibacterial dosing in continuous renal replacement therapy. *Blood Purif.* 2010;30:195–212.

54. Schetz M. Drug dosing in continuous renal replacement therapy: general rules. *Curr Opin Crit Care.* 2007;13:645–651.

55. Böhler J, Donauer J, Keller F. Pharmacokinetic principles during continuous renal replacement therapy: drugs and dosage. *Kidney Int.* 1999;56(Suppl 72): S24–S28.

56. Choi G, Gomersall CD, Tian Q, et al. Principles of antibacterial dosing in continuous renal replacement. *Crit Care Med.* 2009;37:2268–2282.

57. Veltri MA, Neu AM, Fivush BA, Parekh RS, Further SL. Drug dosing during intermittent hemodialysis and continuous renal replacement therapy. Special considerations in pediatric patients. *Pediatr Drugs.* 2004;6:45–65.

58. Roberts JA, Lipman J. Pharmacokinetic issues for antibiotics in the critically ill patient. *Crit Care Med.* 2009;37:840–851.

59. Pallotta K, Manley H. Vancomycin use in patients requiring hemodialysis: a literature review. *Semin Dial.* 2008;21:63–70.

60. Zhanel GG, Wiebe R, Dilay L, et al. Comparative review of the carbapenems. *Drugs.* 2007;67:1027–1052.

61. Mistry GC, Majumdar AK, Swan S, et al. Pharmacokinetics of ertapenem in patients with varying degrees of renal insufficiency and in patients on hemodialysis. *J Clin Pharmacol.* 2006;46:1128–1138.

62. Guskey MT, Tsuji BT. A comparative review of the lipoglycopeptides: orita- vancin, dalbavancin, and telavancin. *Pharmacotherapy.* 2010;30:80–94.

63. Patel JH, Churchwell MD, Seroogy JD, et al. Telavancin and hydroxy propyl- beta-cyclodexrin clearance during continuous renal replacement therapy: an in vitro study. *Int J Artif Organs.* 2009;32:745–751.

64. Wagner CC, Steiner I, Zeitlinger M. Daptomycin elimination by CVVH in vitro; evaluation of factors influencing sieving and membrane absorption. *Int J Clin Pharmacol Ther.* 2009;47:178–186.

65. Burkhardt O, Joukhadar C, Traunmüller F, Hadem J, Welte T, Kielstein J. Elimination of daptomycin in a patient with acute renal failure undergoing extended daily dialysis. *J Antimicrob Chemother.* 2007;60:224–225.

66. Kielstein JT, Eugbers C, Bode-Boeger SM, et al. Dosing of daptomycin in inten- sive care unit patients with acute kidney injury undergoing extended dialysis—a pharmacokinetic study. *Nephrol Dial Transplant.* 2010;25:1537–1541.

67. Dvorchik B, Arbeit RD, Chung J, Lui S, Knebel W, Kastrissios H. Population pharmacokinetics of daptomycin. *Antimicrob Agents Chemother.* 2004;48:2799– 2807.

68. Vilay AM, Grio M, Depestel DD. Daptomycin pharmacokinetics in critically ill patients receiving venovenous hemodialysis. *Crit Care Med.* 2011;39:19–25.

69. Morris MI, Villmann M. Echinocandins in the management of invasive fungal infections, part 1. *Am J Health-Syst Pharm.* 2006;63:1693–1703.

70. Burkhardt O, Kaever V, Burhenne H, Kielstein J. Extended daily doses does not affect the pharmacokinetics of anidulafungin. *Int J Antimicrob Chemother.* 2009;34:282–283.

Chapter 12

Nutrition Support in Critical Illness

Erin Nystrom

LEARNING OBJECTIVES

1. Summarize the clinical consequences of malnutrition.
2. Describe the effect of severe illness on a patient's nutrition status.
3. Compare the risks and benefits of enteral and parenteral nutrition.
4. Identify indications for parenteral nutrition.
5. Estimate a patient's energy and protein requirements, and understand clinical circumstances that may affect these requirements.
6. Calculate a parenteral nutrition formula, including volume and amounts of amino acids, dextrose, and fat.
7. Outline monitoring parameters for parenteral nutrition.

INTRODUCTION

Nutrition support in the intensive care unit (ICU) has traditionally been regarded as a supportive therapy. However, research in the field of nutrition support in critical illness has taken a new direction, focusing on novel modalities and individual nutrients that have disease and inflammation-modulating effects, with intriguing, albeit mixed, results. These newer therapies have yet to gain broad acceptance due to a dearth of quality studies. Likewise, the body of evidence in the field of nutrition support as a whole has been limited to a few randomized controlled trials to guide practice, and as a result, clinical practice may vary considerably from institution to institution.

The purpose of this chapter is to review the use of nutrition support as a supportive therapy in critically ill patients, with a focus on parenteral nutrition (PN). Along with the ICU team, pharmacists play an important role in managing nutrition therapy, especially PN. Practicing nutrition support requires an understanding of the pathophysiology and metabolic alterations that characterize critical illness, and this will also be reviewed. New approaches and controversies will be highlighted briefly.

MALNUTRITION IN CRITICAL ILLNESS

Malnutrition is a common finding in the intensive care unit, affecting up to 40 to 55% of hospitalized patients.[1-4] While no gold standard exists for diagnosis, malnutrition results from either starvation, acute or chronic disease, or a combination of both, and manifests as derangements of body composition, impaired tissue and organ function, and adverse clinical outcomes. While the absolute human and economic costs attributable to malnutrition in hospitalized patients are difficult to quantify, clinical consequences are many; they include increased risk of infectious complications, impaired wound and tissue healing, increased risk of pressure ulcers, loss of muscle mass, impaired cardiac and respiratory muscle function, musculoskeletal weakness, and alterations in gastrointestinal tissue and function. In addition, malnourished patients are more likely to have prolonged lengths of ICU and hospital stay, increased rate of hospital readmissions, and higher mortality.[3-7]

Malnutrition in critical illness is unique from that of pure starvation, such as unstressed anorexia nervosa.[8] In simple starvation, lean muscle mass is relatively preserved in favor of fat oxidation for energy until the malnutrition becomes life-threatening. In contrast, critical illness arising from a pathologic insult is characterized by an acute phase response that results in net protein catabolism. This response is complex and driven by increased circulating levels of counter-regulatory hormones (epinephrine, glucagon, cortisol, and growth hormone, among others) and cytokines (interleukin-1, interleukin-6, tumor necrosis factor-α), along with peripheral tissue resistance to insulin and anabolic hormones.[8,9] In severe metabolic stress, the body's glycogen stores become depleted within 48 hours, and increased proteolysis and lipolysis occur to provide amino acids, glycerol, and free fatty acids for glucose synthesis to fuel tissue function and healing. This occurs primarily at the expense of skeletal muscle breakdown. Furthermore, protein synthesis is impaired by immobility. Critically ill patients' protein requirements are therefore significantly increased, although catabolism will persist despite nutrition provision.[8,10]

It is important to recognize that in critical illness, malnutrition, which may not be present at the time of admission (e.g., previously healthy patient until a trauma), can develop as a result of the catabolic response to the underlying disease state. Therefore, malnutrition of critical illness will not be reversed by nutrition support alone, but by resolution of the underlying inflammatory condition. For this reason, nutrition support in the ICU remains largely a supportive therapy.

NUTRITION ASSESSMENT

There is no consensus definition of malnutrition, and as a result, its diagnosis is subjective. A thorough nutrition assessment by the primary treatment team, nutrition service, or dietitian is necessary to identify the risk for or presence of malnutrition in critically ill patients and is used to assess the need for nutrition support, appropriate timing of initiation, and most appropriate route. Nutrition assessment entails a detailed review of weight history; oral intake and type of intake; use of dietary supplements; comorbid medical conditions and degree of inflammation; medications affecting nutrient intake, absorption, or excretion; gastrointestinal function; and laboratory parameters; as well as a physical exam to assess stores of fat and protein. It has been suggested that severe illness in itself is a state of malnutrition.[8] It is therefore important to discern malnutrition caused by poor intake from that associated with disease, since nutrition intervention alone cannot be expected to significantly improve the metabolic derangements associated with the stress response to severe illness.

Nutrition assessment in critical illness can be challenging, as body weight measurements may be significantly altered by acute changes in fluid status. Furthermore, fluid shifts resulting in edema or ascites may mask weight loss or the physical appearance of malnutrition. If a patient is sedated, unresponsive, or unable to reliably provide information, family or caregiver input may be necessary to obtain relevant history, including both the patient's recent "dry" and usual weights to accurately assess weight history. In addition, a chart review of documented weight history may be useful, if available. Nutritional risk is suggested by an involuntary weight loss exceeding 5% in the preceding month or 10% in the previous 6 months, or a body weight of 20% below ideal body weight. Body mass index (BMI = weight [kg] / height [m]^2) assesses adiposity by scaling a patient's weight to height and is also a useful indicator of nutrition status. Patients with a BMI of less than 18.5 kg/m^2 are considered underweight; a BMI of 25 kg/m^2 or greater is considered overweight, and 30 kg/m^2 or greater is obese. A low BMI is associated with increased mortality.[11,12]

No ideal surrogate marker of malnutrition exists. The use of visceral proteins albumin and prealbumin as nutritional markers is not recommended. In acute or chronic illness, serum levels of albumin and prealbumin are suppressed secondary to reduced hepatic production, increased vascular permeability, hemodilution, and increased clearance and are therefore insensitive to nutrition provision.[13] These visceral proteins are better indicators of the degree of inflammation than of nutrition status and have been found to correlate poorly with clinical outcomes in nutrition intervention trials.[13,14]

SPECIALIZED NUTRITION SUPPORT

Because critically ill patients are often unable to eat safely by mouth, alternate routes of nutrition must be considered once the decision has been made to start nutrition support. Specialized nutrition support entails nutrition via either the enteral or parenteral route. Several factors should be considered in determining the need for enteral or parenteral nutrition, including recent weight loss, ability to eat, gastrointestinal tract function, degree of disease severity, comorbid conditions, adequacy of fat and protein stores, and anticipated duration of suboptimal oral intake. All told, if a patient is anticipated to have suboptimal oral intake lasting at least seven days, specialized nutrition support is indicated.

Enteral nutrition (EN), administered via a feeding tube into the stomach or small intestine, is the preferred route. However, when enteral access is contraindicated or unobtainable, parenteral nutrition (PN) via a central line is necessary.

Enteral Nutrition

Enteral nutrition is the administration of nutrients via a feeding tube and is the preferred route of feeding for patients who cannot meet their nutritional requirement via oral intake alone. Most patients are able to be fed enterally. The common adage "If the gut works, use it!" invokes the economic, safety, physiological, and clinical advantages of using the enteral route when possible. In addition to a considerable cost advantage to using EN over PN, feeding via the enteral route reduces infectious morbidity compared to PN, a benefit thought to be derived from the ability of nutrients in the gut lumen to maintain the structural and functional integrity of the gastrointestinal mucosa.[5] In the gastrointestinal tract, gut-associated lymphoid tissue (GALT) and mucosal-associated lymphoid tissue (MALT), composed of immunoglobulin A-producing immunocytes, play a major role in the gut's immune function, offering a first line of defense against potentially pathogenic enteric organisms.

Enteral feeding tubes are inserted via the nasal, oral, percutaneous, or surgical routes, and the tip ends in the stomach or in the duodenum or jejunum of the small intestine. A number of different types of enteral access devices are available for feeding, depending on a patient's anatomy, condition of the gastrointestinal tract, and anticipated duration of enteral feeding. Nasal feeding tubes (nasogastric, nasoduodenal, or nasojejunal) are the most common tubes used in the ICU setting and are indicated for use when short-term access is needed. Percutaneous feeding tubes inserted directly through the abdominal wall (e.g., percutaneous endoscopic gastrostomy [PEG] or jejunostomy [PEJ]) may be considered when the anticipated need for EN exceeds four weeks.

Enteral nutrition formulas are nutritionally complete and vary in content and clinical application. Caloric density and amount of protein are the primary differences, with most formulas containing between one and two calories per milliliter of formula. The amount of fiber also differs among products. In addition, formulas intended for specific patient populations contain differing electrolyte concentrations (e.g., low electrolytes for renal impairment) and types of protein (e.g., peptides instead of whole protein for pancreatic insufficiency). All of these factors will affect the osmolality of the formula, which can affect tolerance of tube feeding in terms of stool frequency and consistency, electrolyte disturbances, and volume balance. Each of these components should be considered when choosing the most appropriate formula and rate of administration. If adverse events such as diarrhea develop, the type of enteral formula, in addition to other causes—particularly medications—should be evaluated prior to initiating additional drug therapy.

Although EN is undoubtedly the favored route for nutrition support, questions remain about its optimal utilization in the ICU setting: Is early enteral nutrition, started within 24 to 48 hours of ICU admission, beneficial? What is the best position for the feeding tube: gastric or post-pyloric? Are so-called "immune-enhancing" or "immunomodulating" enteral formulas, which include a combination of omega-3 fatty acids, gamma-linoleic acid, glutamine, and/or antioxidants, of benefit in certain patient populations? These questions remain unanswered, and guidelines on nutrition support in critical illness are largely based on expert opinion and limited trial data. Nonetheless, all available guidelines of nutrition support in critical illness advocate EN as the preferred route of nutrition.[4-6,15,16] Enteral nutrition is a practical and less costly alternative to PN, and avoids complications associated with PN; therefore, most critically ill patients receive specialized nutrition support through enteral feedings.

Parenteral Nutrition

Parenteral nutrition (PN) is reserved for moderately to severely ill patients with a nonfunctional or inaccessible GI tract who are anticipated to have suboptimal oral intake of at least seven days.[5] Because PN is associated with numerous complications including infection, thrombosis, electrolyte derangements, hyperglycemia, hypertriglyceridemia, and hepatic abnormalities,[17-21] its use is restricted to a limited patient population. Specific indications for PN include small bowel obstruction, enteric fistula, severe GI bleeding, mesenteric ischemia, chylous effusions, severe mucositis, and severe motility disorders resulting in intolerance to enteral feeding. However, some of these conditions are not absolute contraindications to EN. For example, it may be possible to feed beyond the site of an obstruction or fistula by optimizing the feeding tube tip position. The American Society of Parenteral and Enteral Nutrition provides guidelines for appropriate use of PN.[4,5]

In patients unable to tolerate goal enteral nutrition, delaying PN results in better outcomes than early initiation of PN in the ICU. A large, randomized, controlled trial conducted in over 4,600 adult critically ill patients demonstrated better outcomes in patients for whom PN was withheld until 8 days post admission to the ICU.[22] Deferring PN was associated with earlier discharge from the ICU and hospital, fewer infections, and reduced duration of mechanical ventilation and renal replacement therapy. Unfortunately, although the investigators achieved tight glycemic control, the study was limited by the high amount of calories provided, up to 30 kcal/kg/day, to patients in both early and late PN groups. This potential confounder may account for some of the harm noted in the early PN group and is considered overfeeding by many nutrition experts.

It is clear that PN poses risks. Parenteral nutrition should be initiated with caution in patients with severe metabolic derangements including fluid overload; severe hyperglycemia; severe azotemia; electrolyte abnormalities, particularly hyper- or hypokalemia and hypophosphatemia; and significant metabolic acid–base disturbances. Under these circumstances, PN may exacerbate the underlying condition, and delaying PN initiation until resolution of the metabolic abnormality should be considered. PN is contraindicated in moribund patients.

ENERGY REQUIREMENTS

A number of different methods for estimating energy expenditure in critically ill patients are utilized in clinical practice; however, a single approach has not been formally endorsed in current guidelines.[5] Many advocate the use of predictive equations (e.g., Harris-Benedict, Ireton–Jones, Mifflin–St. Jeor) to estimate basal energy expenditure (BEE) using factors such as sex, age, height, and weight, while others rely on weight-based calculations (e.g., 25 calories [kcal] per kilogram of body weight) to determine daily caloric requirements. All are generally effective when used by a skilled clinician.

Another tool, indirect calorimetry, utilizes measures of gas exchange—oxygen consumption and carbon dioxide production—to measure an individual's resting energy expenditure (REE). Unfortunately, this tool is not widely available and is subject to technical limitations, operator experience, and changes in a patient's clinical condition. Considerable intra-subject variability with this method has also been reported in critically ill patients.[23] Together, these factors limit universal application of indirect calorimetry, although it may be of benefit in patients in whom basal caloric requirements are difficult to estimate. Such cases may include amputation, extremes of weight, and fluid overload. To date, no evidence demonstrates a clear clinical advantage for one single tool or method of measuring or estimating energy expenditure in critically ill patients.

Overall, the trend over the last decade has been to provide fewer calories than in the past, where the use of "stress" factors tended to grossly overestimate caloric requirements in critically ill patients. A review of the relationship between REE, measured via indirect calorimetry, and BEE, estimated using the Harris-Benedict equation, in critically ill patients revealed that measured values do not significantly exceed predicted basal energy expenditure, and therefore do not justify the use of these multipliers.[23,24] It is generally not recommended to feed above 100 to 120% of BEE in critical illness, although patients with burns or traumatic brain injury may require more calories. The Harris-Benedict equation is utilized to estimate BEE, using a patient's actual weight or dry weight estimate:

Females: 655 + 9.6 x weight (kg) + 1.8 x height (cm) – 4.7 x age (years)

Males: 66.5 + 13.8 x weight (kg) + 5 x height (cm) – 6.8 x age (years)

While there is limited data on how to optimally feed overweight and obese patients, hypocaloric, high-protein nutrition program (a.k.a. permissive underfeeding), in the range of 60 to 75% of BEE, is recommended for obese patients (BMI greater than or equal to 30 kg/m^2).[5,23] A handful of studies support the use of hypocaloric regimens that provide aggressive protein in the range of 1.5 to 2.5 g/kg of ideal body weight.[25-27] There is minimal evidence to support the routine use of permissive underfeeding in non-obese, critically ill patients.

In the absence of strong clinical data supporting specific methods to estimate energy requirements, a pragmatic, patient-specific approach that balances nutrition provision with close monitoring of tolerance of exogenous nutrient substrate and good metabolic control is warranted. Table 12–1 outlines suggested caloric and protein goals in specific types of critically ill patients. While these are general starting points, a patient with hyperglycemia or hypertriglyceridemia, for example, may require reduction of dextrose and/or fat calories. Because of insulin resistance and increased gluconeogenesis in metabolic stress, critically ill patients are less tolerant of exogenous carbohydrate and are more susceptible to adverse sequelae of overfeeding. Nutrient substrate must be administered with caution, and regular consideration for the risk versus benefit of nutrition support.

Table 12–1 Daily Energy, Protein, and Unique Requirements in Select Patient Populations

Patient Group	Energy	Protein*	Fat	Comments
Adult critically ill	100–120% of BEE	1.5–2 g/kg	30% of total calories, not to exceed 1 g/kg/day.	Monitor closely tolerance of nutrient substrate, including glucose (to assess dextrose), BUN (to assess protein), and triglycerides (to assess fat provision).
Obesity	60–75% of BEE	1.5–2 g/kg ideal body weight		
Diabetes/ Hyperglycemia	100–120% of BEE	1.5–2 g/kg		Limit dextrose to 150 g on first day of PN; increase to goal after good glycemic control.
				PN insulin: start with 0.05–0.1 units/g dextrose.
				Reducing energy supplied as dextrose may be warranted for patients with refractory hyperglycemia or high insulin requirements.

Table 12-1 Daily Energy, Protein, and Unique Requirements in Select Patient Populations (*Continued*)

Patient Group	Energy	Protein*	Fat	Comments
Liver Failure and Acute Hepatic Encephalopathy	100–120% of BEE	1.5 g/kg, except restrict protein to 0.6–0.8 g/kg for acute hepatic encephalopathy only; titrate to goal protein dose based on patient's neurologic response.	Reduce or hold fat emulsion for triglycerides greater than 300 mg/dl; increasing calories provided by dextrose to compensate for less calories from fat is discouraged.	Alternative amino acid solutions with higher branched chain amino acids (HepatAmine®, Hepatosol®) may be considered for refractory acute hepatic encephalopathy. Remove manganese from PN solutions in patients with severe liver failure or cholestasis.
Refeeding syndrome	75% BEE initially; goal 100–120% BEE	1.5–2 g/kg		Treat electrolyte deficiencies (potassium, phosphorus, magnesium) prior to starting PN. Give intravenous thiamine prior to IV dextrose or initiation of nutrition support and continue replacement for 3–5 days. Monitor potassium, phosphorus, and magnesium levels and fluid status closely.
Renal Failure	100–120% of BEE	Acute renal failure, no dialysis: 0.6–0.8 g/kg Intermittent hemodialysis: 1.2–1.5 g/kg Continuous renal replacement therapy (CRRT): 2 g/kg		Monitor closely electrolytes eliminated by the kidney: potassium, phosphorus, magnesium. For CRRT, minimal PN electrolyte adjustments may be needed; use of "standard" PN electrolyte amounts with CRRT is often acceptable.

*Consider using ideal body weight or adjusted body weight in overweight patients. Adjusted body weight = [0.25 x (actual weight − ideal weight) + ideal weight].

BEE: Basal energy expenditure, as estimated by Harris Benedict

PARENTERAL NUTRITION FORMULATIONS

Parenteral nutrition is the administration of nutrients and fluid—carbohydrate, protein, fat, electrolytes, minerals, vitamins, and water—via a central or peripheral venous catheter. In general, critically ill patients on PN receive central parenteral nutrition (CPN; a.k.a. TPN or total parenteral nutrition). Central venous administration allows infusion of highly osmolar solutions that are too highly concentrated for infusion via a peripheral vein. Peripheral parenteral nutrition (PPN) requires dilution to an osmolarity of less than 900 mOsm/L, and therefore is formulated in a significantly higher volume than CPN. Consequently, PPN is impractical in severely ill patients with cardiac, renal, or hepatic disease who require fluid restriction.

Parenteral nutrition may be administered in either of two forms: a dextrose–amino acid formula (2-in-1) with intravenous fat emulsions (IVFE) given separately from the dextrose, amino acids, and micronutrients, or a total nutrient admixture (TNA or 3-in-1), with dextrose, amino acids, and IVFE included in the same bag for infusion. Advantages of using TNA include convenience and reduced risk of microbial growth in the IVFE; important disadvantages include the need for a larger pore size filter (1.2 vs. 0.22 microns) and increased IVFE compatibility issues.[28] With no clear advantage of one over the other, both formulations are commonly found in practice.

Parenteral Nutrition Components: Macronutrients

Carbohydrates

Carbohydrate in PN is provided in the form of dextrose. Each gram of dextrose monohydrate provides 3.4 calories. This value is less than that of anhydrous dextrose (4 calories/gram) due to the hydration of dextrose for aqueous solution. Dextrose is an efficient source of energy and is required fuel for specific tissues, especially the brain, which requires 100 to 150 grams of glucose daily. Dextrose also has protein-sparing effects, and exogenous administration to provide at least minimal daily requirements limits skeletal muscle breakdown, sparing amino acids for use in gluconeogenesis to meet the body's basal needs.[29] For this reason, dextrose-containing IV fluids may be a good option for patients who are neither eating nor receiving nutrition support.

Critically ill patients are prone to hyperglycemia secondary to insulin resistance, increased hepatic glucose production, and decreased peripheral glucose uptake. Dextrose, while a vital fuel, should be administered carefully and with close monitoring of blood glucose to minimize complications of hyperglycemia, which include impaired immune function and increased risk of infectious complications.[30,31] Carbohydrate overfeeding also increases carbon dioxide production, which may prolong mechanical ventilation in patients with respiratory failure, and increases fatty deposition in the liver (steatosis).[21] In patients who are hyperglycemic or have a history of diabetes, providing no more than 150 grams of dextrose on the first day of PN is recommended.

Fat

Intravenous fat emulsions are an additional, protein-sparing source of energy and provide the essential fatty acids linoleic acid and α-linolenic acid. Commercially available IVFE in the United States contain long-chain triglycerides derived from either soybean oil or a combination of soybean and safflower oil, and are formulated with an egg yolk phospholipid emulsifier and glycerol to make the solution isotonic with plasma. Available IVFE products are 10% (1.1 kcal/mL), 20% (2 kcal/mL), and 30% (3 kcal/mL). The 10% and 20% concentrations may be administered either separately with a 2-in-1 PN or as part of a 3-in-1 solution, while the 30% IVFE is available for use only as a 3-in-1 component. Each fat gram provides 9 calories, but the glycerol component of IVFE is a source of additional calories. As a result, each gram of fat from 10% IVFE has 11 calories, and each gram from 20% and 30% IVFE provides 10 calories.

Use of IVFE permits reduced amounts of dextrose in the nutrition regimen while still meeting energy requirements. Although the optimal percentage of calories to provide as fat is unclear in critically ill patients, about 30% is recommended.[32,33] Fat provision should not exceed 1 g/kg/day.[4] Triglyceride levels should be checked at baseline prior to starting PN and within three days after initiation to assess the patient's fat tolerance. If triglyceride levels exceed 300 mg/dL, consideration should be made for holding IVFE. If this is done, increasing calories from non-fat sources is generally not recommended.[34]

Although the use of IVFE in the ICU is generally considered safe, it remains a source of controversy. Current guidelines and a meta-analysis suggest that fat emulsion should be held for the first week after initiation of PN.[5,35] The rationale for such recommendations is primarily two-fold. First, results from a prospective, randomized trial of 57 trauma patients demonstrated significantly higher rates of infectious complications and lengths of stay in the group of patients who received PN with IVFE compared to patients who did not receive IVFE.[36] However, those patients who received PN with IVFE also received significantly more calories, and it is more likely that the poor outcome in the IVFE group was attributable to overfeeding and hyperglycemia, rather than to the fat emulsion itself.

Secondly, soybean-oil based IVFE, which are the only type available in the United States, is a source of omega-6 fatty acids, which are metabolized to arachidonic acid, a precursor for pro-inflammatory cytokines. The use of large amounts of IVFE may potentially fuel the inflammatory response of critical illness and impair immune function. Alternative fat emulsions from fish oil, a source of anti-inflammatory omega-3 fatty acids, have been developed and are available outside of the United States. Further study is needed to determine the optimal role for fat emulsions in the ICU.

Protein

Protein in parenteral nutrition is provided as crystalline amino acids, and each gram provides 4 calories. Amino acids are a source of nitrogen, which is required for protein synthesis. Protein needs in critical illness are significantly increased as a result of net body catabolism. Nutrition support can decrease, but not prevent, loss of body protein in critically ill patients who are physically immobile and have high circulating levels of inflammatory mediators that drive catabolism. Most critically ill patients with normal renal and hepatic function should receive at least 1.5 to 2 grams of protein per kilogram of body weight per day.[5] This is in contrast to the healthy, well-nourished individual who requires 0.8 grams per kilogram daily. For obese patients, it is reasonable to base protein needs on ideal body weight, targeting 1.5 to 2 grams per kilogram per day.[5,25-27,37] Exceptions where patients require higher amounts of protein include traumatic brain injury, multiple trauma or bone fractures, burns, and continuous renal replacement therapy.[4,38] Patients with renal insufficiency and acute hepatic encephalopathy may require some amount of protein restriction.

Modified amino acid solutions are available for use in specific disease states. For example, amino acid solutions containing higher amounts of branched-chain amino acids are available for use in patients with acute hepatic encephalopathy. Clinical trials thus far do not support routine use for this condition, although it may be considered for patients with refractory hepatic encephalopathy who have not responded to protein restriction.[4,39] There is inadequate data to support the use of other modified amino acid solutions in metabolic stress or renal failure.

Glutamine, a nonessential amino acid present in abundant quantities in the body but relatively deplete in catabolic states, is not a component of parenteral amino acid solutions given its limited stability. However, parenteral glutamine has been the focus of recent study in critically ill patients who require PN for its suggested benefits in immunologic, metabolic, and gastrointestinal function. Clinical trials to date have produced mixed results. While meta-analyses suggest a correlation between use of glutamine-supplemented PN and reduced morbidity and mortality, consistent clinical benefit has not been demonstrated in large, randomized, controlled trials.[40] At this time, a stable intravenous form of parenteral glutamine is not commercially available in the United States.

Parenteral Nutrition Components: Micronutrients

Electrolytes and Minerals

Parenteral nutrition also provides micronutrients essential for life. Electrolytes include sodium and potassium, each of which are added as acetate, chloride, or phosphate salts. Minerals provided are magnesium as sulfate and calcium as the gluconate salt. Phosphorus is provided as the phosphate salt of sodium or potassium. Acetate, a bicarbonate precursor, and chloride salts are provided in amounts suitable for the patient's acid–base status. For example, the proportion of sodium and/or potassium salts given as acetate may be increased in the setting of metabolic acidosis (e.g., diarrhea or renal failure). In patients with metabolic alkalosis (e.g., gastric losses), PN chloride may be increased. Table 12–2 lists daily requirements of parenteral micronutrients.[41]

Modification of PN electrolytes and minerals is required for patients with significant gastrointestinal losses (e.g., nasogastric suctioning or diarrhea), acid–base disorders, renal failure, refeeding syndrome, and use of medications that affect electrolyte excretion. The PN should not be used to manage acute electrolyte disturbances, but rather chronic needs. In general, PN sodium content does not require frequent adjustments

Table 12–2 Daily Parenteral Electrolyte/Mineral Requirement in Healthy Adults[41]

Electrolyte/Mineral	Daily Parenteral Requirement
Sodium (as chloride, acetate, or phosphate in PN)	1–2 mEq/kg
Potassium (as chloride, acetate, or phosphate in PN)	1–2 mEq/kg
Chloride (as sodium or potassium in PN)	As needed for acid–base balance
Acetate (as sodium or potassium in PN)	
Phosphorus (as sodium or potassium in PN)	20–40 mmol
Calcium (as gluconate in PN)	10–15 mEq
Magnesium (as sulfate in PN)	8–20 mEq

beyond that which meets daily maintenance requirements, since disorders of sodium are most commonly fluid-related. Exceptions include severe edema or sodium-losing states such as significant small bowel or stool losses and renal sodium wasting. In addition, frequent modifications of PN calcium beyond the daily requirement are usually not necessary, since serum calcium levels are a poor reflection of total body stores. Exceptions include patients with hypercalcemia, symptomatic hypocalcemia, or clinical reasons for deficiency. Electrolyte and fluid management is discussed in greater detail in Chapter 7.

Vitamins

Vitamin composition of the two most commonly used commercial vitamin products is outlined in Table 12-3.[42-44] These formulations provide the daily requirement of the 13 vitamins, including 4 fat-soluble (A, D, E, K) and 9 water-soluble (B1, B2, B6, niacin, B12, C, folic acid, pantothenic acid, and biotin) vitamins. Unfortunately, the needs of specific vitamins in critical illness are not well-defined. Thiamine stores become depleted relatively

Table 12-3 Adult Parenteral Multivitamin Products[41-43]

Vitamin	Infuvite® Adult or M.V.I. Adult™	M.V.I. – 12™
A (retinol)	3,300 IU	3,300 IU
D (ergo- or cholecalciferol)	200 IU	200 IU
E (alpha-tocopherol)	10 IU	10 IU
K (phytonadione)	150 mcg	—
C (ascorbic acid)	200 mg	200 mg
B_1 (thiamine)	6 mg	6 mg
B_2 (riboflavin)	3.6 mg	3.6 mg
B_6 (pyridoxine)	6 mg	6 mg
B_{12} (cyanocobalamin)	5 mcg	5 mcg
Biotin	60 mcg	60 mcg
Dexpanthenol	15 mg	15 mg
Folic Acid	600 mcg	600 mcg
Niacinamide	40 mg	40 mg

M.V.I. Adult (multi-vitamin infusion) [package insert]. Lake Forest, IL: Hospira; 2007.

M.V.I. – 12 (multi-vitamin infusion without vitamin K) [package insert]. Paramus, NJ: Hospira; 2005.

quickly, and additional thiamine should be provided to patients with poor intake lasting more than two weeks and who are at risk of refeeding syndrome, a potentially life-threatening disorder of malnutrition.

Trace Elements

Commercially available trace element products available for PN compounding contain four or five components: zinc, copper, manganese, and chromium, with or without selenium. If selenium is not included, it must be added separately. Iodine and molybdenum are not included, but additional supplementation is unnecessary as these are thought to be contaminants of other components in PN solutions. Iron is also not a component of PN; for this reason, patients on long-term parenteral nutrition require regular assessment of iron stores.

Like the vitamins, specific trace element requirements in critical illness are not clear. Frequent adjustment of trace element content in PN solutions is unnecessary; however, certain clinical situations may warrant modification. For example, manganese is eliminated in the bile and should be reduced or discontinued in patients with severe liver disease or cholestasis. Copper, also excreted in bile, may also accumulate in this state. Additional zinc may be necessary in patients with significant gastrointestinal losses or those patients receiving a medication with EDTA as a preservative (e.g., some propofol products for several days duration). Changes beyond the standard amount of chromium are not necessary. Selenium has antioxidative properties and has been studied in patients with severe sepsis.[45,46] Further examination is needed to assess potential benefits and risks of supplementation with high-dose selenium.

A STEP-WISE APPROACH TO WRITING A PARENTERAL NUTRITION ORDER

One of the most daunting challenges associated with PN is simply where to start in what can seem to be a complicated evaluation and ordering process. Following a step-wise approach to evaluation and the calculations can be very helpful. The following case outlines an approach to patient assessment and PN prescription development.

> Case: Mary is a 62-year-old female with a history of chronic radiation enteritis following radiation therapy for ovarian cancer 3 years ago. She was admitted to the ICU one day prior with a perforated jejuno-ileal anastomosis and abdominal sepsis following resection of a small bowel obstruction. She is ventilated and hypotensive, and

receiving vasopressors. Her urine output was 1.3 L over the past 24 hours. Her serum creatinine (SCr) is 0.8 mg/dL (reference range 0.8–1.3 mg/dL) and blood urea nitrogen (BUN) is 18 mg/dL (reference range 8–24 mg/dL). Serum electrolytes are within normal limits. Glucose values have ranged from 105 to 140 mg/dL. You have been asked by the surgeon on service to provide recommendations for CPN.

This patient's current weight is 65 kg and she is 168 cm (5'6") tall. She has lost 8 kg in the last month as a result of poor intake, nausea, and vomiting. Using her height and current weight, the Harris-Benedict estimate of basal energy expenditure (BEE) is 1298 calories daily. Her BMI is 23 kg/m^2 and ideal body weight is 59 kg.

Step One: Determine patient's energy and protein and energy requirements.

A reasonable daily caloric goal for this patient, based on the BEE, is about 1300 calories. Given that this patient is critically ill and without renal impairment or acute hepatic encephalopathy, aggressive protein of at least 1.5 g/kg should be provided. This patient is not overweight or obese, and therefore the actual body weight may be used for the protein calculation. In this case 1.5 g/kg × 65 kg (current weight) = 97.5 g protein daily. Therefore, the parenteral nutrition formula should provide about 1300 calories including 100 grams of protein daily.

Step Two: Calculate daily amounts of dextrose, fat, and protein.

The 1300 calories from parenteral nutrition will be provided by dextrose, fat, and amino acids. To calculate necessary calories from each macronutrient, it is easiest to begin with the amino acids. As noted in Step 1, the desired protein provision is 100 grams daily. Each gram of protein provides 4 calories. Therefore:

$$100 \text{ grams/day} \times 4 \text{ kcal/gram} = 400 \text{ calories from protein}$$

Secondly, decide how many calories the patient will receive from fat. Given no history of hypertriglyceridemia, it is reasonable to provide about 30% of total calories from fat. In this case:

$$0.3 \times 1300 \text{ kcal/day} = 390 \text{ calories from fat}$$

Each gram of parenteral fat provides 10 calories (using 20% IVFE). Therefore:

$$390 \text{ kcal/10 kcal/g fat} = 39 \text{ grams of fat}$$

In summary, about 40 grams of fat should be provided in the PN, or 400 calories daily.

Finally, the amount of dextrose is calculated by subtracting the calories provided by amino acids and fat from the total calories. In this case:

$$1300 \text{ kcal} - 400 \text{ kcal (protein)} - 400 \text{ kcal (fat)} = 500 \text{ kcal}$$

Each gram of dextrose is 3.4 calories. Therefore:

$$500 \text{ kcal}/3.4 \text{ kcal/g dextrose} = 147 \text{ grams of dextrose}$$

Rounded, the PN should provide about 150 grams of dextrose, or 510 calories daily.

In summary, the PN should be formulated to provide 100 grams of amino acids, 150 grams of dextrose, and 40 grams of fat.

Step Three: Specify volume of PN to be administered.

Generally, most patients in the ICU should receive a fluid-restricted formula, since patients may be fluid-expanded and this allows easier management of fluids outside of the CPN. To calculate a fluid-restricted PN, one must know what source products are used in the pharmacy's PN compounding process. Stock amino acid solutions for PN compounding are available in concentrations ranging from 8 to 20%. Similarly, dextrose may be compounded from source products ranging in concentrations of 50 to 70% dextrose. Fat emulsion is available as 10, 20, or 30% concentrations.

For this example, assume the pharmacy uses a 70% dextrose solution, a 10% amino acid solution, and 20% fat emulsion. To calculate the minimum-volume PN, determine the volume of each solution needed to provide the desired amounts of dextrose, amino acids, and fat emulsion determined in Step 2.

For dextrose, assuming the source product is 70% dextrose:

$$150 \text{ g dextrose}/x \text{ ml} = 70 \text{ g}/100 \text{ ml}$$
$$x = 214.3 \text{ ml of 70\% dextrose}$$
OR
$$70\% \times (x \text{ ml}) = 150 \text{ g}$$
$$x = 214.3 \text{ ml of 70\% dextrose}$$

Therefore, 215 ml of 70% dextrose provides 150 g of dextrose in the PN.

For protein, assuming the source product is a 10% amino acid solution:

$$100 \text{ g protein}/x \text{ ml} = 10 \text{ g}/100 \text{ ml}$$
$$x = 1000 \text{ ml of 10\% amino acids}$$
OR
$$10\% \times (x \text{ ml}) = 100 \text{ g}$$
$$x = 1000 \text{ ml of 10\% amino acids}$$

Therefore 1000 ml of 10% amino acids will be needed to provide 100 g of amino acids.

Depending on the type of PN used at the hospital (i.e., 2-in-1 or 3-in-1), the fat volume may or may not be included in the PN volume. This hospital utilizes 3-in-1 PN, and so the fat volume should be figured into the total volume. For fat, assuming the source product is 20% concentration:

$$40 \text{ g fat/x ml} = 20 \text{ g/100 ml}$$
$$x = 200 \text{ ml of 20\% fat emulsion}$$
$$\text{OR}$$
$$20\% \text{ fat emulsion} = 2 \text{ kcal/ml}$$
$$400 \text{ kcal/2 kcal/ml} = 200 \text{ ml 20\% fat emulsion}$$

In summary, 215 ml of dextrose solution, 1000 ml of amino acid solution, and 200 ml of fat emulsion will be used to compound this PN.

$$215 \text{ ml} + 1000 \text{ ml} + 200 \text{ ml} = 1415 \text{ ml}$$

This volume should be rounded up to allow for volume from micronutrient additives, which may add 50 to 80 ml of volume. In this case, it is reasonable to order a CPN volume of 1500 ml daily.

Note: If the institution used a 2-in-1 PN, a volume of 1300 ml (215 ml for dextrose and 1000 ml for amino acids) would be acceptable. The fat emulsion would be administered separately as 200 ml infused each day.

Step Four: Finalize parenteral nutrition formula.

Some institutions may order PN components in total daily amounts (e.g., grams of macronutrients daily). If that is the case, the order form may be filled out with the daily amounts of dextrose, amino acids, and fat calculated in Step 2 and the volume determined in Step 3.

However, many institutions order PN components in concentrations. In that case, the concentrations of macronutrients for the final formulation will need to be calculated. In this case, with a final volume of 1500 ml, the concentrations of each macronutrient are:

$$\text{Dextrose: } 150 \text{ g/1500 ml} \times 100 = 10\% \text{ dextrose}$$
$$\text{Amino Acids: } 100 \text{ g/1500 ml} \times 100 = 6.7\% \text{ amino acids}$$
$$\text{Fat: } 40 \text{ g/1500 ml} \times 100 = 2.7\% \text{ fat}$$

Again, it is important to know what base product your institution uses for PN compounding, since several concentrations of dextrose, amino acids, and fat are commercially available. When using more concentrated base solutions, for example, total PN volume and macronutrient concentrations can be easily modified with the addition of sterile water for injection. Further, stability of the final compounded solution is very important, and it may be necessary to adjust the choice of stock solutions to ensure final solution stability. Stability tables and compounding automation software will help guide the pharmacist to produce a safe product.

Some hospitals use premade PN solutions where the amino acids and dextrose are typically prepared in dual chambered bags that are mixed at the point of use. These solutions have set dextrose and amino acid concentrations and ratios, and in this case, the pharmacist will need to determine the solutions available for use and modify the ultimate prescription from the base calculations outlined in steps 1 through 3 above to match the available products. Therefore, it is important for a pharmacist to be very familiar with the pharmaceutical calculations involved in parenteral nutrition compounding so that they can work within any system.

MONITORING

Recommended monitoring parameters for patients on parenteral nutrition are provided in Table 12-4.[47] Parenteral nutrition monitoring is individualized based on patient needs, but at a minimum, baseline weight; electrolytes, including phosphorus and magnesium; SCr; BUN; glucose; and triglycerides should be measured. Following initiation of PN, electrolytes should be evaluated daily until stable. Glucose should be monitored at least daily, but every 6 hours or even more frequently is common in the ICU. Triglycerides should be measured within three days of initiation and then at least once weekly. Fluid status should be monitored closely by assessing daily weights, SCr, BUN, serum sodium, urine output, and reviewing fluid intake and other losses from gastrointestinal or wound sources. Evaluating fluid losses will also aid in assessment of electrolyte and acid–base status. Arterial blood gases should be reviewed when available. Regular monitoring of trace elements is not recommended unless there is clinical reason to suspect deficiency or toxicity. Overall, the degree and frequency of monitoring should be individualized to each patient's needs.

Unfortunately, no reliable laboratory parameter exists to assess overall adequacy of the nutrition program. Prealbumin and measured nitrogen balance have been commonly referenced as parameters to assess the adequacy of protein provision; however, several factors limit their application in critical illness. Since these values do not correlate with clinical outcomes, routine use is not recommended.[13,14]

In addition to the parameters mentioned above, daily PN monitoring should include a thorough review of the medication profile to identify medications that may affect electrolytes (e.g., insulin, diuretics, ACE inhibitors,

Table 12–4 Parenteral Nutrition Monitoring Parameters[47]

Parameter	Baseline	Post-Initiation	Comment
Electrolytes (Sodium, potassium, phosphorus, chloride, and bicarbonate)	X	Daily until stable	May reduce frequency once stable Patients at risk of refeeding syndrome require more frequent monitoring of potassium and phosphorus
Calcium, Magnesium	X	Magnesium: Twice weekly until stable	May follow magnesium and calcium less closely; serum levels are not good indicators of total body stores
		Calcium: as needed, based on symptoms	Both magnesium and calcium are bound to albumin and may be low in the setting of hypoalbuminemia
SCr/BUN	X	Daily with electrolyte panel	May reduce frequency once stable
Blood glucose	X	One to four times daily	May reduce frequency once stable
Triglycerides	X	Within 3 days of PN start, then every 2 weeks	Patients with hypertriglyceridemia require more frequent assessment
AST, ALT, alk phos, bilirubin	X	Once every two weeks	
Weight	X	Daily	Weight gain of more than 0.25 kg from day to day is reflective of fluid shifts
Intake and output	X	Daily	In: IV fluids, fluid from medication infusions, blood products, oral or enteral intake Out: Urine, dialysis, stool, fistula(s), other gastrointestinal losses, and wound output
CBC	X	Weekly	Check if signs of line infection
Temperature	X	Daily	Check if signs of line infection
Trace elements (copper, selenium, manganese, zinc)		With clinical signs/ symptoms of deficiency or toxicity	Manganese accumulates with liver disease, cholestasis, and long-term PN use Zinc is lost in gastrointestinal secretions (e.g., stool and ostomy output)

Table 12–4 Parenteral Nutrition Monitoring Parameters[47] (*Continued*)

Parameter	Baseline	Post-Initiation	Comment
			Consider assessing copper, selenium, and zinc levels in severely malnourished patients
Iron		With long-term PN use	Iron studies (total iron binding capacity, % saturation, ferritin) do not reliably assess iron deficiency in acute illness
Medication profile	X	Daily	Medications that affect electrolyte, mineral, and glucose values (furosemide, amphotericin, ACE inhibitors, corticosteroids, etc.)
			Propofol (formulated in 10% fat emulsion providing 1.1 kcal/ml)
			Dextrose- or sodium-containing IV fluids or with medication infusions/piggybacks

amphotericin, foscarnet), acid–base and fluid status (e.g., furosemide), and glycemic control (e.g., steroids, octreotide, insulin). Intravenous fluids should be reviewed to assess fluid and acid–base status (e.g., hyperchloremic acidosis related to high rates of 0.9% sodium chloride infusion). There is no need for dextrose-containing IV fluids in patients who are receiving goal nutrition support. Calories from medication infusions formulated in D5W (5% dextrose in water) and from propofol, which is formulated in a 10% fat emulsion providing 1.1 calories/mL, should be accounted for every day, with adjustments made to the nutrition program as needed.

Finally, the patient's indication for PN and gastrointestinal function should be regularly assessed for the opportunity to transition from PN to nutrition via the oral or enteral routes.

Complications of parenteral nutrition may be categorized as metabolic (e.g., hypercarbia, hypertriglyceridemia, hyperglycemia, refeeding syndrome), catheter-related (e.g., infection, thrombosis), or gastrointestinal (parenteral-nutrition- or intestinal-failure-associated liver disease).[17-19] While a detailed review of PN-associated complications is beyond the scope of this chapter, adverse effects can be minimized with avoidance of overfeeding, careful monitoring, and good catheter site care.

SUMMARY

Pharmacists play a significant role in the assessment and provision of nutrition support in the ICU, as appropriate nutrition provision is an essential part of supportive care of the critically ill patient. Because quality trials of nutrition support in critical illness are scarce, clinical practice in nutrition support, to date, is based heavily on expert opinion and may vary from institution to institution. Available nutrition support studies are unfortunately limited by heterogeneity, and small study populations, inconsistencies in nutrition support provided (timing, nutrition composition, control nutrition support), lack of intention-to-treat analysis, and variable metabolic control (e.g., hyperglycemia). Additional research is necessary to further define the best timing, amount, and route of nutrition support, as well as to demonstrate clinical utility of specific nutrition support modalities, including new fat emulsions, glutamine, and antioxidants. As research on such components as these continues, nutrition may evolve from supportive to active therapy in critically ill patients.

KEY POINTS

- Critical illness is characterized by a state of net protein catabolism. Nutrition support limits, but does not stop, protein breakdown and prevents adverse effects of malnutrition.
- Target daily calorie provision is 100 to 120% of BEE in critical illness. Protein requirements are 1.5 to 2 grams/kg. Hypocaloric, high-protein feeding in obese patients is recommended.
- Enteral nutrition is the preferred route of nutrition. Parenteral nutrition should be reserved for patients with inaccessible or non-functional GI tracts.
- Protein restriction may be necessary in some patients with renal failure and acute hepatic encephalopathy.
- Parenteral nutrition should be monitored closely, with regular, individualized assessment of relevant clinical and laboratory parameters and with the goal of attaining metabolic control.
- Nutrition support is a supportive therapy. The routine use of nutrition support therapies with immunomodulating effects cannot be recommended at this time given lack of strong clinical data.

SELECTED SUGGESTED READINGS

- Ziegler T. Parenteral nutrition in the critically ill patient. *N Engl J Med.* 2009;361:1088–1097.

- McClave SA, Martindale RG, Vanek VW, et al. Guidelines for the provision and assessment of nutrition support therapy in the adult critically ill patient: Society of Critical Care Medicine (SCCM) and American Society for Parenteral and Enteral Nutrition (A.S.P.E.N.). *JPEN J Parenter Enteral Nutr.* 2009;33:277–316.
- Btaiche IF, Khalidi N. Metabolic complications of parenteral nutrition in adults, part 1. *Am J Health-Syst Pharm.* 2004;61: 1938–1949.
- Btaiche IF, Khalidi N. Metabolic complications of parenteral nutrition in adults, part 2. *Am J Health-Syst Pharm.* 2004;61:2050–2059.
- The NICE-SUGAR Study Investigators. Intensive versus conventional glucose control in critically ill patients. *N Eng J Med.* 2009;360:1283–1297.
- Casaer MP, Mesotten D, Hermans G, et al. Early versus late parenteral nutrition in critically ill adults. *N Eng J Med.* 2011;365:506–517.

REFERENCES

1. Bistrian BR, Blackburn GL, Hallowell E, et al. Protein status of general surgical patients. *JAMA.* 1974;230:858–860.
2. Bistrian BR, Blackburn GL, Vitale J, et al. Prevalence of malnutrition in general medical patients. *JAMA.* 1976;235:1567–1570.
3. Ziegler T. Parenteral nutrition in the critically ill patient. *N Engl J Med.* 2009;361:1088–1097.
4. A.S.P.E.N. Board of Directors, Clinical Guidelines Task Force. Guidelines for the use of parenteral and enteral nutrition in adult and pediatric patients. *J Parenter Enteral Nutr.* 2002;26:1SA–138SA.
5. McClave SA, Martindale RG, Vanek VW, et al. Guidelines for the provision and assessment of nutrition support therapy in the adult critically ill patient: Society of Critical Care Medicine (SCCM) and American Society for Parenteral and Enteral Nutrition (A.S.P.E.N.). *J Parenter Enteral Nutr.* 2009;33:277–316.
6. Singer P, Berger MM, Van den Berghe G, et al. ASPEN guidelines on parenteral nutrition: intensive care. *Clin Nutr.* 2009;28:387–400.
7. National Alliance for Infusion Therapy and the American Society for Parenteral and Enteral Nutrition Public Policy Committee and Board of Directors. Disease-related malnutrition and enteral nutrition therapy: a significant problem with a cost-effective solution. *Nutr Clin Pract.* 2010;25:548–554.
8. Jensen GL, Mirtallo J, Compher, et al. Adult starvation and disease-related malnutrition: a proposal for etiology-based diagnosis in the clinical practice setting from the International Consensus Guideline Committee. *J Parenter Enteral Nutr.* 2010;34:156–159.
9. Pomposelli JJ, Flores EA, Bistrian BR. Role of biochemical mediators in clinical nutrition and surgical metabolism. *J Parenter Enteral Nutr.* 1988;12:212–218.

10. Shaw JHF, Wildbore M, Wolfe RR. Whole body protein kinetics in severely septic patients: the response to glucose infusion and total parenteral nutrition. *Ann Surg.* 1987;205:288–294.

11. Landi FOG, Gambassi G, et al. Body mass index and mortality among hospitalized patients. *Arch Intern Med.* 2000;160:2641–2644.

12. Galano A, Pieper C, Kussin P, et al. Relationship of body mass index to subsequent mortality among seriously ill hospitalized patients. *Crit Care Med.* 1997;25:1962–1968.

13. Johnson AM, Merlini G, Sheldon J, et al. Clinical indications for plasma protein assays: transthyretin (prealbumin) in inflammation and malnutrition. *Clin Chem Lab Med.* 2007;45:419–426.

14. Koretz RL. Death, morbidity and economics are the only end points for trials. *Proc Nutr Soc.* 2005;64:277–284.

15. Cerra FB, Rios Benitez M, Blackburn GL, et al. Applied nutrition in ICU patients: a consensus statement of the American College of Chest Physicians. *Chest.* 1997;111:769–778.

16. Kreymann KG, Berger MM, Deutz NEP, et al. ESPEN guidelines on enteral nutrition: intensive care. *Clin Nutr.* 2006;25:210–223.

17. Btaiche IF, Khalidi N. Metabolic complications of parenteral nutrition in adults, part 1. *Am J Health-Syst Pharm.* 2004;61:1938–1949.

18. Btaiche IF, Khalidi N. Metabolic complications of parenteral nutrition in adults, part 2. *Am J Health-Syst Pharm.* 2004;61:2050–2059.

19. Ghabril MS, Aranda-Michel J, Scolapio JS. Metabolic and catheter complications of parenteral nutrition. *Curr Gastroenterol Rep.* 2004;6:327–334.

20. Veterans Affairs Total Parenteral Nutrition Cooperative Study Group. Perioperative total parenteral nutrition in surgical patients. *N Engl J Med.* 1991;325:525–532.

21. Klein CJ, Stanek GS, Wiles CE. Overfeeding macronutrients to critically ill adults: metabolic complications. *J Am Diet Assoc.* 1998;98:795–806.

22. Casaer MP, Mesotten D, Hermans G, et al. Early versus late parenteral nutrition in critically ill adults. *N Engl J Med.* 2011;365:506–517.

23. Miles JM. Energy expenditure in hospitalized patients: implications for nutritional support. *Mayo Clin Proc.* 2006;81:809–816.

24. Kinney JM. History of parenteral nutrition, with notes on clinical biology. In: Rombeau JL, Rolandelli RH, eds. *Clinical Nutrition: Parenteral Nutrition.* 3rd ed. Philadelphia: W.B. Saunders; 2001:1–20.

25. Dickerson RN, Rosato EF, Mullen JL. Net protein anabolism with hypocaloric parenteral nutrition in obese stressed patients. *Am J Clin Nutr.* 1986;44:747–755.

26. Burge JC, Goon A, Choban PS, et al. Efficacy of hypocaloric total parenteral nutrition in hospitalized obese patients: a prospective, double-blind randomized trial. *J Parenter Enteral Nutr.* 1994;18:203–207.

27. Choban PS, Burge JC, Scales D, et al. Hypoenergetic nutrition support in hospitalized obese patients: a simplified method for clinical application. *Am J Clin Nutr.* 1997;66:546–550.

28. Rollins CJ. Total nutrient admixtures: stability issues and their impact on nursing practice. *J Intraven Nurs.* 1997;20:299–304.

29. Driscoll DF, Bistrian BR. Parenteral nutrition (macronutrient fuels). In: Shikora SA, Martindale RG, Schwaitzberg SD, eds. *Nutritional Considerations in the Intensive Care Unit: Science, Rationale and Practice. 1st ed.* Dubuque, Iowa: Kendal/Hunt; 2002:39–49.

30. Van den Berghe G, Wouters P, Weekers F, et al. Intensive insulin therapy in critically ill patients. *N Eng J Med.* 2001;345:1359–1367.

31. The NICE-SUGAR Study Investigators. Intensive versus conventional glucose control in critically ill patients. *N Eng J Med.* 2009;360:1283–1297.

32. Jeejeebhoy KN, Anderson GH, Nakhooda AF, et al. Metabolic studies in total parenteral nutrition with lipid in man. *J Clin Invest.* 1976;57:125–136.

33. Driscoll DF, Adolph M, Bistrian BR. Lipid emulsions in parenteral nutrition. In: Rombeau JL, Rolandelli RH, eds. *Clinical Nutrition: Parenteral Nutrition. 3rd ed.* Philadelphia:W.B. Saunders; 2001:35–59.

34. Paluzzi M, Meguid MM. A prospective, randomized study of the optimal source of nonprotein calories in total parenteral nutrition. *Surgery.* 1987;102:711–717.

35. Heyland DK, MacDonald S, Keefe L, et al. Total parenteral nutrition in the critically ill patient: a meta-analysis. *JAMA.* 1998;280:2013–2019.

36. Battistella FD, Widergren JT, Anderson JT, et al. A prospective, randomized trial of intravenous fat emulsion administration in trauma victims requiring total parenteral nutrition. *J Trauma.* 1997;43:52–60.

37. McMahon MM, Farnell MB, Murray MJ. Nutritional support of critically ill patients. *Mayo Clin Proc.* 1993;68:911–920.

38. Brown RO, Compher C, American Society for Parenteral and Enteral Nutrition (A.S.P.E.N.) Board of Directors. A.S.P.E.N. clinical guidelines: nutrition support in adult acute and chronic renal failure. *J Parenter Enteral Nutr.* 2010;34:366–377.

39. Als-Nielsen B, Koretz RL, Gluud LL, et al. Branched-chain amino acids for hepatic encephalopathy. *Cochrane Database Syst Rev.* 2003;Issue 1. Art. No.: CD001939. DOI: 10.1002/14651858.CD001939.

40. Wischmeyer PE. Glutamine: role in critical illness and ongoing clinical trials. *Curr Opin Gastroenterol.* 2008;24:190–197.

41. Mirtallo J, Canada T, Johnson D, et al. Safe practices for parenteral nutrition. *J Parenter Enteral Nutr.* 2004;28:S39–S70.

42. Infuvite Adult (multiple vitamins for infusion) [package insert]. Deerfield, IL: Baxter Healthcare; 2007.

43. M.V.I. Adult (multi-vitamin infusion) [package insert]. Lake Forest, IL: Hospira; 2007.

44. M.V.I. – 12 (multi-vitamin infusion without vitamin K) [package insert]. Paramus, NJ: Hospira; 2005.

45. Angstwurm MWA, Enggelmann L, Zimmermann T, et al. Selenium in intensive care (SIC): results of a prospective randomized, placebo-controlled, multiple-center study in patients with severe systemic inflammatory response syndrome, sepsis, and septic shock. *Crit Care Med.* 2007;35:118–126.

46. Berger MM, Shenkin A. Selenium in intensive care: probably not a magic bullet but an important adjuvant therapy. *Crit Care Med.* 2007;35:306–307.

47. Mirtallo J. Overview of Parenteral Nutrition. In: Gottschlich MM, ed. *The ASPEN Nutrition Support Core Curriculum: A Case-based Approach—The Adult Patient.* Silver Spring, MD: American Society for Enteral and Parenteral Nutrition; 2007:274.

Chapter 13

Fundamentals of Antimicrobial Therapy in the Critically Ill

Brad Laible

LEARNING OBJECTIVES

1. Identify likely microbial pathogens associated with common infections in critically ill patients.
2. Discuss institution-specific and patient-specific factors that must be considered in the selection of antimicrobial agents for infections in the critically ill.
3. Describe strategies employed in the treatment of common multi-drug resistant pathogens, specifically methicillin-resistant *Staphylococcus aureus* (MRSA) and *Pseudomonas aeruginosa*.
4. Recommend antimicrobial regimens for common infections in critically ill patients based on current guidelines and related literature.
5. Define and discuss strategies for de-escalation.
6. Identify potential adverse consequences of antimicrobial therapy.

INTRODUCTION

The purpose of this chapter is to familiarize the reader with the most essential concepts of infectious disease (ID) pharmacotherapy in the intensive care unit (ICU) setting. A careful institution- and patient-specific approach is paramount, with an emphasis on early and aggressive empiric antimicrobial therapy when infection is suspected.

Many factors must be taken into account when choosing the most appropriate antimicrobial regimen. For example, institution-specific pathogen resistance patterns must be considered. This may require careful review of current institution-specific or even ICU-specific antimicrobial susceptibilities to guide agent selection. Antimicrobial formulary is another institution-specific factor that must be considered, as treatment decisions must generally be made within the confines of the approved formulary. Patient-specific factors must also be evaluated and may include, but are not limited to: suspected site of infection and associated microbial flora, recent antimicrobial use, known history of infection and past culture results, allergy history, organ system function, immune function, and body habitus. Finally, antimicrobial regimens can be broadly grouped into empiric or definitive therapy. Empiric regimens are given based upon suspected infection site and multiple other known factors prior to identifying a specific pathogen(s). These regimens often include broad spectrum agents administered while awaiting results from cultures or other diagnostic studies. Definitive therapy is then developed by tailoring antimicrobial regimens based on culture results, diagnostic studies, and patient response, otherwise known as de-escalation, and is vital for reducing the emergence of resistance and potential adverse consequences of antimicrobial use, such as *Clostridium difficile*-associated disease (CDAD).

This chapter first describes several specific considerations for antimicrobial selection in the critically ill. An understanding of these specific issues allows the pharmacist to provide a reasoned approach to antimicrobial therapy and helps provide understanding of the applicable guidelines for treatment of infections based upon the site of infection. The remainder of the chapter describes some of the common treatment regimens associated with infection by organ system or site of infection. Adverse events associated with antimicrobial therapy are also described.

Complete textbooks could be and have been written on the management of severe infectious diseases. Treatment of infectious diseases is highly driven by guideline statements and emerging primary literature, but since these can change rapidly, care must be taken to follow the most current version of treatment protocols and dosing guidelines for all therapies, and this is particularly true with antimicrobial agents. This overview chapter should serve as a summary of the most important ID-related topics, and the reader is referred to current guidelines and primary literature for definitive current recommendations for therapy.

FACTORS AFFECTING INITIAL ANTIMICROBIAL SELECTION

Likely Pathogens Based on Site of Infection

Most severe ICU infections occur when microorganisms are able to bypass host defenses at three main sites: respiratory tract, intra-abdominal compartment, and urinary tract. Bacteremia may also occur, with the infecting pathogen usually originating from these three main sites or due to foreign devices such as intravascular catheters. Severe infection can result in sepsis, end organ damage, shock, and ultimately death. Knowledge of site-specific pathogens most likely to cause infection is imperative to appropriate initial antimicrobial selection. Recent antimicrobial history and other patient-specific factors, such as immune suppression and place of residence prior to admission, are just a few risk factors for multi-drug resistant pathogens that need to be considered when deciding which pathogens to target. Ultimately, appropriate empiric therapy, typically defined as at least one agent found to be active against the responsible pathogen based on culture and susceptibility results, is essential, as inappropriate empiric therapy is associated with higher mortality.[1,2] Achieving this goal often requires broad multi-agent empiric therapy, using rapidly bactericidal agents when possible, with subsequent de-escalation when culture and susceptibility results are available.

Respiratory Tract

Severe community-acquired infection of the lower respiratory tract (usually referred to as community-acquired pneumonia or CAP) is most often caused by *Streptococcus pneumoniae*, although other pathogens such as *Haemophilus influenzae* and *Moraxella cattarhalis* commonly cause this infection in patients with underlying broncopulmonary disease. *Staphylococcus aureus* (especially during an influenza outbreak) and atypical pathogens (*Legionella species, Mycoplasma pneumoniae, Chlamydia pneumoniae*) are also common causes and should be considered when selecting initial antimicrobial therapy.[3] *Enterobacteriaceae* and *Pseudomonas aeruginosa* may need to be considered as a cause of CAP if the patient has a history of chronic oral steroid use, severe bronchopulmonary disease, alcoholism or frequent antibiotic use.[3,4] Severe nosocomial infection of the lower respiratory tract, including hospital-acquired pneumonia (HAP), ventilator-associated pneumonia (VAP), and healthcare-associated pneumonia (HCAP), is often caused by multi-drug resistant pathogens, such as *P. aeruginosa*, *S. aureus*, particularly methicillin-resistant *S. aureus* (MRSA), and aerobic enteric Gram-negative bacilli, including *Escherichia coli*, *Klebsiella pneumoniae*, and *Acinetobacter* species.[5] Other Gram-negative bacilli to consider include *Enterobacter* species, *Serratia* species, and *Stenotrophomonas maltophilia*.

Intra-Abdominal Compartment

Intra-abdominal infections generally occur due to penetration of normal gastrointestinal tract flora into sterile spaces. *Escherichia coli*, an enteric Gram-negative bacilli, is the most commonly associated pathogen causing community-acquired infection.[6] Other common flora that reside within the gastrointestinal tract include *Klebsiella* species, viridans streptococci, *Bacteroides* species (an anaerobic bacteria) and to a lesser extent, *P. aeruginosa*. *Enterococcus* species, MRSA, and fungal species, most commonly *Candida albicans* and *C. glabrata*, may also play a role. This is particularly true in the setting of severe and/or healthcare-associated infection.

Urinary Tract

Urinary tract infections can be both community- and hospital-acquired, with most hospital-acquired infections resulting from catheterization of the urinary tract. Similar to intra-abdominal infection, pathogens responsible for urinary tract infection generally originate from the gastrointestinal tract. These infections are most commonly caused by *E. coli*, although many other organisms, such as *Klebsiella* species, *Enterobacter* species, *P. aeruginosa*, and *Enterococcus* species may be responsible pathogens.[7] *Candida* species are also commonly isolated in urine cultures, particularly in those patients with urinary catheterization and/or recent antibiotic use.[8] Positive urine cultures may represent colonization rather than true infection, and therefore positive cultures should be evaluated in the context of clinical symptoms; patients with asymptomatic colonization should not be treated with antimicrobials in most situations. Finally, polymicrobial infection is common in patients with long-term catheterization.[9] The negative adverse events associated with urinary catheterization have lead to initiatives to minimize the overall duration of use of urinary catheters.

Other Sites of Infection

Although less common, infections of the central nervous system, such as meningitis, may be life-threatening, primarily when bacterial in origin. Responsible bacterial pathogens can be anticipated based on age. For example, *Streptococcus agalactiae* and *E. coli* commonly cause meningitis in neonates, while *S. pneumoniae* is the most common cause in adults.[10] Meningitis may also result as a complication of neurosurgery or head trauma, where organisms such as staphylococci and Gram-negative bacilli are the predominant pathogens.

Intravascular catheter and skin and soft tissue infections (SSTIs) may also be seen in the ICU. Intravascular catheter infections are primarily caused by coagulase-negative staphylococci, although *S. aureus*, Gram-negative bacilli, and *Candida* may play a role.[11] *Staphylococcus aureus* and streptococci species (usually *S. pyogenes*) are the most common causes of SSTIs.[12] A careful assessment of risk factors for MRSA must be performed when selecting treatment for these infections, with addition of empiric MRSA therapy for high-risk patients.

Finally, pseudomembranous colitis is a common complication of antimicrobial use in the ICU. This condition is primarily caused by the release of toxin from an anaerobic pathogen, *C. difficile*, and is a major infection control problem resulting from both antimicrobial overuse and poor hand hygeine.[13]

Diagnostic Testing

While diagnostic testing alone does not provide the clinical insight necessary for most treatment decisions, these pieces of information may help in the process. Abnormal white blood cell count (generally < 4,000 or > 11,000 WBC/mm^3) and fever (temperature > 100.4° F) are commonly identified signs of potential infectious disease. Unstable blood pressure, tachycardia, and tachypnea may also result from serious infectious disorders. The following section details further diagnostic testing employed in making infection-related diagnoses.

Radiography

While pharmacists are generally not asked to order and evaluate radiographical testing, the knowledge of the appropriate use of these diagnostic testing methods is essential for understanding when and when not to initiate antimicrobial therapy. For example, chest radiography (X-ray) results are an essential component of making a diagnosis of pneumonia. The presence of pulmonary infiltrates on a chest X-ray in correlation with clinical symptoms is generally diagnostic for pneumonia and antimicrobial therapy is warranted.[3,5] Computed tomography (CT scan) is useful to identify severe gastrointestinal infections, such as diverticulitis or intra-abdominal abscesses.[6] Finally, ultrasonography may be particularly useful for the diagnosis of certain biliary infections, such as acute cholecystitis and ascending cholangitis. Additional radiological testing methods may also be used, but are beyond the scope of this chapter and the reader is encouraged to review other medical texts and resources.

Gram Stains

Gram stains of potentially infected fluid and/or tissue may be valuable in decisions regarding empiric antimicrobial use. Gram staining can identify the presence of bacteria and leukocytes, indicating possible infection. Gram stains should be critically evaluated, however, as improperly collected specimens can be misleading. For example, the presence of an excessive amount of squamous epithelial cells (generally defined as greater than 10 cells per high-powered field) may represent a respiratory specimen contaminated by oral flora, potentially leading to inappropriate antimicrobial therapy.[14] Gram stains can be useful for identifying the shape and spatial arrangement of potential bacterial pathogens, information that may be used to direct empiric antimicrobial therapy for infections such as pneumonia and meningitis while awaiting final culture results. For example, respiratory specimens with Gram-positive cocci arranged in pairs may direct empiric therapy specific for *S. pneumoniae*. Gram staining of blood cultures positive for Gram-positive cocci in clusters may indicate *S. aureus* or coagulase-negative staphylococci. While Gram stains may be helpful, it must be recognized that not all causative pathogens will be identified via the Gram staining procedure,[15,16] and therefore, it is important to provide empiric therapy for the most likely causative pathogens for a specific infection until final culture results are obtained. It is also important to note that not all pathogens can be identified by standard Gram staining. For example, an atypical pathogen, *M. pneumoniae*, lacks a cell wall and cannot be identified by Gram staining technique. Alternative staining methods may be necessary for some pathogens. Acid fast staining, for example, may be performed to help identify *Mycobacterium tuberculosis*.

Cultures

Although not always definitive, cultures may be used to determine the presence of infection. Cultures can be procured from most sites of potential infection, including blood, urine, respiratory secretions, cerebrospinal fluid, peritoneal fluid, and purulent discharge from wounds. Once again, the clinician must always consider the quality of the specimen when making decisions based on culture results. One of the most important considerations is determining colonization versus true infection. Bacterial pathogens identified from normally sterile sites, such as cerebrospinal fluid and peritoneal fluid, are easier to interpret, as these sites do not generally harbor non-pathogenic bacteria and usually reflect true infection. Conversely, chronic wounds and the upper respiratory tract of critically ill patients commonly become colonized with bacteria and positive cultures from these sites do not always represent true infection. For example, wound cultures are more reliable when deep tissue cultures are obtained aseptically in the operative setting as compared to superficial wound swabbing done at the bedside. In a similar fashion, deep respiratory cultures obtained by bronchoscopy may be more reliable than expectorated sputum or tracheal aspirates. While negative cultures of lower respiratory tract secretions generally rule out infection, false negative results may occur when recent (within 72 hours) antimicrobial changes have been made.[17] It is important to note that not all potential respiratory pathogens culture well in standard growth media. *Legionella pneumophilia*, for example, requires special media for adequate growth and alternative methods are generally used to identify this pathogen, such as a urine antigen test. Finally, positive or negative cultures must always be evaluated in the context of the patient's clinical situation. Positive cultures in the absence of symptoms may represent colonization, while negative cultures in the context of severe illness may represent a false negative result.

Other Laboratory Testing

Antigen detection methods are primarily used to identify pathogens rapidly and in some cases, when growth in culture takes too long to be practical. For example, immunoassays for the detection of urinary *Legionella pneumophilia* antigen are typically preferred over culture in the diagnosis of severe CAP, as this organism is slow growing (3 to 5 days for culture to become positive).[18] *Legionella pneumophilia* antigen can be detected in the urine of patients with current or recent (within weeks) infection. The *L. pneumophilia* antigen test only detects serogroup 1, although this subgroup represents about 80 to 95% of infections. This test has a reported sensitivity of 70 to 90% and specificity of nearly 99% for this serogroup.

Pneumococcal urinary antigen tests are also available to aid in the diagnosis of CAP, providing results within about 15 minutes. This test may be helpful when respiratory specimens cannot be obtained in a timely fashion or when antimicrobial therapy has already been initiated (which decreases the yield of *S. pneumoniae* in culture). This test has a reported sensitivity of 50 to 80% and specificity of greater than 90%. Drawbacks to these tests include the fact that pneumococcal and *Legionella* urine antigen testing does not provide susceptibility information and that the results of these tests commonly do not lead to changes in antimicrobial therapy for CAP, as currently recommended regimens already provide coverage for these organisms. Finally, immunoassays are also available for the detection of group A streptococci (*S. pyogenes*) and *C. difficile*.

Molecular techniques, such as polymerase chain reaction (PCR) and peptide nucleic acid fluorescent in situ hybridization (PNA FISH) are rapidly expanding tools that may prove useful in treatment decisions. These techniques rapidly identify microorganism-specific DNA, RNA, or proteins in a specimen, with results usually available within hours (within 1 hour with some PCR tests).[19] For example, PCR testing is now available for MRSA, *C. difficile*, and viral pathogens such as influenza, herpes simplex virus, and human immunodeficiency virus, among others. Certain PCR tests can also rapidly differentiate between methicillin susceptible *S. aureus* (MSSA) and MRSA in a specimen. Multiple PNA FISH tests are also now available, and include rapid testing for Gram-positive, Gram-negative, and fungal pathogens immediately upon detection of positive cultures. PNA FISH assays, for example, may differentiate between *S. aureus* and other staphyloccocci, or between *C. albicans* and other yeasts faster than standard culture techniques. Emerging data suggests improvement in antimicrobial utilization with these techniques.[20] While molecular methods appear to be helpful, at this time they supplement, rather than replace, standard identification and susceptibility methods. A detailed discussion of the specific methodology and clinical use of these emerging technologies is beyond the scope of this text.

Finally, procalcitonin, a biomarker currently being investigated in the management of sepsis, appears to have a role in determining patient specific antimicrobial treatment duration. The role of serum procalcitonin concentrations in the diagnosis and treatment of sepsis is further discussed in Chapter 10.

Institution-Specific Considerations

Antibiograms

Each medical institution should collect pathogen-specific susceptibility data for selected antimicrobials and create an antibiogram report for annual or semi-annual distribution; unit-specific antibiograms are desirable, but not always available. These antibiograms should be reviewed for trends in susceptibility and utilized as an aid in decisions regarding appropriate empiric antimicrobial selection for disease-specific pathways. For example, *P. aeruginosa* susceptibilities should be tracked, with adjustment of recommendations for empiric nosocomial pneumonia therapy as appropriate. Pharmacists should ensure that they have access to and a thorough knowledge of local antibiograms to optimize recommendations.

Antimicrobial Formulary

Antimicrobial formularies are used for multiple reasons. First, formularies can be used to direct prescribers to the most appropriate antimicrobials based on current disease-specific treatment guidelines and institution-specific patterns of resistance. The formulary can be further enhanced if formal written protocols are implemented to direct antimicrobial use. Formularies may also be used to encourage use of the narrowest spectrum antimicrobials and antimicrobials with the most optimal cost-to-benefit ratio. Formulary restrictions for certain agents (for example: anti-pseudomonal carbapenems, or newer agents with specific limited indications), may limit overuse of broad-spectrum agents or reduce antimicrobial costs. However, while antimicrobial acquisition cost is clearly an important consideration, it is necessary to recognize that the most expensive medication is the one that leads to an adverse drug reaction or that does not result in the intended outcome or cure.

Patient-Specific Considerations

Drug Allergies

Patient drug allergies are commonly reported and often create a dilemma for the critically ill. Due to limited treatment options for many common organisms encountered in the ICU such as *P. aeruginosa* and MRSA, every effort must be made to clarify the nature and severity of reported antimicrobial allergies. This should be done proactively, ideally at admission when possible. Penicillin allergies are among the most commonly reported antimicrobial reactions, although many of these "allergies" actually represent gastrointestinal intolerance or minor rash or pruritis. Severe IgE-mediated anaphylactic reactions are rare but typically result in diffuse erythema, pruritis, urticaria, angioedema, hyperperistalsis, bronchospasm, hypotension, and/or arrhythmia.[21] Such reactions should be investigated thoroughly and clearly documented.

Cross reactivity between penicillin-derived products and other beta-lactam-based antimicrobials, such as cephalosporins and carbapenems, is controversial. Historical estimates indicated approximately a 10% rate of cross-reactivity between penicillin and cephalosporins. This rather high rate of cross-reactivity may have resulted from early cephalosporins having similar side chains to penicillin and the fact these compounds were also often known to be contaminated with trace amounts of penicillin.[21] Current cephalosporins (especially second through fifth generation agents) typically have dissimilar side chains compared to penicillin and are free of penicillin contamination, which likely results in a lower cross-reactivity risk than historically reported. Carbapenems have a similar structure to penicillin and would be expected to have some degree of cross-reactivity. While previous retrospective data suggested an allergic cross-reactivity rate of approximately 10%,[22,23] recent prospective data based on skin testing suggests this rate may be as low as 1%.[24,25] Aztreonam, a monobactam, has minimal reported cross-reactivity with other beta-lactams and may be used as an alternative agent for most patients with beta-lactam allergies. Allergic reactions to aztreonam are thought to be related to a side chain similar to one found on ceftazidime, so aztreonam should be used with caution in patients with allergies specific to this agent.[21]

For patients with a history of minor adverse effects from penicillin, such as gastrointestinal intolerance or minor rash/pruritis, it is generally reasonable to trial a cephalosporin or carbapenem. For patients with a history of severe penicillin allergy or anaphylaxis (bronchospasm, hypotension, arrhythmia, etc.), the potential risk versus benefit must be carefully considered before agent selection. If non-beta-lactam antimicrobials are not an option, careful selection of a carbapenem or a cephalosporin with dissimilar side chains may be appropriate. If a patient has few or no alternatives, a process called "desensitization" may also be considered. Desensitization involves administration of incrementally higher doses of antimicrobial at specified intervals until the goal dose of antimicrobial is reached. This process takes about one day.

Vancomycin may cause a syndrome called "Red Man's" (pruritis and facial, neck, and upper torso flushing) caused by direct release of mast cell mediators due to administration of vancomycin at an excessive infusion rate.[21] This does not represent a true allergy and can be alleviated by infusing each dose of vancomycin over a longer duration, such as extending a one gram dose from a 60-minute to 90-minute infusion. Premedication with diphenhydramine may be given to patients that continue to have symptoms despite prolongation of the vancomycin infusion.

Recent Antimicrobial History

Careful investigation of recent antimicrobial use is an important component of empiric agent selection for infections in the ICU. Recent antimicrobial therapy may give resistant pathogens a selective advantage at the site of infection. Therefore, when recent antimicrobial use is confirmed, it is generally advisable to choose an agent (or agents) from an alternate antimicrobial class. In the case of severe healthcare-associated infections, for example, recent antimicrobial use may increase the risk of infection with resistant pathogens such as *P. aeruginosa* and MRSA.[5] Non-bacterial pathogens such as *Candida* should also be considered in this situation depending on the site of infection and duration of previous antimicrobial therapy.[6,11]

Immune Function

Current immune status is a crucial consideration when selecting an empiric or definitive antimicrobial regimen. Host immune function plays a major role in eradication of microorganisms. For those patients with poor immune function due to cancer, chemotherapy, diabetes mellitus, or other immunosuppressive conditions, more of the burden of microbial eradication is placed on the antimicrobial agent. This commonly requires high doses of agents with a high level of bactericidal activity. Patients with poor immune function are also more susceptible to infection with multi-drug resistant pathogens, such as *P. aeruginosa*. For these reasons, aggressively dosed bactericidal anti-pseudomonal beta-lactam antimicrobials, such as cefepime or carbapenems, are generally preferred for critically ill neutropenic patients with fever (neutropenic fever).[26,27]

Renal Function

Many commonly used antimicrobials in the ICU require dose adjustment for renal function. Although the methods used to estimate renal function are sometimes controversial, the pharmacist is commonly asked to make this estimate and adjust antimicrobial doses accordingly. The most common pitfall in this decision process is inadequate dosing due to excessively conservative estimates of renal function or decisions made without considering enough patient specific factors such as urine output. For example, a serum creatinine concentration may be elevated in response to significant dehydration, yet quickly correct to the normal range with fluid resuscitation. If a hasty dosing decision was made based on a renal function estimate with the initial creatinine measurement, significant underdosing may occur. Careful attention to all data elements that indicate kidney function will result in the most appropriate recommendations regarding dosing in these patients.

Patients with significant renal impairment often require renal replacement therapies, such as hemodialysis, sustained low-efficiency dialysis (SLED), and continuous veno-venous hemodialysis (CVVHD), as discussed in Chapter 11. These renal replacement therapies have varying effects on the elimination of many antimicrobials and therefore may affect selection of antimicrobial dose.

Finally, it is also important to note that certain antimicrobials may impair renal function. Amphotericin, aminoglycosides, and vancomycin are well-known for their nephrotoxic potential, and this is particularly true when used in combination. Beta-lactam antimicrobials have also been known to impair renal function by causing interstitial nephritis.

Patient Size/Weight

Patient size and weight may be important considerations when selecting antimicrobial agents. Most antimicrobial agents are dosed on a milligram per kilogram basis for the neonatal or pediatric population, and certain antimicrobial agents used in the adult ICU population are dosed in this manner as well. Knowing whether to use actual, lean, or an adjusted weight for calculations can be controversial and generally antimicrobial-specific. For example, vancomycin is usually dosed based on actual body weight, while intravenous acyclovir should be dosed based on lean body weight. For those patients with morbid obesity, evidence for the most appropriate antimicrobial dosing is lacking for many agents. In general, aggressive dosing at the upper end of dosage ranges is recommended for these patients, particularly for agents that are not typically dosed based on body weight.

Pharmacokinetic and Pharmacodynamic Considerations

Knowledge of the fundamentals of antimicrobial pharmacokinetics (PK) (what the body does to the drug) and pharmacodynamics (PD) (what the drug does to the body or microorganism) is essential for pharmacists working in the critical care setting. Recognizing relevant, drug-specific PK and PD parameters is vital in selecting not only the most appropriate antimicrobial, but also the dose. Appropriate antimicrobial dosing is important, as inadequate dosing may result in the development of resistance and potentially treatment failure.

Pharmacists are commonly asked to provide PK services by calculating patient-specific dosage regimens to achieve target antimicrobial concentrations, and this is most easily accomplished for medications with readily available testing for serum concentrations. For example, pharmacists commonly calculate vancomycin dosage regimens to achieve a goal vancomycin trough concentration or aminoglycoside regimens that provide peak and trough concentrations within specified ranges. Pharmacists are also often asked to provide dosing recommendations for antimicrobial agents in which serum concentration measurements are not readily available, such as beta-lactams and fluoroquinolones.

The expected concentration of an antimicrobial at the infection site may also be an important consideration in both antimicrobial selection and dosing. Carbapenems, for example, are commonly used for infected pancreatic necrosis, as carbapenems achieve high concentrations in pancreatic tissue. Similarly, ceftriaxone or cefotaxime are considered first line agents for bacterial meningitis, as these antimicrobials may achieve therapeutic concentrations in the central nervous system if high doses are used (for example, ceftriaxone 2 gm IV every 12 hours).[10] Interestingly, the differences in tissue concentrations achieved by specific agents can lead to clinical controversy for certain infections. Linezolid, for example, typically achieves epithelial lining fluid concentrations similar to or higher than concomitant serum values, while levels of vancomycin in lung tissue and epithelial lining fluid may be only a fraction of the serum value.[28] The therapeutic implications of the difference in lung tissue concentrations between these two agents in the treatment of MRSA pneumonia will be discussed later in this chapter.

The PK and PD activity of antimicrobials can generally be categorized as time-dependent, concentration-dependent, or dependent on the ratio of area under the drug concentration-time curve to minimum inhibitory concentration (AUC/MIC). An illustration of these PK/PD parameters is found in Figure 13–1.

Time-Dependent Antimicrobials

Beta-lactam agents, such as penicillins, cephalosporins, and carbapenems, are classic time-dependent antimicrobials. To achieve optimal bactericidal activity, concentrations of these antibacterials should exceed the MIC of the causative pathogen for at least 40% of the dosing interval for carbapenems, 50% for penicillins, and 70% for cephalosporins.[29,30] This generally requires administration of standard doses of the selected beta-lactam agent at specified intervals, often requiring multiple daily doses for the desired time-dependent effect. Recent MIC increases with certain organisms (for example, *P. aeruginosa*) have lead to the use of unique dosing strategies with beta-lactams to ensure drug concentrations exceed the MIC for the desired percentage of the dosing interval.[30] Such strategies may include extended

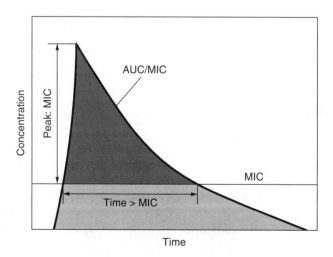

Figure 13–1 Pharmacokinetic/Pharmacodynamic Parameters

infusions over 2 to 6 hours or continuous infusions to achieve this target as opposed to standard 30- to 60-minute infusions.[31]

Concentration-Dependent Antimicrobials

Aminoglycosides are examples of concentration-dependent antimicrobials used in clinical practice. In general, the higher the peak concentration achieved with these agents, the higher the rate of antimicrobial kill. Because of this property, these agents are ideally suited for high doses (e.g., 5 to 7 mg/kg/dose with gentamicin or tobramycin) given at extended intervals of 24 hours or longer. This strategy maximizes the rate of antimicrobial kill, while potentially minimizing the risk of toxicity (primarily renal) by allowing for a period of time at the end of the dosing interval in which serum concentrations are low or unmeasurable. Such doses of aminoglycosides also provide a substantial post-antibiotic effect (bacterial growth suppression following brief antimicrobial exposure). Daptomycin is another concentration-dependent antimicrobial commonly used in the ICU.

Agents Influenced by AUC/MIC

The AUC/MIC ratio can be thought of as the amount of exposure of antimicrobial exceeding the MIC of the organism. Maximizing AUC/MIC with certain antimicrobials, such as fluoroquinolones,[32] vancomycin,[33] and linezolid (although this agent also appears to demonstrate time-dependent properties),[34] may optimize efficacy while limiting the potential for resistance. Optimization of this ratio in the setting of renal impairment may require careful dose adjustment, utilizing high doses of renally eliminated antimicrobials with reduced frequency (e.g., reduce from every 24 to 48 hours with levofloxacin) to maximize the AUC/MIC ratio while minimizing the risk of adverse effects. Application of AUC/MIC principles in the use of vancomycin will be discussed later in this chapter.

Antimicrobial Resistance Considerations

Methicillin-Resistant Staphylococcus Aureus

Staphylococcus aureus is an ever-increasing cause of serious bacterial infection in ICU patients. In fact, some studies indicate *S. aureus* has become the leading cause of nosocomial pneumonia, with isolates reported as methicillin-resistant in more than 50% of cases.[35] Based on the relatively high incidence of MRSA infection in many ICUs, antimicrobial activity against this pathogen is often an important consideration when determining empiric regimens.

MRSA results from acquisition of the *mecA* gene, which encodes for an altered penicillin binding protein (PBP2a) with reduced affinity for beta-lactam antimicrobials. This organism can infect nearly any tissue or organ system and is commonly responsible for not only nosocomial pneumonia, but also catheter-associated bacteremia, SSTI, and less commonly, intra-abdominal infection. While traditionally a pathogen of nosocomial acquisition only, community-associated MRSA (CA-MRSA) infections are becoming more common. CA-MRSA is most often responsible for SSTIs,[12] but may also cause other infections, such as necrotizing community-acquired pneumonia severe enough to warrant ICU admission.[3]

MRSA Risk Factors   Major risk factors for nosocomial MRSA infection include prolonged hospitalization, recent hospital admission or surgery, residence in a long-term care facility, indwelling catheters or devices, dialysis, recent antimicrobial use, and colonization with MRSA prior to or during hospital stay, among others.[36-38] Risk factors for CA-MRSA are less clearly defined, but patients infected with this organism are usually relatively young and with few chronic medical conditions.[38] This pathogen seems most prevalent in pediatric and neonatal populations, prisoners, indigenous populations, intravenous drug abusers, or in persons of low socioeconomic status. Patients placed in situations of close physical contact, such as those that participate in contact sports or the military, also seem at higher risk of CA-MRSA.

MRSA Treatment Options   Vancomycin binds to the D-alanyl-D-alanine portion of peptidoglycan precursors, preventing synthesis of the bacterial cell wall. This agent is generally considered the "gold standard" for treatment of serious infections caused by MRSA, including pneumonia, SSTIs, bacteremia, and meningitis. Although vancomycin continues to be recommended among first line agents for the treatment of MRSA infections,[28] serious concerns have developed regarding the efficacy of this agent in recent years. A new phenomenon, referred to as "MIC creep," has been reported.[39] Isolates exhibiting "MIC creep" have minimum inhibitory concentration values at the high end of the susceptibility range (MIC = 1.5 or 2 mcg/mL). Infections caused by MRSA isolates with MICs at this level have been associated with a higher rate of treatment failure and mortality when compared to infections caused by isolates with lower vancomycin MIC values.[40,41]

An important consideration in the utilization of vancomycin for severe MRSA infections is the target AUC/MIC ratio. This ratio can be approximated with the equation below. A recent review of vancomycin dose optimization describes the use of this equation in further detail.[42]

$$AUC_{0-24} = (\text{Total vancomycin dose over 24 hours}) / Cl_{vanco}$$

Animal and limited human studies indicate an AUC/MIC ratio of 400/1 is optimal for the treatment of serious MRSA infections.[33,43] Selection of appropriate dose and goal trough is imperative in achieving this target ratio. Loading doses of 25 to 30 mg/kg, with subsequent maintenance doses of 15 to 20 mg/kg every 8 to 12 hours, generally will produce a trough of 15 to 20 mcg/mL in most patients with normal renal function. A vancomycin trough of 15 mcg/mL is considered a reasonable surrogate marker of achievement of an AUC/MIC ratio of 400 if the MRSA isolate has an MIC of 1 mcg/mL or less.[33,43] Unfortunately, it is unlikely that such a dosing strategy and subsequent expected trough (15 to 20 mcg/mL) will achieve the optimal AUC/MIC target of 400/1 if the MRSA isolate has a vancomycin MIC of 2 mcg/mL or greater. Furthermore, the aggressive vancomycin dosing strategies often required to achieve this optimal 400/1 ratio in this situation (often 4 grams or more per day) appear to result in unacceptable rates of nephrotoxicity.[44] Alternative antimicrobials should be considered for isolates at this MIC level (2 mcg/mL or greater), or any time patients are not responding to therapy.

Currently available alternatives to vancomycin for the treatment of serious MRSA infections include linezolid, daptomycin, tigecycline, quinupristin/dalfopristin, telavancin, and ceftaroline. Linezolid, a protein synthesis inhibitor at the 50S ribosome, has been extensively studied for the treatment of nosocomial pneumonia and SSTI. A retrospective MRSA subgroup analysis of combined results from two major nosocomial pneumonia trials indicated a potential mortality advantage with linezolid when compared to vancomycin.[45] However, a meta-analysis comparing linezolid to glycopeptides (including vancomycin) did not confirm this mortality benefit.[46] A yet unpublished prospective, randomized, double-blind, multicenter trial[47] comparing linezolid versus vancomycin for the treatment of confirmed MRSA nosocomial or healthcare-associated pneumonia may provide more definitive information regarding the potential superiority of linezolid compared to vancomycin for this infection.

Serious adverse effects of linezolid include thrombocytopenia and myelosuppression. Peripheral and optic neuropathy have also been reported with long-term use. Linezolid inhibits monoamine oxidase, resulting in reduced metabolism of serotonin. The concomitant use of linezolid and serotonergic agents, such as selective serotonin reuptake inhibitors (SSRIs) or tricyclic antidepressants (TCAs), may result in serious and sometimes fatal serotonin syndrome reactions characterized by hypertension, hyperthermia, myoclonus, arrhythmias, and confusion.

Daptomycin is a concentration-dependent intravenous antimicrobial with bactericidal activity caused by rapid depolarization of bacterial cell membrane potential, resulting in inhibition of DNA, RNA, and protein synthesis, ultimately leading to cell death but without cell lysis. This agent is primarily used in the treatment of SSTI and bacteremia with or without right-sided endocarditis. Daptomycin has the advantage of once-daily dosing and relatively few side effects, although myopathy and rhabdomyolysis have been reported. Creatinine phosphokinase (CPK) should be monitored weekly during daptomycin use, with therapy discontinued if CPK levels are greater than 1,000 U/L with symptoms, or greater than 2,000 U/L regardless of the presence of symptoms, according to product labeling.[48] In addition, withholding other agents with the potential to cause rhabdomyolysis, such as statins, should also be considered. Case reports of pulmonary eosinophilia have been reported with this agent.[49] It should be noted that daptomycin is inactivated by pulmonary surfactant, and is therefore not appropriate for treatment of pulmonary infections.[48]

Tigecycline is a glycylcycline antimicrobial structurally similar to minocycline, but with a broad range of antimicrobial activity, including activity against pathogens resistant to antimicrobials from the tetracycline class. This agent is a primarily bacteriostatic protein synthesis inhibitor that exhibits advanced binding to the 30S ribosomal subunit due to side chain modification, resulting in a broad spectrum of activity that includes most aerobic Gram-positive organisms (including MRSA and VRE) and many aerobic Gram-negative organisms (*Pseudomonas* and *Proteus* are notable exceptions). This agent is also active against most clinically relevant anaerobic and atypical organisms. The wide spectrum of activity with tigecycline makes this agent most appropriate when MRSA is a component of a polymicrobial infection. Tigecycline has a large volume of distribution, resulting in high tissue concentrations but relatively low serum concentrations. The relevance of low tigecycline serum concentrations in critically ill patients with bacteremia is unclear, but selection of an alternative agent in this situation may be warranted. In fact, the Food and Drug Administration (FDA) released a safety announcement based on a pooled analysis of clinical trial data showing higher mortality with tigecycline compared to alternative treatments in patients with serious infections.[50] This increased risk was most clearly seen in patients treated for ventilator-associated pneumonia (not an FDA-approved indication). The most common adverse effect with tigecycline is severe nausea and vomiting, which may lead to discontinuation of therapy in some patients.

Quinupristin/dalfopristin, a combination of streptogramin, telavancin, a lipoglycopeptide, and ceftaroline, a new anti-MRSA cephalosporin, are also potential options for severe MRSA infections in the ICU. While quinupristin/dalfopristin has proven efficacy in the treatment of SSTI and pneumonia, adverse effects of this agent (thrombophlebitis, arthralgias, and myalgias) limit its use. Telavancin is a relatively new agent with proven activity against SSTI, but limited clinical experience and the potential risk of nephrotoxicity[51] do not encourage first line use at this time. Ceftaroline, a novel compound with high affinity for PBP2a (resulting in MRSA activity) and PBP2x (resulting in enhanced activity against *S. pneumoniae*, including drug-resistant strains), has been recently approved for the treatment of skin and soft tissue infections and CAP. The role of this agent in treatment guidelines is yet to be determined. Ceftobiprole, another anti-MRSA cephalosporin investigated for the treatment of complicated skin and soft tissue infections, is unavailable in the United States at the time of this writing.

Vancomycin-Resistant Enterococcus

Vancomycin-resistant enterococcus (VRE) is among the leading causes of nosocomial infection in the United States, and infections with this pathogen are most commonly found in the ICU. This organism commonly causes bacteremia (especially central vascular catheter-related), infected surgical wounds, intra-abdominal infections, and urinary tract infections, among others.[52] Positive cultures do not always represent true infection, however, as colonization with this organism in non-sterile sites, such as the peri-rectal or rectal area, often occurs. Vancomycin-resistant enterococcus develops as a result of changes in penicillin binding proteins due to acquisition of VanA, VanB, or VanD genes that encode for ligases that produce D-alanyl-D-lactate, which replaces D-alanyl-D-alanine at the terminal end of peptidoglycan cell wall precursors. Vancomycin has poor affinity for D-alanyl-D-lactate, resulting in vancomycin resistance. Vancomycin resistance is most common among *E. faecium* strains. Most VRE strains are multi-drug resistant, often exhibiting resistance to penicillin, ampicillin, aminoglycosides, and fluoroquinolones. Risk factors for VRE infections include patient colonization, contaminated environments, and selective pressure due to antimicrobials. Other risk factors include renal insufficiency, corticosteroid use, neutropenia, or cancer. Treatment options for VRE are limited, but may include linezolid, daptomycin, or tigecycline.

Pseudomonas Aeruginosa and Other Multi-Drug Resistant Gram-Negative Organisms

Pseudomonas aeruginosa is an important ICU pathogen. This organism commonly causes hospital-acquired urinary tract and wound infections, and is the most common multi-drug resistant (MDR) Gram-negative organism associated with hospital-acquired or ventilator-acquired pneumonia.[5] This organism is virtually everywhere (soil, air, water, animals), but does not usually cause community-acquired infections in otherwise healthy people. *Pseudomonas aeruginosa* is an opportunistic pathogen that generally establishes colonization of epithelium first, with subsequent infection only when normal host defenses are impaired or bypassed.

Risk Factors   Risk factors for *P. aeruginosa* are numerous, and often involve compromise of mechanical or immune defenses. For example, endotracheal intubation bypasses normal mechanical defenses of the upper airways, such as cough and mucociliary clearance, which may allow a significant bacterial inoculum of colonizing bacteria to enter the lower airways of the lungs and establish infection. By day five of mechanical ventilation, the upper airways of most patients become colonized with Gram-negative bacilli (potentially *P. aeruginosa*) and therefore these patients are at risk of pneumonia due to this pathogen.[53] Patients with cystic fibrosis or other severe bronchopulmonary diseases may also become chronically colonized with *P. aeruginosa* and become infected in a similar manner due to compromised mechanical or immune function.

Broad-spectrum antimicrobial therapy may eradicate protective normal flora, allowing *P. aeruginosa* to proliferate and ultimately develop serious infection. Treatments such as chemotherapy and conditions such as human immunodeficiency virus (HIV) may impair host immune defenses, allowing for establishment of *P. aeruginosa* infection.[5] Chronic oral corticosteroid use and alcoholism also pose a risk.[3] Finally, skin is another mechanical barrier that can be bypassed due to burns, trauma, or indwelling devices, resulting in infection with this pathogen.

Treatment   Treatment for serious infections caused by *P. aeruginosa* can be challenging, as there is no uniformly active agent. *Pseudomonas aeruginosa* exhibits multiple resistance mechanisms, both intrinsic and acquired in nature. Intrinsic mechanisms, such as beta-lactamases and efflux pumps, commonly render narrow-spectrum beta-lactam and non-beta-lactam agents ineffective. Acquired mechanisms of resistance are constantly developing and may include porin mutations or deletions (which reduces drug penetration), target enzyme mutations, drug modifying enzymes, or mutations resulting in broad-spectrum beta-lactamase production.[54]

Because there is a high risk of acquired resistance, combination therapy for empiric treatment of presumed *P. aeruginosa* infection is generally recommended, at least until culture and susceptibility results have been reported, although there are minimal data to support this practice. Although data suggest there may be synergistic activity against *P. aeruginosa* with certain antimicrobial combinations, evidence regarding outcomes with this approach is limited for immunocompetent patients, commonly resulting in marginal to no benefit.[55-58] When combination regimens are selected, they generally involve agents with different mechanisms of action. For example, an antipseudomonal beta-lactam (e.g., cefepime, piperacillin, or meropenem) is commonly paired with either an antipseudomonal fluoroquinolone (ciprofloxacin or levofloxacin) or an aminoglycoside (tobramycin, gentamicin, or amikacin). De-escalation to monotherapy is generally recommended when susceptibility data is available and the patient is improving. Agents with potential activity against *P. aeruginosa* are listed in Table 13–1.

Other potentially MDR Gram-negative pathogens causing serious ICU infections include *Acinetobacter, E. coli, Enterobacter, Klebsiella*, and *Serratia* species, among others. Resistance in these organisms often involves production of some type of broad spectrum beta-lactamase.[54] These broad spectrum beta-lactamases may include plasmid-mediated extended spectrum beta-lactamases (ESBLs), which inactivate penicillins, cephalosporins, and aztreonam, although carbapenems usually remain active. Plasmids responsible for ESBLs often contain additional resistance determinants that result in resistance to non-beta-lactam agents. AmpC beta-lactamase and carbapenemases are also examples of broad-spectrum beta-lactamases. AmpC beta-lactamase is an inducible broad-spectrum beta-lactamase which may be hyperproduced by mutated strains. Hyperproduction of AmpC beta-lactamase often renders many beta-lactam agents ineffective. Cefepime and carbapenems tend to remain active if hyperproduction of AmpC beta-lactamase is the

Table 13–1 Antimicrobial Agents with Clinically Relevant Activity Against Pseudomonas Aeruginosa

Antimicrobial Class	Agent(s)
Extended-spectrum Penicillins	Piperacillin
	Ticarcillin
Third-generation Cephalosporin	Ceftazidime
Fourth-generation Cephalosporin	Cefepime
Carbapenems	Imipenem
	Meropenem
	Doripenem
Fluoroquinolones	Ciprofloxacin
	Levofloxacin
Aminoglycosides	Tobramycin
	Gentamicin
	Amikacin
Monobactams	Aztreonam
Polymyxins	Colistin

sole mechanism of resistance. Carbapenemases hydrolyze most beta-lactam agents to some degree, but may go undetected without appropriate laboratory testing, as carbapenem MICs may remain in the susceptible range. Full resistance to carbapenems due to carbapenemases does not usually occur unless outer membrane permeability has also been altered. Antimicrobial options may be limited for carbapenemase-producing pathogens. Non-beta-lactam agents, such as amikacin, tigecycline, or colistin, for example, may retain clinically relevant activity.

Fungi

Fungal infections can be a significant source of morbidity and mortality in the critically ill. Risk factors such as immune suppression and use of broad-spectrum antibacterials, central venous catheters, parenteral nutrition, renal replacement therapy, and prosthetic implantable devices can allow for fungal infections to take hold.[59] Fungal infections can be especially hard to treat, and the antifungal agents used can be associated with significant toxicity. Fungus can also be a common contaminant of cultures, and the clinician must determine if a positive fungal culture represents an active pathogen or not. While a full description of antifungal treatments is beyond the scope of this chapter, a brief description of common pathogens and preferred treatments is provided here.

Candida species comprise the most common fungal pathogens, with *C. albicans* and *C. glabrata* being most frequently associated with severe disease.[60] Increasing resistance to fluconazole has lead to recommendations for the use of the echinocandin drug class in clinically unstable patients with proven or suspected invasive candidiasis, especially for those patients with recent azole exposure.[59,60] The echinocandin class includes micafungin, caspofungin, and anidulafungin, and all three are given intravenously. These agents provide fungicidal activity against most *Candida* species, with relatively few side effects and drug interactions in comparison to other antifungal agents. Transitioning from an echinocandin to fluconazole is reasonable when the patient becomes clinically stable and the identified isolate is likely to be susceptible to fluconazole (for example, *C. albicans*). Fluconazole is available both intravenously and orally (high bioavailability), and is relatively well tolerated by most patients, although hepatotoxicity and rash can occur. All azoles inhibit the cytochrome P450 enzyme system and have the potential to cause significant drug interactions when combined with agents metabolized by this system. It is important to note that fluconazole is poorly active against *C. krusei* and some *C. glabrata*. Current recommendations suggest patients with *C. glabrata* infections should not be treated with fluconazole unless isolate susceptibility can be confirmed.[59] Current guidelines do state, however, that if a patient improves with empiric fluconazole therapy (prior to knowledge of species identification) and subsequent follow-up cultures have been negative, it is considered reasonable to continue fluconazole.[59] An alternative azole agent, voriconazole, and amphotericin B can also be considered for the treatment of invasive candidiasis in selected circumstances, but these agents have their own toxicity issues. Voriconazole causes visual disturbances in addition to the adverse effects and drug interactions common to the azole class. Adverse effects are particularly problematic with amphotericin B and include nephrotoxicity, electrolyte disturbance (magnesium and potassium wasting), and infusion reactions resulting in fever, chills, and rigors. Lipid amphotericin B formulations help to attenuate these adverse effects, but they remain a concern.

Additional organisms, such as *Aspergillus, Histoplasma, Blastomyces, Cryptococcus, Cocidiodes,* and *Pneumocystis,* can also result in critical illness. Serious infections caused by these fungal species are most often identified with immunocompromised patients.[60] Medications used to treat infections caused by these pathogens (exluding *Pneumocystis*) include voriconazole, itraconazole, posaconazole, amphotericin B, and the echinocandins. Trimethoprim-sulfamethoxazole is the treatment of choice for *Pneumocystis* pneumonia.

EMPIRIC THERAPY APPROACHES

Empiric therapy options for specific infections are guided by many factors, most of which have already been discussed in this chapter, but suspected site of infection is one of the most important. Treatment guidelines are available for many infections common to the ICU, and these guidelines are usually written by professional organizations with various areas of expertise and are often frequently updated. The recommendations within these guidelines can be a valuable resource in making not only patient-specific treatment decisions, but also in developing institution-specific empiric treatment guidelines or protocols.

Sepsis

Sepsis is the most serious life-threatening infection-related complication found in the ICU. Appropriate empiric antimicrobial selection is a key component in reducing mortality with this condition and is typically directed at the site of infection. The most common sources of infection that leads to sepsis are pulmonary, intra-abdominal, urinary tract, and bacteremia.

Appropriate therapeutic approaches for the treatment of sepsis are discussed in Chapter 10, and antimicrobial therapy should target the suspected site of infection and pathogens as described below.

Pneumonia

Community-Acquired Pneumonia

Guideline-recommended empiric antimicrobial therapy for CAP in the ICU is designed to ensure adequate activity primarily against *S. pneumoniae* and the atypical pathogens (*Mycoplasma, Chlamydia,* and *Legionella*), as well as additional pathogens previously described,[3] with combination therapy.[3,61] Guidelines for the treatment of MRSA also suggest adding empiric coverage for MRSA in patients with CAP that is severe enough to warrant ICU admission.[28] This coverage spectrum can be accomplished through the use of an antipneumococcal beta-lactam (cefotaxime, ceftriaxone, or ampicillin-sulbactam) used in combination with either azithromycin or an antipneumococcal fluoroquinolone (levofloxacin or moxifloxacin).[3] Vancomycin or linezolid may also be added for MRSA coverage.[28] In CAP patients with significant pseudomonal risk factors (immune suppression, recent broad spectrum antimicrobial use, severe bronchopulmonary disease, chronic oral corticosteroid use),[3] regimens should include a combination of two agents active against *P. aeruginosa*, while maintaining adequate activity against *S. pneumoniae* and the atypicals. A combination of piperacillin/tazobactam and levofloxacin is one example of this type of regimen.

Optimal duration of therapy for CAP is determined based on patient response. Current guidelines suggest patients should be treated for a minimum of 5 days, with therapy discontinuation recommended when the patient has been afebrile for 48 to 72 hours and is clinically stable.[3] Longer durations of therapy may be necessary if the initial regimen was not active against the identified pathogen or if extrapulmonary infection is present. Tigecycline and ceftaroline have also recently received CAP indications, but older therapies remain the mainstay of treatment.

Nosocomial Pneumonia

Nosocomial pneumonia is now divided into three major categories: hospital-acquired (HAP), ventilator-associated (VAP), or healthcare-associated (HCAP).[5] Hospital-acquired pneumonia is defined as pneumonia that occurs 48 hours or more after admission, but was not incubating at the time of admission. Similarly, VAP is defined as pneumonia occurring 48 to 72 hours after endotracheal intubation. Patients with HCAP usually develop pneumonia outside the hospital setting, but have specific risk factors for infection with nosocomial pathogens that include hospitalization for at least 2 days in the previous 90 days, residence in a nursing home or long-term care facility, home infusion therapy or wound care, and chronic dialysis.

Treatment decisions for nosocomial pneumonia are generally based on the presence of risk factors for MDR pathogens, which include antimicrobial therapy within the previous 90 days, current hospitalization of 5 days or more, high frequency of antibiotic resistance within the community or specific hospital unit, or immunosuppressive disease and/or therapy.

Patients developing HAP or VAP within the first 3 to 4 days of hospital admission are termed to have "early onset" disease if risk factors for MDR pathogens are not present. Pathogens responsible for early onset HAP or VAP are similar to those responsible for CAP, although atypical organisms rarely play a role. Limited spectrum antimicrobials are recommended for "early onset" HAP or VAP, and must provide adequate activity against *S. pneumoniae, H. influenzae*, methicillin-susceptible *S. aureus* (MSSA), and susceptible enteric Gram-negative bacilli such as *E. coli* and *K. pneumoniae*. Monotherapy is generally recommended and may include ceftriaxone, levofloxacin or moxifloxacin, or ertapenem, according to current guidelines.[5]

Patients developing HAP or VAP on or after day 5 of admission or have previous MDR risk factors are categorized as having "late onset" disease. Because of MDR risk, empiric antimicrobial therapy should be broad, as inappropriate empiric regimens are associated with increased mortality in critically ill patients. In general, these empiric regimens should be designed to promote appropriate therapy for *P. aeruginosa* and MRSA. Because *P. aeruginosa* is generally a MDR pathogen, two-agent combination regimens with potential activity against this organism are recommended as part of initial therapy. The two antipseudomonal agents should have different mechanisms of action to increase the likelihood of selecting at least one agent to which the organism is ultimately found susceptible. Recent antimicrobial therapy (within the past 2 weeks) should also be considered, avoiding recently used agents due to risk of resistance. A third agent with activity against MRSA (vancomycin or linezolid most commonly) is also recommended if MRSA risk factors are present or if there is a high incidence of MRSA locally.[5] Recommended empiric treatment options for late onset HAP, VAP, or HCAP are listed in Figure 13–2.

De-escalation, or narrowing the spectrum of antimicrobial selection, can generally be achieved within 48 to 72 hours after initiation of the empiric regimen when respiratory culture results are available. For example, if an empiric regimen of piperacillin/tazobactam, ciprofloxacin, and vancomycin

Antipseudomonal cephalosporin (ceftazidime, cefepime) **OR**
Antipseudomonal carbapenem (imipenem/cilastatin, meropenem, or doripenem)
OR
Antipsuedomonal Beta-lactam/Beta-lactamase inhibitor (piperacillin/tazobactam)

Plus
Antipseudomonal fluoroquinolone (ciprofloxacin, levofloxacin) **OR**
Aminoglycoside (tobramycin, gentamicin, or amikacin)

Plus
Vancomycin or Linezolid

Figure 13–2 Treatment recommendations for hospital-acquired (HAP), ventilator-associated (VAP), or healthcare-associated pneumonia (HCAP)[5]

is used and the sputum culture does not identify MRSA, vancomycin may be discontinued. If this same sputum culture reveals *P. aeruginosa* susceptible to both piperacillin/tazobactam and ciprofloxacin, de-escalation to mono-therapy may be recommended.

Duration of therapy for HAP, VAP, or HCAP depends on the infecting organism, adequacy of empiric therapy, and patient response. Evidence suggests therapy can be limited to 7 days as long as empiric therapy was adequate and *P. aeruginosa* is not the infecting organism.[5,62] Due to data showing a higher risk of relapse with disease caused by *P. aeruginosa*, traditional regimens of 14 days or longer may be advisable.

Intra-Abdominal Infections

Community-acquired infections of the intra-abdominal compartment are generally caused when normal gastrointestinal flora are allowed to penetrate normally sterile tissues or fluids and establish infection. Source control, as well as early and aggressive antimicrobial treatment, is recommended for most patients with intra-abdominal infection. Source control may involve drainage of infected fluid collections or abscesses or other surgical procedures necessary to restore normal gastrointestinal function. Most empiric antimicrobial regimens are broad spectrum, but designed specifically to provide adequate coverage for enteric Gram-negative bacilli, such as *E. coli*, viridans streptococci, and anaerobic bacilli such as *Bacteroides*.[6] For high-severity community-acquired infections or hospital-acquired infections, empiric coverage of enterococci is also recommended. Piperacillin/tazobactam and specific carbapenems, such as imipenem/cilastatin, meropenem, and doripenem, would be appropriate empiric monotherapy approaches. Combination therapy with ceftazidime or cefepime with metronidazole is also recommended. The combination of levofloxacin or ciprofloxacin with metronidazole may also be considered as empiric therapy, although these regimens are not recommended unless local *E. coli* susceptibility to fluoroquinolones exceeds 90%. Guideline recommended options for high-severity community-acquired intra-abdominal infections are listed in Figure 13–3.

While not recommended for routine use as empiric therapy, the addition of an antifungal agent may be considered when *Candida* is grown from intra-abdominal cultures. Empiric therapy against MRSA may also be considered in patients with healthcare-associated infection and known colonization or recent antimicrobial therapy with treatment failure.

De-escalation in the setting of intra-abdominal infection can be difficult, as these infections are generally polymicrobial. Cultures from abdominal specimens may be useful, although not all gastrointestinal organisms (anaerobes, for examples) grow well in culture. In general, regimens may be adjusted based on culture results as long as the chosen regimen still provides reasonable coverage against the most common pathogens (*E. coli*, viridans streptococci, and *Bacteroides*). According to current guidelines, duration of antimicrobials should be limited to 4 to 7 days in most situations. When source control (drainage of an abscess, for example) is difficult to achieve, duration of therapy may need to be longer and ultimately is determined by patient response.

Monotherapy options
Imipenem/cilastatin
Meropenem
Doripenem
Piperacillin/tazobactam

Combination options
Cefepime plus metronidazole
Ceftazidime plus metronidazole
Ciprofloxacin[a] plus metronidazole
Levofloxacin[a] plus metronidazole

Figure 13–3 Treatment recommendations for community-acquired intra-abdominal infections of high severity[6]

[a]Fluoroquinolones should only be used as empiric therapy if local antibiograms indicate >90% susceptibility of *Escherichia coli* to fluoroquinolones.

Urinary Tract Infections

Severe urinary tract infections are common in the ICU setting. *Escherichia coli* is the most common pathogen responsible, although other Enterobacteriaceae, such as *K. pneumoniae* and *Proteus mirabilis*, and *Staphylococcus saprophyticus* may also be involved in otherwise healthy women with uncomplicated cystitis or pyelonephritis.[7,63] Recommended empiric therapy for hospitalized women in this situation consists of an intravenous fluoroquinolone, aminoglycoside with or without ampicillin, extended spectrum cephalosporin or extended spectrum penicillin with or without an aminoglycoside, or a carbapenem.[63] Patients with short-term catheterization are usually infected with a single organism, most often *E. coli*, but other Enterobacteriaceae, such as *Klebsiella, Serratia, Citrobacter,* and *Enterobacter*; non-fermenters such as *P. aeruginosa*; and Gram-positive cocci such as coagulase-negative staphylococci and enterococci may also be responsible pathogens.[9] Additionally, *Candida* species may also be involved.[8] Patients with chronic urinary catheters are at risk for the above pathogens, but their infections are commonly polymicrobial.[9] Although specific antimicrobial treatment recommendations for catheter-associated urinary tract infections are not made in current guidelines,[9] empiric coverage against Enterobacteriaceae, *P. aeruginosa*, and enterococci seems reasonable. This may include treatment with agents such as piperacillin/tazobactam or an antipseudomonal carbapenem. Recommended duration of therapy ranges from 3 to 14 days depending on the agent chosen, ability to remove the urinary catheter, and patient response to therapy.[9] Although *Candida* is a common colonizer of urinary catheters in the hospital setting, therapy should generally only be initiated (in addition to catheter exchange or removal when possible) when urine cultures are positive for *Candida* and patients demonstrate clinical symptoms.[8]

Other Infections in the Intensive Care Unit

Numerous infections may require treatment and monitoring in the ICU. In addition to the infections already discussed, infections common to ICU patients also include meningitis, severe SSTI, and endocarditis.

Meningitis is a neurologically devastating disease and prompt recognition of the signs and symptoms, diagnostic testing, and initiation of antimicrobial therapy is paramount. The most common pathogen causing meningitis in critically ill patients is *S. pneumoniae*, although varying pathogens can be expected based on the patient's age and predisposing conditions.[10] The reader is encouraged to consult current guidelines for specific details. Following lumbar puncture to obtain a cerebrospinal fluid specimen for analysis and culture, in community-acquired infection, prompt initiation of a high dose intravenous ceftriaxone or cefotaxime (for example, ceftriaxone 2 g every 12 hours) plus intravenous vancomycin (target trough 15 to 20 mcg/mL) should be initiated according to current guidelines. Vancomycin is generally included in this regimen to provide activity against penicillin-resistant *S. pneumoniae*. Ampicillin should also be added to the empiric regimen for infants less than one month of age due to risk of *Streptococcus agalactiae* and *Listeria*, as well as for adults over 50 years of age for coverage of *Listeria*. When culture and susceptibility information is available, vancomycin (and possibly ampicillin) may be discontinued if the pathogen is found to be susceptible to the third generation cephalosporin. Finally, while adjunctive systemic corticosteroid therapy may reduce inflammation-related penetration of antimicrobials such as vancomycin across the blood–brain barrier into the cerebrospinal fluid, systemic corticosteroids may attenuate the destructive inflammatory response associated with bacterial meningitis and have been found to reduce mortality when used in empiric treatment in adults, particularly those cases caused by *S. pneumoniae*.[64] Corticosteroid therapy has also been associated with a reduction of hearing loss in infants and children with bacterial meningitis caused by *H. influenzae*.[10] Systemic corticosteroids should therefore be considered as part of empiric therapy for both adults and infants/children with this condition. Intravenous dexamethasone is the recommended agent (0.15 mg/kg every 6 hours) and should be administered 10 to 20 minutes prior to or with the first dose of antibiotic and continued for 48 to 96 hours.[10]

Aggressive streptococcal, staphylococcal, or clostridial skin and soft tissue infections may occasionally require treatment in the ICU. These infections often require debridement of infected tissue and initiation of a beta-lactam agent in combination with vancomycin or linezolid until culture results are available. The use of ribosomal-active agents, such as clindamycin or linezolid, may also reduce toxin production by these pathogens and limit tissue destruction. Depending upon the patient's co-morbid conditions and extent of infection, SSTIs may require prolonged antibiotic therapy, adjunctive wound treatment measures such as wound vac therapy and hyperbaric oxygen, and extensive debridement and reconstruction surgeries. Pain control can be a significant component of the overall care of these patients as well.

Acute bacterial endocarditis caused by staphylococci can present as severe sepsis and prompt initiation of antimicrobial therapy is necessary. Acute bacterial endocarditis due to Gram-negative bacteria must also be considered. Endocarditis due to other pathogens, such as viridans streptococci, also commonly occurs, although infection with this pathogen is generally subacute in nature, with a more indolent course and lower severity of illness on presentation. A majority of patients with acute bacterial endocarditis will have positive blood cultures if these cultures are drawn before antimicrobial administration, and initial empiric therapy should include activity against *S. aureus* (including coverage for MRSA with risk factors) and Gram-negatives, with de-escalation to definitive therapy when culture results are available. For patients with native valves, this may require the use of vancomycin plus gentamicin and ciprofloxacin until culture results are known. For patients with prosthetic valves, this may require the use of vancomycin in combination with gentamicin, rifampin, and possibly cefepime according to current guidelines.[65] If a pathogen is identified, guidelines recommend specific agents and durations of therapy based on the identified pathogen and susceptibilities, and patient-specific factors, such as the presence of native or prosthetic heart valve, duration of symptoms, and history of intravenous drug use.

POTENTIAL ADVERSE CONSEQUENCES OF ANTIMICROBIAL THERAPY

Clostridium Difficile-Associated Disease

One of the most notorious and immediately apparent consequences of antimicrobial use, overuse, and lack of hand hygiene is *Clostridium difficile*-associated disease (CDAD). *Clostridium difficile*-associated disease develops when normal gastrointestinal flora are eliminated and *C. difficile* is allowed to proliferate unimpeded within the gastrointestinal tract. *Clostridium difficile* produces a potent tissue toxin resulting in gastrointestinal tissue destruction described as pseudomembranous colitis. The most severe presentation, toxic megacolon, can lead to sepsis and ultimately death. Therapy for CDAD generally requires cessation of current antimicrobials (if possible) and treatment with metronidazole or oral vancomycin. Current recommendations suggest utilization of oral vancomycin (125 mg orally 4 times daily) for initial treatment of patients with severe disease manifested by significant leukocytosis (white blood cell count ≥ 15,000 cells/mL) and acute renal insufficiency (serum creatinine ≥1.5 times the premorbid level).[13] For patients with severe CDAD complicated by hypotension, shock, ileus, or megacolon, high dose oral vancomycin (500 mg orally 4 times daily) should be used with or without intravenous metronidazole (500 mg IV every 8 hours). Rectal vancomycin (given as a retention enema) may also be considered in patients with severe CDAD complicated by complete ileus. Colectomy may be required for patients with a high severity of illness. The usual duration of antimicrobial therapy for an initial episode of CDAD should be 10 to 14 days.

Induction of Resistance

Antimicrobial resistance is a well known, but not readily apparent, consequence of antimicrobial use and overuse. Unfortunately, restriction of antimicrobials with problematic resistance often results in overuse and subsequent resistance to alternative antimicrobials or classes of antimicrobials, a phenomenon referred to as "squeezing the balloon."[66] It appears as though the only sure method to limit resistance is by limiting antimicrobial use whenever prudent to do so. A detailed description of specific mechanisms of resistance is beyond the scope of this chapter, but the reader is encouraged to consult the many well-written reviews on this topic.[54]

Other Consequences of Antimicrobial Therapy

Beyond the risk of CDAD and resistance, most antimicrobials have a risk of adverse effects. Classic examples of toxicity that must be anticipated are nephrotoxicity with aminoglycosides and vancomycin, and rash with beta-lactams. Many antibiotics have been associated with thrombocytopenia, and the pharmacist should ensure that antibiotic and other potential causes have been evaluated. Other less-widely known adverse effects include hyperkalemia with trimethoprim-sulfamethoxazole and interstitial nephritis with penicillin-based drugs. The potential risks for these adverse effects should be anticipated and considered when determining recommendations for drug selection and monitoring.

SUMMARY

Knowledge of infectious diseases and their management is an essential component in critical care pharmacotherapy. Many institutional and patient-specific factors must be considered in the selection of appropriate antimicrobial agents based on indication and risk factors for resistance and toxicity. Appropriate de-escalation and treatment duration is paramount in reducing resistance and limiting adverse effects of antimicrobial therapy.

KEY POINTS

- Providing appropriate empiric antimicrobial therapy is vital for reducing mortality in critically ill patients with severe infections. This may require empiric broad-spectrum antimicrobial therapy while awaiting culture results and other diagnostic testing.

- Institution-specific factors (e.g., antimicrobial resistance patterns) and patient-specific factors (e.g., site of infection, recent antimicrobial use, allergy history, infection history, immune function, and organ system function) should be considered when selecting antimicrobial therapy in the critically ill.
- A careful assessment of risk factors for multi-drug resistant pathogens, specifically methicillin-resistant *Staphylococcus aureus* and *Pseudomonas aeruginosa*, should be made when selecting empiric antimicrobial therapy.
- Narrowing antimicrobial regimens based on culture results and diagnostic studies, otherwise known as de-escalation, is recommended for reducing the emergence of resistance and other potential adverse consequences of antimicrobial use (e.g., *Clostridium difficile*-associated disease).

SELECTED SUGGESTED READINGS

- Solomkin JS, Mazuski JE, Bradley JS, et al. Diagnosis and management of complicated intra-abdominal infection in adults and children: guidelines by the Surgical Infection Society and the Infectious Diseases Society of America. *Clin Infect Dis.* 2010;50: 133–164.
- Baddour LM, Wilson WR, Bayer AS, et al. Infective endocarditis: Diagnosis and management. *Circulation.* 2005;111:3167–3184.
- Limper AH, Knox KS, Sarosi GA, et al. An official American Thoracic Society Statement: Treatment of fungal infections in adult pulmonary and critical care patients. *Am J Respir Crit Care Med.* 2011;183:96–128.
- Cohen SH, Gerding DN, Johnson S, et al. Clinical practice guidelines for Clostridium difficile infection in adults: 2010 update by the Society for Healthcare Epidemiology of America (SHEA) and the Infectious Diseases Society of America (IDSA). *Infect Control Hosp Epidemiol.* 2010;31(5):431–455.
- Liu C, Bayer A, Cosgrove SE, et al. Clinical practice guidelines by the Infectious Diseases Society of America for the treatment of methicillin-resistant Staphylococcus aureus infections in adults and children. *Clin Infect Dis.* 2011;52:1–38.
- Mandell LA, Wunderink RG, Anzueto A, et al. Infectious Diseases Society of America/American Thoracic Society consensus guidelines on the management of community-acquired pneumonia in adults. *Clin Infect Dis.* 2007;44(Suppl 2):S27–S72.

- Rybak M, Lomaestro B, Rotschafer JC, et al. Therapeutic monitoring of vancomycin in adult patients: a consensus review of the American Society of Health-System Pharmacists, the Infectious Diseases Society of America, and the Society of Infectious Disease Pharmacists. *Am J Health-Syst Pharm.* 2009;66:82–98.

REFERENCES

1. Kollef MH, Sherman G, Ward S, et al. Inadequate antimicrobial treatment of infections: a risk factor for hospital mortality among critically ill patients. *Chest.* 1999;115:462–474.
2. Ibrahim EH, Sherman G, Ward S, et al. The influence of inadequate antimicrobial treatment of bloodstream infections on patient outcomes in the ICU setting. *Chest.* 2000;118:146–155.
3. Mandell LA, Wunderink RG, Anzueto A, et al. Infectious Diseases Society of America/American Thoracic Society consensus guidelines on the management of community-acquired pneumonia in adults. *Clin Infect Dis.* 2007;44(Suppl 2): S27–S72.
4. Arancibia F, Bauer TT, Ewig S, et al. Community-acquired pneumonia due to Gram-negative bacteria and Pseudomonas aeruginosa: incidence, risk and prognosis. *Arch Intern Med.* 2002;162:1849–1858.
5. American Thoracic Society; Infectious Diseases Society of America. Guidelines for the management of adults with hospital-acquired, ventilator-associated, and healthcare-associated pneumonia. *Am J Respir Crit Care Med.* 2005;171:388–416.
6. Solomkin JS, Mazuski JE, Bradley JS, et al. Diagnosis and management of complicated intra-abdominal infection in adults and children: guidelines by the Surgical Infection Society and the Infectious Diseases Society of America. *Clin Infect Dis.* 2010;50:133–164.
7. Ward TT, Jones SR. Genitourinary tract infections. In: Betts RF, Chapman SW, Penn RL, eds. *Reese and Betts' A practical approach to infectious diseases.* 5th ed. Philadelphia: Lippincott Williams & Wilkins; 2003:493–540.
8. Pappas PG, Rex JH, Sobel JD, et al. Guidelines for treatment of candidiasis. *Clin Infect Dis.* 2004;38:161–189.
9. Hooton TM, Bradley SF, Cardenas DD, et al. Diagnosis, prevention, and treatment of catheter-associated urinary tract infection in adults: 2009 international clinical practice guidelines from the Infectious Diseases Society of America. *Clin Infect Dis.* 2010;50:625–663.
10. Tunkel AR, Hartman BJ, Kaplan SL, et al. Practice guidelines for the management of bacterial meningitis. *Clin Infect Dis.* 2004;39:1267–1284.
11. Mermel LA, Allon M, Bouza E, et al. Clinical practice guidelines for the diagnosis and management of intravascular catheter-related infection: 2009 update by the Infectious Diseases Society of America. *Clin Infect Dis.* 2009;49:1–45.
12. Stevens DL, Bisno AL, Chambers HF, et al. Practice guidelines for the diagnosis and management of skin and soft-tissue infections. *Clin Infect Dis.* 2005;41: 1373–1406.

13. Cohen SH, Gerding DN, Johnson S, et al. Clinical practice guidelines for Clostridium difficile infection in adults: 2010 update by the Society for Healthcare Epidemiology of America (SHEA) and the Infectious Diseases Society of America (IDSA). *Infect Control Hosp Epidemiol.* 2010;31(5):431–455.

14. Engelkirk PG, Duben-Englekirk J. *Laboratory diagnosis of infectious diseases: essentials of diagnostic microbiology.* Baltimore: Lippincott Williams & Wilkins; 2008.

15. Raghavendran K, Wang J, Belber C, et al. Predictive value of sputum gram stain for the determination of appropriate antibiotic therapy in ventilator-associated pneumonia. *J Trauma.* 2007;62:1377–1382.

16. Albert M, Friedrich JO, Adhikari NK, et al. Utility of Gram stain in the clinical management of suspected ventilator-associated pneumonia. Secondary analysis of a multicenter randomized trial. *J Crit Care.* 2008;23:74–81.

17. Souweine B, Veber B, Bedos JP, et al. Diagnostic accuracy of protected specimen brush and bronchoalveolar lavage in nosocomial pneumonia: impact of previous antimicrobial treatments. *Crit Care Med.* 1998;26:236–244.

18. Murray PR, Rosenthal KS, Kobayashi GS, et al. *Medical Microbiology. 4th ed.* St. Louis: Mosby, Inc.; 2002.

19. Procop GW. Molecular diagnostics for the detection and characterization of microbial pathogens. *Clin Infect Dis.* 2007;45;S99–S111.

20. Parta M, Goebel M, Thomas J, et al. Impact of an assay that enables rapid determination of Staphylococcus species and their drug susceptibility on the treatment of patients with positive blood culture results. *Infect Control Hosp Epidemiol.* 2010;31:1043–1048.

21. Robinson JL, Hameed T, Carr S. Practical aspects of choosing an antibiotic for patients with a reported allergy to an antibiotic. *Clin Infect Dis.* 2002; 35:26–31.

22. Sodhi M, Axtell SS, Callahan J, et al. Is it safe to use carbapenems in patients with a history of allergy to penicillin? *J Antimicrob Chemother.* 2004;54: 1155–1157.

23. Prescot WA, DePestel DD, Ellis JJ, et al. Incidence of carbapenem-associated allergic-type reactions among patients with versus patients without a reported penicillin allergy. *Clin Infect Dis.* 2004;38:1102–1107.

24. Atanaskovic-Markovic M, Gaeta F, Mdjo B, et al. Tolerability of meropenem in children with IgE-mediated hypersensitivity to penicillins. *Allergy.* 2008;63: 237–240.

25. Romano A, Viola M, Gueant-Rodriquez RM, et al. Imipenem in patients with immediate hypersensitivity to penicillins. *N Engl J Med.* 2006;354:2835–2837.

26. de Naurois J, Novitsky-Basso I, Gill MJ, et al. Management of febrile neutropenia: ESMO clinical practice guidelines. *Ann Oncol.* 2010;(Suppl 5):252–256.

27. Hughes WT, Armstrong D, Bodey GP, et al. 2002 guidelines for the use of antimicrobial agents in neutropenic patients with cancer. *Clin Infect Dis.* 2002;34:730–751.

28. Liu C, Bayer A, Cosgrove SE, et al. Clinical practice guidelines by the Infectious Diseases Society of America for the treatment of methicillin-resistant Staphylococcus aureus infections in adults and children. *Clin Infect Dis.* 2011;52:1–38.

29. Craig WA. Interrelationship between pharmacokinetics and pharmacodynamics in determining dosage regimens for broad-spectrum cephalosporins. *Diagn Microbiol Infect Dis.* 1995;22:89–96.

30. Burgess DS, Frei CR. Comparison of beta-lactam agents for the treatment of Gram-negative pulmonary infections in the intensive care unit based on pharmacokinetics/pharmacodynamics. *J Antimicrob Chemother.* 2005;56:893–898.

31. Kim A, Sutherland CA, Kuti JL, et al. Optimal dosing of piperacillin-tazobactam for the treatment of Pseudomonas aeruginosa infections: prolonged or continuous infusion? *Pharmacotherapy.* 2007;27:1490–1497.

32. Madras-Kelly KJ, Ostergaard BE, Hovde LB, et al. Twenty-four-hour area under the concentration-time curve/MIC ratio as a generic predictor of fluoroquinolone antimicrobial effect by using three strains of Pseudomonas aeruginosa and an in vitro pharmacodynamic model. *Antimicrob Agents Chemother.* 1996;40:627–632.

33. Moise-Broder PA, Forrest A, Birmingham MC, et al. Pharmacodynamics of vancomycin and other antimicrobials in patients with Staphylococcus aureus lower respiratory tract infections. *Clin Pharmacokinet.* 2004;43:925–942.

34. Andes D, van Ogtrop ML, Peng J, et al. In Vivo pharmacodynamics of a new oxazolidinone (linezolid). *Antimicrob Agents Chemother.* 2002;46:3484–3489.

35. Klevens RM, Edwards JR, Tenover FC, et al. Changes in the epidemiology of methicillin-resistant Staphylococcus aureus in intensive care units in US hospitals, 1993–2003. *Clin Infect Dis.* 2006;42:389–391.

36. Rehm SJ, Tice A. Staphylococcus aureus: Methicillin-susceptible S. aureus to methicillin-resistant S. aureus and vancomycin-resistant S. aureus. *Clin Infect Dis.* 2010;51(S2):S176–S182.

37. Honda H, Krauss MJ, Coopersmith CM, et al. Staphylococcus aureus nasal colonization and subsequent infection in intensive care unit patients: does methicillin resistance matter? *Infect Control Hosp Epidemiol.* 2010;31:584–591.

38. David MZ, Daum RS. Community-associated methicillin-resistant Staphylococcus aureus: epidemiology and clinical consequences of an emerging epidemic. *Clin Microbiol Rev.* 2010;23;616–687.

39. Steinkraus G, White R, Friedrich L. Vancomycin MIC creep in non-vancomycin-intermediate Staphylococcus aureus (VISA), vancomycin-susceptible clinical methicillin-resistant S. Aureus (MRSA) blood isolates from 2001–05. *J Antimicrob Chemother.* 2007;60:788–794.

40. Sakoulas G, Moise-Broder PA, Schentag J, et al. Relationship of MIC and bactericidal activity to efficacy of vancomycin for treatment of methicillin-resistant *Staphylococcus aureus* bacteremia. *J Clin Microbiol.* 2004;42:2398–2402.

41. Lodise TP, Graves J, Evans A, et al. Relationship between vancomycin MIC and failure among patients with methicillin-resistant *Staphylococcus aureus* bacteremia treated with vancomycin. *Antimicrob Agents Chemother.* 2008;52:3315–3320.

42. DeRyke CA, Alexander D. Optimizing vancomycin dosing through pharmacodynamic assessment targeting area under the concentration-time curve/minimum inhibitory concentration. *Hosp Pharm.* 2009;44:751–765.

43. Rybak M, Lomaestro B, Rotschafer JC, et al. Therapeutic monitoring of vancomycin in adult patients: a consensus review of the American Society of Health-System Pharmacists, the Infectious Diseases Society of America, and the Society of Infectious Disease Pharmacists. *Am J Health-Syst Pharm.* 2009;66:82–98.
44. Lodise TP, Lomaestro B, Graves J, et al. Larger vancomycin doses (at least four grams per day) are associated with an increased incidence of nephrotoxicity. *Antimicrob Agents Chemother.* 2008;52:1330–1336.
45. Wunderink RG, Rello J, Cammarata SK, et al. Linezolid vs vancomycin: analysis of two double-blind studies of patients with methicillin-resistant Staphylococcus aureus nosocomial pneumonia. *Chest.* 2003;124:1789–1797.
46. Kalil AC, Murthy MH, Hermsen ED, et al. Linezolid versus vancomycin or teicoplanin for nosocomial pneumonia: a systematic review and meta-analysis. *Crit Care Med.* 2010;38:1802–1808.
47. Kunkel M, Kollef M, Niederman M, et al. Linezolid vs vancomycin in the treatment of nosocomial pneumonia proven due to methicillin-resistant *Staphylococcus aureus*. Abstract presented at the 48th Annual Meeting of the Infectious Disease Society of America; October 21–24, 2010; Vancouver, BC.
48. Daptomycin for injection [package insert]. Lexington, MA: Cubist Pharmaceuticals, Inc.; 2010.
49. Lal Y, Assimacopoulous AP. Two cases of daptomycin-induced eosinophilic pneumonia and chronic pneumonitis. *Clin Infect Dis.* 2010;50:737–740.
50. U.S. Food and Drug Administration. FDA drug safety communication: Increased risk of death with Tygacil (tigecycline) compared to other antibiotics used to treat similar infections. www.fda.gov/drugs/drugsafety/ucm224370.htm. Accessed July 20, 2011.
51. Stryjewski ME, Graham DR, Wilson SE, et al. Assessment of telavancin in complicated skin and skin structure infections study. *Clin Infect Dis.* 2008;46:1683–1693.
52. Cetinkaya Y, Falk P, Mayhall CG. Vancomycin-resistant enterococci. *Clin Micrbiol Rev.* 2000:687–707.
53. Chandler RE. Pulmonary infections. In: Starlin R, Lin TL, eds. *The Washington Manual Infectious Diseases Subspecialty Consult.* Philadelphia: Lippincott Williams & Wilkins; 2005:31–46.
54. Nicasio AM, Kuti JL, Nicolau DP. The current state of multi-drug resistant Gram-negative bacilli in North America. *Pharmacotherapy.* 2008;28:235–249.
55. Hilf M, Yu VL, Sharp J, et al. Antibiotic therapy for Pseudomonas aeruginosa bacteremia: outcome correlations in a prospective study of 200 patients. *Am J Med.* 1989;87;540–546.
56. Fowler RA, Flavin KE, Barr J, et al. Variability in antibiotic prescribing patterns and outcomes in patients with clinically suspected ventilator-associated pneumonia. *Chest.* 2003;123:835–844.
57. Paul M, Benuri-Silbiger I, Soares-Weiser K, et al. Beta lactam monotherapy versus beta-lactam–aminoglycoside combination therapy for sepsis in immunocompetent patients: systematic review and meta-analysis of randomized trials. *BMJ.* 2004;328:668.

58. Heyland DK, Dodek P, Muscedere J, et al. Randomized trial of combination versus monotherapy for the empiric treatment of suspected ventilator-associated pneumonia. *Crit Care Med.* 2008;36:737–744.

59. Pappas PG, Kauffman CA, Andes D, et al. Clinical practice guidelines for the management of candidiasis: 2009 update by the Infectious Diseases Society of America. *Clin Infect Dis.* 2009;48:503–535.

60. Limper AH, Knox KS, Sarosi GA, et al. An official American Thoracic Society Statement: Treatment of fungal infections in adult pulmonary and critical care patients. *Am J Respir Crit Care Med.* 2011;183:96–128.

61. Weiss K, Low DE, Cortez L, et al. Clinical characteristics at initial presentation and impact of dual therapy on the outcome of bacteremic Streptococcus pneumoniae pneumonia in adults. *Can Respir J.* 2004;11:589–593.

62. Chastre J, Wolff M, Fagon J, et al. Comparison of 8 vs 15 days of antibiotic therapy for ventilator-associated pneumonia in adults. *JAMA.* 2003;290:2588–2598.

63. Gupta K, Hooton TM, Naber KG, et al. International clinical practice guidelines for the treatment of acute uncomplicated cystitis and pyelonephritis in women: a 2010 update by the Infectious Diseases Society of America and the European Society for Microbiology and Infectious Diseases. *Clin Infect Dis.* 2011;52:e103–e120.

64. De Gans J, Vand De Beek D. Dexamethasone in adults with bacterial meningitis. *N Engl J Med.* 2002;347:1549–1556.

65. Baddour LM, Wilson WR, Bayer AS, et al. Infective endocarditis: diagnosis and management. *Circulation.* 2005;111:3167–3184.

66. Rahal JJ, Urban C, Segal-Maurer S. Nosocomial antibiotic resistance in multiple Gram-negative species: experience at one hospital with squeezing the resistance balloon at multiple sites. *Clin Infect Dis.* 2002;34:499–503.

Chapter 14

Hematologic Diseases and Bleeding Complications of Critical Illness

Bradley Beck

LEARNING OBJECTIVES

1. Understand the importance of bleeding and thrombosis in the critical care setting.
2. List treatment options for reversing anticoagulation in life-threatening bleeding.
3. Compare and contrast parenteral anticoagulants available for use in the critical care setting.
4. Recall treatment options for heparin-induced thrombocytopenia (HIT).
5. List maternal and fetal complications from HELLP syndrome.
6. Describe important treatment strategies for managing patients with sickle cell anemia.
7. List important laboratory markers to monitor in patients with acute leukemia who are undergoing induction chemotherapy.

INTRODUCTION

Hematologic complications affect nearly all patients in the critical care setting, can include everything from uncontrollable bleeding to thromboembolism with an unknown cause, and range from the reason for admission to the intensive care unit (ICU) (bleeding or infection in a leukemia patient) to a related complication (venous thromboembolism in a patient admitted for a chronic obstructive pulmonary disease (COPD) exacerbation).[1] Sites of bleeding can be obvious, such as a forehead abrasion or a major liver laceration in a trauma patient, or not, such as a chronic gastrointestinal bleed in an elderly nursing home patient. Critically ill patients are also at significant risk for thrombosis due to all of the factors identified in Virchow's triad (hypercoagulable states, vascular injury, and decreased blood flow), manifesting through the presence of lines and tubes, disease processes, and many other conditions.[1] The focus of this chapter will be to review hematologic conditions affecting critically ill patients in two basic discussions: bleeding and clotting. While these two aspects of critical illness may be difficult to visualize, patients are evaluated by the medical team on a daily basis for bleeding and thromboembolism risk and the risks and benefits associated with treatment regimens.

BLEEDING

Typically defined as minor or major bleeding, complications of bleeding can range from insignificant to life-threatening. While there is no standard definition of major bleeding, it has been considered to be any of the following in clinical trials: fatal or life-threatening bleeding, reduction of the hemoglobin by a set number (often 2 to 3 gm/dL), a specified number of transfusions required, or other specific criteria.[2] Bleeding can present from multiple causes: pharmacologic anticoagulation, medication therapy due to adverse events, disease processes, traumatic injury, and surgical complications. These causes of bleeding and their correction will be explored in the following discussion.

A patient receiving anticoagulation therapy presents unique management concerns in a critical care setting due to the inherent risks associated with anticoagulation therapy. Critically ill patients on anticoagulants often require achievement of rapid hemostasis prior to invasive procedures or surgery, and there are several ways to achieve this, including blood product replacement, prothrombin concentrate complexes, recombinant clotting factors, tranexamic acid, and vitamin K replacement.[2-4] Patients with significant bleeding who are not on anticoagulation therapy are typically managed with blood product replacement unless there are laboratory markers that would indicate other pharmacologic therapy as mentioned above.[2,3] Table 14-1 lists common blood products and their make-up. Table 14-2 lists several products used for the reversal of anticoagulant medications.

Table 14–1 Blood Products for Use in Hemorrhaging Patient[3]

Blood Product	What It Provides	Dosing Unit	Indication	Limitations
Packed Red Cells	Hemoglobin	Units (about one pint)	Bleeding, Anemia	Different blood types must be matched, supply, transfusion reactions
Platelets	Platelets	Units (six-pack)	Thrombocytopenia	Supply, transfusion reactions
Plasma	Clotting factor replacement	Units (300–400 ml per unit)	Bleeding, elevated INR	Supply, thawing time (stored frozen)
Cryoprecipitate	Specific plasma components (factor VIII, fibrinogen, factor XIII, von Willebrand factor)	Units (bags)	Factor VIII and von Willebrand factor deficiency, fibrinogen replacement	Specific factors only, thawing time (stored frozen), supply
Whole Blood	All components (red cells, white cells, and platelets)	Unit (about one pint)	Requirements for red blood cells, plasma, and platelets	Not readily available (under study protocols only)

INR = international normalized ratio.

Table 14-2 Pharmacologic Clotting Factor Replacement for Use in Anticoagulation Reversal[3,4]

Product	What It Provides	Dosing Unit	Indication	Benefits	Limitations
Phytonadione (Vitamin K)	Cofactor for production of factors II, VII, IX, and X	1–10 mg IV, Sub-q, oral	Reversal of elevated INR	Cheap, effective reversal of warfarin	Slow: takes 6–12 hours to work and infusion reactions possible
Prothrombin Concentrate Complex (Berliplex, Profilnine SD)	Factors II, VII, IX, and X	Product dependent	Supplement in patients with Factor IX deficiency (anticoagulation reversal is off-label use)	Replaces clotting factors inhibited by warfarin, reverses elevated INR, works in 5–10 minutes	Possible infusion reactions, transmission of viral pathogens
Recombinant Activated Factor VII (Novoseven RT)	Activated factor VII	20–160 mcg/kg (40–80 mcg/kg for trauma)	Hemophilia patients with bleeding episodes (anticoagulation reversal and traumatic hemorrhage are off-label use)	Provides activated clotting factor responsible for activating the extrinsic clotting cascade	Thromboembolic complications (arterial and venous)

For patients who suffer acute hemorrhagic events secondary to anticoagulant therapy, withholding any anticoagulation to prevent further expansion of the hematoma is of the utmost importance.[5,6] After the bleeding event is controlled, the clinician must decide when it is appropriate to (1) provide pharmacological thromboembolism prophylaxis to such patients, and (2) resume therapeutic anticoagulation if it is still indicated. These questions are complicated; the somewhat simplified answer is that pharmacological prophylaxis and therapeutic anticoagulation should only be restarted after evaluation of the risks and benefits and it is determined that the benefits of such treatment outweigh the risks, as a re-bleeding event into the same area that caused the initial event can be fatal.[2]

The guidelines for management of spontaneous intracranial hemorrhage in adults discuss both of the questions asked above.[7] For the first question of prophylaxis, careful evaluation of the benefits and risks for the patient must be completed and thoroughly evaluated prior to starting therapy, but therapy can be safely considered in most patients at 3 to 4 days after bleeding has stopped.[5,6] Regarding the second question of restarting therapeutic anticoagulation, the risks and benefits must be even more closely scrutinized for appropriateness of restarting therapy. Unfortunately the decision isn't all that simple. Historically, the attitude of "Anticoagulation caused this event, so the patient can never be anticoagulated again" was common, but probably inappropriate. A thorough review of the patient's past medical history, a review of the event itself, evaluation of the patient's current status, and other pertinent evaluations should be completed. In some cases, changes of therapy from warfarin to aspirin or clopidogrel may be appropriate.[2,5,7] In other cases, therapy with a vitamin K antagonist or similar therapeutic anticoagulant may still be indicated.[2,5] According to the guidelines for management of spontaneous intracranial hemorrhage, consideration for restarting warfarin 7 to 10 days after the bleeding event occurred is appropriate.[7]

There are many indications for blood product replacement in the intensive care unit, including acute hemorrhage as described above, trauma, anemia of critical illness, anemia of chronic disease, anemia due to medications, hemolysis, and others. In the absence of cardiac disease and early goal-directed therapy for severe sepsis and septic shock, a general threshold for transfusion of packed red blood cells is a hemoglobin of 7 g/dL.[8-10] The reasons for this are two-fold: the risks involved with transfusions and the cost and availability of products.[8,9] Table 14–3 contains a detailed list of risks involved with the transfusion of blood products. Hemoglobin replacement with blood products helps provide the oxygen-carrying capacity necessary to supply all the cells of the body with the products for aerobic metabolism and help carry

Table 14–3 Risks Related to Blood Product Transfusions[8,9]

Risks Related to Blood Product Transfusions	
Viral transmission	Fever
Anaphylaxis	Lung injury
Rash/Pruritis	Hemolysis

Table 14–4 Types of Red Blood Cell Preparations[8]

Blood Product	Difference from Packed Red Cells	Indication
Leukoreduced	Near elimination of leukocytes to reduce cytokine release when transfused	Chronic transfusions, transplant patients, history of reactions to transfusions
Irradiated	Irradiation eliminates presence of T-cells	Reduce reactions when transfused
Washed	Red cells washed to eliminate plasma proteins	Severe reactions to transfusions, some immune globulin deficiencies

away byproducts that are harmful to living cells.[8-10] Furthermore, there are several different types of red blood cell preparations available. Table 14–4 has a description of each type of red blood cell preparation and the role that it plays in the critical care setting.

Aside from packed red cells, which are processed and preserved with a citrate solution to prevent coagulation, other options include whole blood and autologous blood harvesting. Whole blood is a product that has been primarily studied and utilized in the combat trauma setting, where access to processed blood products can take up precious time that does not exist. Whole blood has also been evaluated in the massive transfusion protocol setting for use when a blood bank may be critically low on a specific type of blood product. The autologous blood harvesting process is the least-commonly used of all types of transfusions. This process involves removing red blood cells from fluid collections that have copious amounts of blood present and reinfusing this product after minimal processing. The process of reinfusing blood products that have leaked into fluid collections is not frequently done in the critical care setting, but it is of interest for patients that refuse blood product transfusions for personal or spiritual reasons (i.e., Jehovah's Witness or patients who do not tolerate cross-matched blood products).[8-10]

Finally, cryoprecipitate is a blood product that has specific indications for its use. Cryoprecipitate is a product that is rich in fibrinogen, von Willebrand factor, factor VIII, and factor XIII and gets its name because the production process includes the freezing of blood product to collect and separate these factors. This product is primarily utilized in patients with fibrinogen deficiencies or von Willebrand factor deficiencies, although there are other products specifically marketed for these indications (i.e., Humate P, Alphanate P, etc.). Cryoprecipitate is commonly used in patients with underlying hematologic disease and patients who have a deficiency of fibrinogen due to causes such as consumptive coagulopathies (severe trauma, ongoing hemorrhage).

Certain settings in the treatment of bleeding due to a von Willebrand deficiency can also be treated with a trial of desmopressin acetate.[11] Desmopressin acetate increases levels of factor VIII through action on vasopressin receptors, thus affecting platelet function. This activity can be especially useful in patients who are uremic. Desmopressin acetate is dosed at 0.3 mcg/kg and usually given once, as repeat doses are ineffective.

There are several medication products that can be used to aid in hemostasis. The two most commonly studied include recombinant activated factor VII (rFVIIa) and prothrombin complex concentrate (PCC); both products are described in Table 14-2. The rFVIIa product works by providing a coagulant "burst" at any area that has exposed tissue factor. Tissue factor is typically expressed at the site of an injury, which has made the use of rFVIIa particularly interesting in the area of traumatic injury. After initial success with the product, use has somewhat declined because of the risk of thromboembolism and uncertainty over the most appropriate dose. Several studies have attempted to find the "correct" dose of rFVIIa for subsets of patients (e.g., trauma, liver disease, anticoagulation reversal).[12] Doses between 20 and 60 mcg/kg have been studied with varying levels of success and adverse events. To date, there has not been any single study that has proven one dose superior to another dose when safety and efficacy are concerned. Because rFVIIa will form clots at any site of exposed tissue factor, adverse events, including both venous thromboembolism and arterial thromboembolic events, have occurred in patients receiving rFVIIa; therefore, each patient's risks and benefits of using such an agent should be weighed carefully. PCC is a collection of either three (II, IX, and X) or four factors (II, VII, IX, and X), depending upon the specific product, and it has been found to be particularly useful in reversing the effects of warfarin. Dosing is dependent upon the degree of anticoagulant reversal that is needed, along with patient size.

Medications that exert their pro-coagulant activity through inhibition of fibrinolysis have been utilized in the treatment of bleeding, specifically tranexamic acid and aminocaproic acid. Tranexamic acid has also been used in the setting of refractory hemorrhage due to traumatic injury and for prevention of bleeding peri-operatively with cardiac surgery. Tranexamic acid exerts its pro-coagulant activity through inhibition of fibrinolysis. Studies of tranexamic acid in traumatic injury have been limited, but have produced statistically significant results for reduction of death from bleeding events when compared to placebo.[13] Tranexamic acid may be administered intravenously or orally, but studies in patients with traumatic injury have primarily used the intravenous route. Aminocaproic acid has also been used to control or prevent bleeding in situations where systemic medications for coagulation are not desired. Aminocaproic acid exerts its mechanism of action through competitive inhibition of the activation process for plasminogen. An advantage of aminocaproic acid is that it can be used orally or topically, as well as via parenteral administration. Aminocaproic acid has been primarily utilized topically (oral route) for cases of refractory bleeding in patients undergoing oral surgery and for patients on systemic anticoagulation undergoing dental extraction. Aminocaproic acid has also been evaluated for use in preventing post-operative hemorrhage following cardiovascular surgery.[14] These medications are not without their risks, however, as they have both been associated with case reports of massive arterial and venous thromboembolic complications.[15]

Another set of hemostatic agents includes topical thrombin products. There are two marketed products that are used as topical hemostatic agents during and after surgical procedures, which differ only in their source: one is bovine in origin and the other is recombinant. The primary difference between the two is increased risk of antibody formation to the bovine product, leading to decreased efficacy in producing hemostasis.[16] The two products were compared head-to-head in a phase III study, which showed a decreased immunologic response to recombinant human thrombin and led to its ultimate approval.[17]

HYPERCOAGULABLE STATES

Daily patient evaluation for venous thromboembolism (VTE) prophylaxis is necessary in every critical care setting, as changes in hypercoagulable states, vascular injury, and blood flow occur constantly. Fluctuation in patient variables makes pharmacologic anticoagulation a complicated therapeutic adventure fraught with the potential for severe adverse events. Multiple agents are available for the prevention and treatment of VTE disease in the ICU, including both mechanical devices and pharmacologic options. Mechanical devices are useful when medication prophylaxis is contraindicated. Different agents have compelling indications for use and also reasons to avoid routine use. The following is a brief discussion of each medication and the risks and benefits of therapy. Doses for prevention of VTE will be referred to as prophylactic dosing, while doses that are used for the treatment of active thromboembolism (venous or arterial) will be referred to as treatment dosing.[18,19]

When clotting factor replacement is given, some patients experience systemic hypercoagulability.[3,4,20] Any surface on which tissue factor is exposed provides the correct ingredients for formation of a thromboembolic event (i.e., if the exposed tissue factor is in the brachial vein, then an upper extremity thrombosis may occur, and if the exposed tissue factor is located in one of the coronary arteries, then an acute myocardial infarction may occur, etc.). These unintended adverse events associated with clotting factor replacement have been evaluated extensively in safety and efficacy studies in an attempt to maximize dosing of clotting factor replacement to provide maximal hemostasis while also achieving reduced unintended therapeutic effects.[3,4,20]

Heparin

Heparin exerts its primary anticoagulant activity through the inactivation of thrombin by interacting with antithrombin and inactivating activated factor X.[19] Antithrombin is a natural anticoagulant, but when bound to heparin, antithrombin inactivates thrombin at a much faster rate than occurs naturally. Heparin ranges in molecular weight from 3,000 to 30,000 Daltons. Higher molecular weight heparin is necessary for catalyzing the inactivation of thrombin, and lower molecular weight heparin molecules are responsible for heparin's activity on factor X. Heparin is only available for parenteral administration. Table 14–5 describes heparin dosing for various indications.[18,19]

Heparin therapy is monitored with the activated partial thromboplastin time (aPTT), the activated clotting time (ACT), or the anti-Xa assay.[19,21] The aPTT is used for routine laboratory monitoring of heparin activity, while the ACT is used in cardiac catheterization procedures and cardiac surgery for bedside anticoagulation monitoring. The therapeutic aPTT range within a specific institution is created based upon a regression curve correlated to an anti-Xa activity level of 0.3 to 0.7 units/mL. A more direct measure of heparin activity is the heparin anti-Xa assay.[21] The heparin anti-Xa assay is a measure of the amount of factor Xa that has been inhibited in a laboratory specimen; heparin therapy is then titrated to a "therapeutic range" of anti-Xa values. This anti-Xa assay is generally considered to be a more accurate reflection of heparin activity than the aPTT and is becoming more commonly used

Table 14–5 Heparin Dosing for Various Indications[19]

Indication	Bolus Dose	Maintenance Infusion
DVT prophylaxis	N/A	5000 units subcutaneously every 8 hours
DVT/PE treatment	80 units/kg intravenously	18 units/kg/hr intravenously
ST segment elevation myocardial infarction (STEMI) with thrombolytic therapy	60 units/kg intravenously (maximum of 4000 units)	16 units/kg/hr intravenously (maximum of 1000 units/hr)
Non-ST segment elevation myocardial infarction (non-STEMI) or unstable angina	60–70 units/kg intravenously (maximum of 5000 units)	12–15 units/kg/hr intravenously (maximum of 1000 units/hr)

in clinical practice. One drawback of the heparin anti-Xa assay is that there are few outcome studies using anti-Xa level as a direct monitoring tool, or regarding the risk of recurrent venous thromboembolism or adverse effects (bleeding), whereas this data is more readily available for the aPTT.[21] It is important to clearly understand the laboratory testing in place for heparin at any institution to ensure appropriate dosing and monitoring.

Heparin antithrombin activity is irreversible, but with a systemic half-life of only 90 minutes, the anticoagulant effect dissipates fairly quickly. Unbound heparin can be rapidly neutralized with protamine sulfate at a dose of 1 mg of protamine for every 100 units of heparin, to a maximum of 50 mg of protamine. The dose of protamine for heparin reversal is adjusted based on the amount of time that has passed since the heparin was administered, due to the rapid elimination of heparin in the plasma.[2,19] It should be noted that heparin is metabolized and inactivated by the liver. It is important to remember that the heparin dose needed for anticoagulation is very dependent upon specific patient factors including age, sex, size, and clot burden, to name a few. Specific dose adjustments are not necessary in patients with impaired kidney function; dose adjustments for patients with liver dysfunction are non-specific, as adjustment of dosing based upon aPTT or anti-Xa levels will be better markers of systemic anticoagulation.[19]

Adverse effects of heparin include bleeding, bone loss (in long-term use), and heparin-induced thrombocytopenia. Regular (at least daily) checks of the anti-Xa level or aPTT, depending upon institution protocols, are necessary for monitoring heparin therapy. Levels outside of the therapeutic range increase the risk of adverse events from either a subtherapeutic heparin effect, leading to increasing thrombus size, to a supratherapeutic heparin effect, increasing the risk of bleeding. Other important monitoring items include hemoglobin, platelets, and signs and symptoms of bleeding or thrombosis.[19]

Low-Molecular Weight Heparins

Heparin can be modified by chemical or enzymatic depolymerization to produce a purified selection of heparin molecules that have a lower average molecular weight. These products have been classified as low-molecular weight heparins (LMWH) and have distinct advantages over unfractionated heparin; for example, the LMWH products have higher affinity for factor Xa and lower affinity for factor IIa than heparin. Table 14-6 lists LMWH and doses that are available in the United States. For each specific LMWH, doses for therapeutic anticoagulation have been studied for efficacy and safety up to maximum weights. A current drug reference source should be consulted for individualized and up-to-date recommendations.[19]

The primary improvement of LMWH over unfractionated heparin lies in dosing. LMWH has set doses that require little monitoring in patients who are not pregnant, without renal insufficiency, and are not extremely under or overweight. Doses for patients free of these characteristics need monitoring of blood counts (hemoglobin and platelets) every 1 to 3 days, assessment of kidney function, and physical examination for signs of bleeding and thrombosis daily while on therapy. Patients with the listed characteristics are appropriate for monitoring of the anti-Xa activity for the LMWH prescribed. Anti-Xa activity for LMWH is typically evaluated through use of peak anti-Xa levels drawn 4 to 6 hours after a dose of LMWH is given. Routine use of anti-Xa levels for most or all patients on LMWH greatly reduces their cost–benefit ratio of therapy when compared to unfractionated heparin (UFH).[19] Critically ill patients have often been shown to fall outside of the pharmacokinetic/pharmacodynamic profile for LMWH therapy that would be expected for "normal" patients. There are no unique adverse effects of LMWH over heparin, but the risks of bleeding and heparin-induced thrombocytopenia (HIT) persist, although HIT rates are lower than with heparin. LMWHs also have a longer half-life than heparin—on average, the elimination half-life of LMWH approaches 2 to 3 times that of heparin, allowing for doses to be given once or twice daily.[19] One concern with the LMWHs is that they take longer to clear from the body than UFH, and therefore take longer to reverse without a specific intervention should a bleeding event occur. Therefore, it is important to consider many factors when choosing whether to use heparin or a LMWH for anticoagulation in the critically ill patient.

Table 14-6 Indications and Dosing of LMWH Products and Fondaparinux[19]

Generic Name	Trade Name	Indication	Dose*	CrCl to Adjust Dose	Adjusted Dose*
Dalteparin	Fragmin	Deep vein thrombosis (DVT) prophylaxis for low-risk patients	2500 units daily	†	†
		DVT prophylaxis for high-risk patients	5000 units daily	†	†
		Acute Coronary Syndrome	120 units/kg twice daily (max 10,000 units/dose)	Mild to moderate renal impairment	‡
		VTE treatment	200 units/kg/day (max 18,000 units/dose)	Mild to moderate renal impairment	‡
Enoxaparin	Lovenox	DVT prophylaxis	40 mg daily	Less than 30 ml/min	30 mg daily
		DVT prophylaxis (trauma)	30 mg twice daily	Less than 30 ml/min	30 mg daily
		STEMI (>75 years of age)	0.75 mg/kg twice daily	Less than 30 ml/min	0.75 mg/kg daily
		DVT/Pulmonary embolism (PE)	1 mg/kg twice daily	Less than 30 ml/min	1 mg/kg daily
		DVT/PE	1.5 mg/kg once daily	Less than 30 ml/min	1 mg/kg daily
		Unstable angina	1 mg/kg twice daily	Less than 30 ml/min	1 mg/kg daily
Tinzaparin	Innohep	DVT	1.75 mg/kg daily	Less than 20 ml/min	†
Fondaparinux	Arixtra	Acute STEMI	2.5 mg IV x1, then 2.5 mg sub-q daily	Less than 80 ml/min	†
		DVT/PE (once daily dosing)	< 50kg = 5mg	Less than 80 ml/min	†
			50–100kg = 7.5mg		
			> 100kg = 10mg		
		Non-STEMI	2.5 mg daily	Less than 80 ml/min	†
		DVT prophylaxis	2.5 mg daily	Less than 80 ml/min	†

*All doses sub-cutaneous unless indicated
†Not applicable/available
‡Manufacturer recommends dose adjustment based on anti-Xa level

Because of the difference in molecule size and action, reversal of LMWH is not the same as heparin. LMWH occasionally will respond favorably to reversal with protamine, and the dose of protamine is related to the amount of time that has passed since administration of the LMWH.[2,19] The dosing of protamine for LMWH is controversial, but a dose of 1 mg protamine for each 100 units of dalteparin or 1 mg of enoxaparin is generally recommended.

LMWHs are metabolized, but not inactivated, by the liver and elimination occurs through the kidney.[19] Therefore, patients with renal dysfunction will need reduced doses of LMWH for prophylaxis and treatment; otherwise, LMWH will accumulate in patients with renal dysfunction and can potentially cause increased and unintended supratherapeutic anticoagulation.[19] Dose adjustments are unclear, although reducing the dose of enoxaparin by about 50% is recommended for creatinine clearance levels of 20 to 30 ml/min. Table 14–6 lists common LMWH doses and suggested changes for patients with renal impairment.[19] There is at least one small study that indicates that dalteparin does not need dosage adjustment for a duration of treatment of less than 7 days, but confirmatory studies are needed.[22]

Fondaparinux

Fondaparinux is a synthetic pentasaccharide with affinity only for factor Xa.[19] Fondaparinux is unique in that its half-life approaches 20 hours and is thus given once daily via the subcutaneous route. There is negligible metabolism in the body for fondaparinux, with the primary method of elimination from the body through the kidneys. At the time of this writing, fondaparinux has no specific dosing adjustments for any degree of kidney dysfunction and is thus recommended to be used with caution in creatinine clearance less than 80 ml/min and contraindicated in creatinine clearance less than 30 ml/min.[19] Unlike LMWH, there is no known method of reversing the effects of fondaparinux, so once a dose is given, the patient will be anticoagulated for at least the next 24 hours.[2] Also differing from the LMWH medications is the relative inability to monitor fondaparinux with the standard anti-Xa assay.[19] Many institutions will have the laboratory equipment to monitor LMWH but not fondaparinux due to lack of use, cost, and need to calibrate laboratory equipment more frequently and specifically for fondaparinux.

In the ICU setting, a patient's renal function can fluctuate frequently, making dosing of LMWH or fondaparinux difficult. Consideration for changing therapy to intravenous heparin can help to eliminate concerns over poor distribution from subcutaneous sites of administration, accumulation due to renal dysfunction, reversibility of anticoagulant effect, and others.

Anticoagulation Adverse Events

Another item of concern with parenteral anticoagulation in the critical care setting is the risk of spinal hematoma occurring in patients who have epidural, spinal, intrathecal, or other manipulation with puncture of the vertebral space. This includes intrathecal injection of chemotherapy, spinal taps for cerebrospinal fluid sampling, and placement of epidural catheters for pain control.[2] Neuraxial hematoma can cause paralysis, but this is preventable when parenteral anticoagulation is allowed to reverse prior to the procedure commencing (when possible). Anticoagulation, including prophylaxis, should be held a minimum of two hours following removal of the epidural catheter.[5]

Fibrinolytics

Once a clot is formed, it may be necessary to direct therapy at dissolving the clot. Specific indications for fibrinolysis with medications such as alteplase or reteplase exist, with the primary indication in the critical care setting being for arterial thrombotic events such as acute myocardial infarction (see Chapter 9) or acute ischemic stroke (see Chapter 15). A select set of other indications for fibrinolysis in the ICU include treatment of venous thromboembolism or pulmonary embolism. Fibrinolytics are typically reserved for unique situations where other options for anticoagulation have been exhausted and the outcome is expected to be poor (i.e., fatality or loss of limb).[23] Treatment of a deep venous thrombosis with fibrinolytics is a specialized interventional procedure using low doses of fibrinolytics infused continuously through a catheter that has been placed distal to the thrombus. Fibrinolytic therapy for pulmonary embolism is considered when cardiovascular collapse is present or imminent, defined as hypotension and right ventricular failure. In such situations for PE, alteplase is typically dosed at 100 mg, given intravenously over 2 hours.

Warfarin

The use of warfarin can be difficult in the ICU setting. Changes in type and amount of nutritional intake, fluctuation in liver function due to factors such as hypotension or medications, and a multitude of other factors can adversely affect the transition from therapeutic parenteral anticoagulation to oral warfarin therapy. Warfarin therapy done carefully, monitored closely, and without complications can be less costly than parenteral anticoagulation, but in a constantly changing patient, therapy with warfarin can be unpredictable. Warfarin therapy can be initiated most safely in a stable patient who is tolerating a diet and has recovered from their critical illness.

Heparin-Induced Thrombocytopenia

Heparin-induced thrombocytopenia is a pathological condition characterized by thrombocytopenia in the setting of anticoagulation, occasionally associated with new thrombotic events, that is dependent on both clinical presentation and pathological examination (presence of antibodies) for diagnosis.[24] Heparin-induced thrombocytopenia occurs when antibodies form to the complex of heparin and platelet factor 4.[23] These antibodies recognize the heparin/platelet factor 4 complex on the surface of platelets and destroy the bound platelets.[24,25] This destruction of the platelets causes platelets to become activated and thus, despite thrombocytopenia, widespread clotting can occur in both veins and arteries (anywhere tissue factor is present).[24-27] HIT has been associated with the administration of heparin, low-molecular weight heparin, and fondaparinux exposure, in decreasing order of incidence.[24-33] Literature shows that patients in whom true HIT develops have a 30 to 75% increased risk of new thrombus formation, which can be life and/or limb threatening events.[26]

Heparin-induced thrombocytopenia is an uncommon occurrence, but due to the severe consequences and "labeling" associated with the diagnosis of HIT, further discussion on the incidence of this disease process is warranted.[24-28] "Labeling" of patients as positive for HIT must be done with caution, as this limits therapeutic options for anticoagulation and presents problems for future practitioners that will care for the patient. Patients that are diagnosed with HIT must be counseled of their condition and informed that they should never again receive heparin.[26] Debate exists about whether or not heparin can be re-instituted in patients with HIT after the event has been completely resolved, but in clinical practice with an often unclear history of allergies, re-trials of heparin in a patient with a history of HIT are rare.[24-28]

Patients at high risk of developing HIT fit into the following groups: post-cardiac surgery, previous heparin exposure within 100 days, and therapy with heparin greater than 7 days.[26-28] The risks of developing HIT are 1 to 5% for heparin, approximately 1% for LMWH, and less than 0.1% for fondaparinux.[26,29,30,32,33] It should be noted that HIT is a clinical diagnosis using evaluation of platelet counts (any drop of 30 to 50% should be investigated for HIT), signs of new thrombosis or skin lesion, and, if strongly suspected based on these initial factors, by evaluation of a HIT antibody titer.[28]

HIT antibody titers are evaluated primarily by use of platelet activation assays and enzyme immunoassay (EIA), which have distinct advantages and disadvantages that will not be discussed here.[26,27] HIT antibodies are a source of confusion for many clinicians due to imperfect specificity associated with both the platelet activation assay and EIA. Both mechanisms of analysis are sensitive (can detect the presence of antibodies), but poorly specific, thus causing a positive result to be essentially useless for diagnosis of HIT without other clinical symptoms and work-up. While a positive result on a HIT antibody titer is not diagnostic on its own, a negative HIT antibody titer is useful for ruling out a true HIT syndrome.[26–28]

Lo and colleagues[34] published a clinical scoring system, based on four factors, to assist clinicians in the diagnosis of HIT. The four factors accounted for in the clinical scoring system are: degree of thrombocytopenia, timing of developing thrombocytopenia, development of thrombosis, and whether or not other causes are present that could be responsible for the thrombocytopenia.[34] This clinical scoring system, often referred to as the 4T score, can be found in Table 14–7. The 4T score evaluates risk factors that patients present with at the time of questioning HIT and categorizes the patient into high, intermediate, or low risk. Recommendations for treatment or watchful waiting are also found in Table 14–7.

Treatment of HIT requires therapeutic anticoagulation to prevent further thrombosis from occurring until the antibody-mediated allergic reaction has passed.[26] As shown above, unfractionated heparin, LMWH, and fondaparinux have all been associated with HIT, so they cannot be options for anticoagulation of HIT due to their potential to worsen the situation and they must be stopped immediately. Patients with a HIT diagnosis are at elevated risk of clotting due to HIT and underlying disease processes. The direct thrombin inhibitors argatroban, bivalirudin, and lepirudin are the only agents that have not been associated with antibody formation and HIT; thus, they are the anticoagulants of choice for a patient with HIT or history of HIT.[24–26] Due to lack of frequent use, many clinicians struggle with dosing and monitoring the direct thrombin inhibitors, so therapy with these agents is often protocolized to each specific institution. Direct thrombin inhibitors are monitored with serial aPTT measurements and institution-specific protocols define a set aPTT target. The goal range for a therapeutic aPTT is 1.5 to 3 times the baseline aPTT range for the patient in question.

Much research and data have been published advocating the use of fondaparinux in HIT.[29,30] These data are intriguing, as the longer chains of heparin and LMWH have been shown to be the culprits of HIT development, and fondaparinux is a small-molecule pentasaccharide that, in theory,

Table 14-7 4T Scoring System for HIT[34]

Category	2 points	1 point	0 points
Degree of thrombo-cytopenia	Platelet drop >50%	Platelet drop by 30–50%	Platelet drop <30%
Timing of thrombocytopenia	Within 5–10 days or ≤1 day with heparin exposure within 30 days	Not clearly within 5–10 days, onset after 10 days, or ≤1 day with heparin exposure 30–100 days prior	Platelet fall <4 days without recent (within 100 days) heparin exposure
Thrombus formation	New thrombus, skin necrosis, systemic reaction to heparin bolus	Progressive thrombus, non-necrotizing skin lesions, or suspected thrombus	None
Other factors responsible for thrombocytopenia	None	Possible	Definite

Clinical Significance of 4T Score

0–3	Low probability
4–5	Intermediate probability
6–8	High probability

should not be associated with the same problems as UFH and LMWH. Case reports exist, however, detailing the association of HIT with fondaparinux, leading to the lack of use in patients with strong suspicion of HIT.[31,32] Data do exist supporting the use of fondaparinux in patients with a history of HIT, in patients who have recovered platelet counts to baseline after HIT occurrence, and when a low suspicion of HIT exists.[29,30] Careful monitoring of platelet counts, bleeding, and new thrombosis is definitely warranted in all of the above circumstances.

Because patients who develop HIT were being anticoagulated when HIT occurred, and because HIT is a procoagulant disease, patients typically require warfarin therapy after the platelet count has recovered. The *Chest* guidelines[26] describe transition to warfarin therapy from direct thrombin inhibitors in the chapter on Prevention and Treatment of Heparin-Induced Thrombocytopenia, and the reader is referred there for assistance with transitioning patients from therapeutic anticoagulation to warfarin therapy as this most commonly is accomplished outside of the ICU setting.

DISSEMINATED INTRAVASCULAR COAGULOPATHY

Another major hematologic complication encountered in the critical care setting is disseminated intravascular coagulopathy (DIC). Appropriate management of the underlying illness with early goal-directed therapy has been shown to be the best method for reversal of DIC.[35,36] DIC is a second-ary syndrome that is always a result of an underlying condition, and the condition that brings about DIC is responsible for activation of cytokines, which then adversely affect the clotting cascade.[37,38] The primary clotting factors involved in DIC are thrombin (factor II) and activated factor VII.[36] Activated factor VII complexes to tissue factor that is expressed on the surface of cells that have been exposed to cytokines, which then cleaves pro-thrombin to thrombin and subsequently causes localized fibrin formation and clotting. As the term DIC would suggest, this happens throughout the body (disseminated) and uses nearly all of the clotting factors available. As such, patients have poor circulation to capillary beds because of systemic clotting (thus worsening hypoperfusion and leading to organ system fail-ure), are at risk for bleeding from multiple locations (due to clotting factor deficiencies), and have elevated coagulation studies (due to utilization of clotting factors and the inability of the liver to regenerate clotting factors rapidly).[35-38]

Untreated, the condition that causes DIC lessens the body's ability to compensate for the multiple problems associated with both the underly-ing illness and DIC. As both progress, the liver and other major organs are further hypoperfused and the liver especially is unable to regenerate enough clotting factors to slow and stop any hemorrhage. Through this process of DIC, platelets are consumed in the massive numbers of small clots that have formed rapidly, causing thrombocytopenia on laboratory evaluation. This type of thrombocytopenia and clotting factor deficiency is often re-ferred to as a consumptive coagulopathy, and it is often observed in septic patients.[35-38]

On review of the pathophysiology of DIC, several observations can be made on the potential treatment of this condition.[35-38] First, reversal of the underlying cause is the most important factor in a positive outcome when DIC occurs. Secondly, recombinant activated factor VII would be expected as a potentially devastating choice of therapy for a patient with DIC and its use is contraindicated in such patients. Third, platelet transfusions will be of little benefit and could result in harm in DIC, as the systemic clotting may actually worsen with such an intervention. Platelets and other plasma products are only recommended if life-threatening bleeding is present or an immediate surgical procedure is necessary. Finally, despite the bleeding that is often present with DIC, anticoagulation may actually be of benefit to these patients. Some agents that have been studied for treatment of DIC include heparin, drotrecogin alfa, tissue factor pathway inhibitor, and antithrombin concentrates. The results of all studied products have been encouraging at times, but ultimately have not resulted in specific therapies.

OTHER SPECIFIC HEMATOLOGIC CONDITIONS IN CRITICAL CARE

Bleeding and thrombosis are potentially devastating reasons for admission to the ICU, as well as complications of other disease states. The following are less common, though still important, conditions that occur in the intensive care unit that are hematology based. Brief descriptions of the disease states, their importance to the ICU, and common pharmacologic treatments follow.

Liver Disease

The liver is vitally important in all aspects of hematologic homeostasis in the human body. Responsible for production of nearly all clotting factors, proteins affecting the coagulation cascade, and the factors that inhibit clotting, liver disease can be incredibly difficult to manage from a hematologic perspective due to the major bleeding and clotting problems that can arise.[39,40] Elevated liver function tests, prolonged clotting times, and other markers of liver failure all are important when considering the degree of liver disease, which is valuable information for understanding the level of severity of hematologic disorders.[39] Factors such as decreased production of clotting factors, poor nutrition (vitamin K deficiency), systemic fibrinolysis, platelet destruction, and dysfunctional platelets can cause major bleeding that is difficult, if not impossible, to stop without massive blood product replacement and pharmacologic therapy. Disseminated intravascular coagulation is a common cause of thrombosis and bleeding in the liver failure patient and is associated with high morbidity and mortality due to limited treatment options.[39,40] Pharmacologic options for major bleeding due to liver disease include: vitamin K (due to malnutrition), recombinant activated factor VII (due to decreased production), and PCC (due to decreased production of clotting factors).[39] Anticoagulation is difficult to manage in patients with liver disease, as clotting times are often elevated at baseline due to underlying disease. Improvement in liver function may allow for improvement in hematologic status and anticoagulation therapy initiation.

HELLP Syndrome

The HELLP syndrome is an obstetric and gynecologic emergency associated with hemolysis (H), elevated liver enzymes (EL), and low platelets (LP).[41] HELLP occurs most commonly in pregnant women who have been diagnosed with preeclampsia or eclampsia (preeclampsia is a condition that occurs after 20 weeks of gestation that is signified by development of hypertension and proteinuria, while eclampsia is a condition that follows preeclampsia, in which seizures occur that are not due to a history of a seizure disorder or another brain condition). Women that develop HELLP are at heightened risk of developing several severe complications that are shown in Table 14-8. Intracranial hemorrhage and hepatic hematoma are the most severe complications of HELLP syndrome, usually occurring when the platelet count falls below 20 K/μL.[41]

HELLP most commonly develops in the third trimester of pregnancy and can usually be successfully treated with delivery of the infant.[41] Before and after delivery of the infant, corticosteroids can be utilized to treat the symptoms of HELLP, with the most common being dexamethasone (10 or 12 mg IV every 12 hours) and betamethasone (12 mg IM every 12 hours), both for a total of two doses. Both corticosteroids are considered equivalent for prevention of complications from HELLP, but have not been compared head-to-head in clinical trials. Treatment with corticosteroids has virtually eliminated the most severe complications of HELLP (hepatic rupture and intracranial hemorrhage), but complications still do occur. Surgical methods of hemostasis are required for resolution of the bleeding event, as platelet transfusions alone are usually ineffective for treatment of the hemorrhaging

Table 14-8 Maternal and Fetal Complications of HELLP[39]

Organ System	Complication	Patient Affected
Hematologic	DIC/Bleeding	Mother
Hematologic	Thrombocytopenia	Mother and Child
Cardiovascular	Pulmonary Edema	Mother
Central Nervous System	Stroke	Mother
Central Nervous System	Visual (Retinal Detachment, etc.)	Mother
Renal	Acute Kidney Injury	Mother
Hepatic	Liver Hemorrhage	Mother
Infectious (Systemic)	Sepsis	Mother and Child

HELLP patient. Pharmacologic options for hemostasis in hemorrhage related to HELLP may be appropriate in conjunction with surgical methods. Recombinant activated factor VII has been considered the treatment of choice in conjunction with surgery in this patient population.

Sickle Cell Anemia

Sickle cell anemia is an inherited blood disorder characterized by increased blood viscosity and inflexible red blood cells that have a tendency to adhere to other red blood cells and blood vessel walls.[42] As blood cells mature, they tend to form sickle-shaped cell membranes and pass slowly through capillaries and irritate vascular endothelium. The most severe complications of sickle cell disease are veno-occlusive disorders such as stroke and myocardial infarction caused by decreased blood flow, causing ischemia in these important areas. Up to 11% of patients with sickle cell disease will have a stroke by 20 years of age.[43,44]

Sickle cell anemia severity is associated with the amount of fetal hemoglobin present on laboratory evaluation.[42] A low percentage of fetal hemoglobin is associated with organ damage and early death. Hydroxyurea is a medication that has been shown to increase fetal hemoglobin concentrations in patients with sickle cell anemia, although the mechanism for this increase is not completely known.[45,46]

Patients experiencing intense pain, acute chest syndrome (hypoxia, cough, etc.), severe infections, severe anemias, or cerebrovascular events that require intervention are experiencing major clinical complications of sickle cell disease, sometimes called sickle cell crisis. Important considerations in the treatment of sickle cell anemia crises are pain control and infection treatment or prevention.[42,47] Pain occurs through pathways involving both the vascular beds, which become irritated due to abnormally formed cells causing veno-occlusion, and bone marrow expansion in response to erythropoietin production.[47] Patients commonly require narcotic therapy to manage pain and high doses can be required to manage acute flares of sickle cell disease. Infection prophylaxis is required due to continual immune suppression from chronic hydroxyurea therapy.[43-46] These patients have compromised immune systems due to their spleen being overloaded with red blood cells to filter; as a result, patients with sickle cell anemia are especially susceptible to infections due to encapsulated bacteria (i.e., pneumococcal infections, neisseria infections, etc.).[43,44] As an important adverse effect, hydroxyurea suppresses and induces apoptosis in neutrophils, thus compromising the immune system, and the dose of hydroxyurea must be titrated to fetal hemoglobin percentage balanced with neutrophil count.[45,46]

Acute Leukemia

Acute leukemias can present in a variety of fashions, ranging from pancytopenia with a low white blood cell count to a relatively normocytopenic situation with elevated blast (immature cells) cell counts. Either situation represents a condition where the immune system responsible for fighting infection is compromised. The acute leukemias with the most potential to involve an ICU stay involve either high lymphoblast counts or leukemia with concomitant infectious etiology.[48]

When dealing with leukemia with a concomitant infectious etiology, the spectrum of pathogens that need to be considered seems endless, from bacteria to viruses and even fungi and molds. Aggressive broad-spectrum therapy needs to be started at first signs of infection because of both the underlying immune-compromised status (leukemia) and prolonged duration of neutropenia after chemotherapy has been initiated.[48]

Leukemias with high lymphoblast (referred to commonly as blast) cell counts present different issues than previously discussed in this chapter. Patients with high lymphoblast counts will often be pancytopenic, have an extremely high or low white blood cell count, and have highly viscous plasma.[48] To prevent adverse events from the increased viscosity of the plasma caused by excessive blast cells, either chemotherapy and plasmapheresis or chemotherapy alone may be indicated to eliminate the blast cells and achieve control over the disease process. In either treatment scenario, blood and platelet transfusions are generally contraindicated unless symptoms of poor perfusion exist (chest pain, extreme weakness, etc.). Plasmapheresis is a specialized procedure where blood is processed through a machine calibrated for removal of appropriately sized molecules. Plasmapheresis can be utilized to rapidly remove blast cells from the plasma without rupturing the undesired cells and exposing the patient to potentially toxic molecules released from cell lysis.[48]

Induction chemotherapy is the most effective method for inducing remission from the underlying disease and normalizing the blood counts, but rapid killing of blast cells with chemotherapy can cause the quick release of intracellular proteins and electrolytes from blast cells into the systemic circulation.[48] This release of intracellular products from tumor cells is referred to as tumor lysis syndrome.[49]

Tumor lysis syndrome occurs most commonly in rapidly proliferating malignancies such as leukemias and lymphomas, but can also occur with other malignancies such as myelomas and small cell lung cancer.[49] Tumor lysis syndrome can have devastating effects on the heart, kidneys, and lungs. Rapid release of intracellular electrolytes such as potassium and phosphorous can cause cardiac conduction abnormalities. Phosphorous and calcium can bind and precipitate in high concentrations and, while generally benign acutely, tissue ischemia can occur from this precipitant being present. Electrolyte abnormalities associated with lysis syndrome are managed through typical algorithms described in Chapter 7.

Furthermore, cytokine release during tumor lysis syndrome can cause high fevers, which can be mistaken for infection and lead to early and unnecessary antibiotic administration which can have adverse effects of their own. Cytokines can also be responsible for capillary leak syndrome, causing peripheral edema, hypotension, and pulmonary edema.[49]

Acute kidney injury due to tumor lysis results from the release and breakdown of the most commonly found product inside of cells, protein. Protein catabolism is rapid and responsible for the formation of uric acid, which is insoluble in the plasma and precipitates in joints and the renal tubules if it is not excreted rapidly. Normally, proteins are broken down to hypoxanthine. Hypoxanthine is metabolized to xanthine by xanthine oxidase, and xanthine is then broken down to uric acid by the same enzyme. Hypoxanthine and xanthine are much more soluble in the plasma than uric acid and do not precipitate like uric acid. The class of medications called the xanthine oxidase inhibitors (allopurinol and febuxostat) can be utilized to slow the accumulation of uric acid and attenuate the acute kidney injury process. Xanthine oxidase inhibitors are most effective when utilized before uric acid begins to accumulate in the plasma, but can have some effect in slowing the accumulation of uric acid at any point of initiation during induction chemotherapy. Allopurinol is the less expensive agent of the two xanthine oxidase inhibitors available in the United States, though no studies have been undertaken to directly compare the use of allopurinol and febuxostat in tumor lysis syndrome. Allopurinol is typically dosed at 300 mg by mouth daily for the treatment and prevention of tumor lysis syndrome.[49]

Rasburicase is an enzyme that breaks down uric acid to allantoin, which is also much more soluble than uric acid and can then be excreted.[49] Rasburicase is a recombinant enzyme, so the potential for hypersensitivity reaction exists. Rasburicase is administered intravenously at a dose of 3 to 6 milligrams for prevention of tumor lysis syndrome when used with urinary alkalinization and allopurinol. More aggressive dosing or repeat dosing of rasburicase may be needed based on the clinical situation (higher uric acid levels, higher degree of renal dysfunction, etc.).

Induction chemotherapy will generally lead to pancytopenia lasting between two and three weeks. During this time, patients are susceptible to hemorrhage, complications from anemia, and infection. Fortunately, complications from hemorrhage and anemia are lessened by transfusion of platelets and packed red blood cells. Neutropenia, however, is a more difficult problem to handle.

Infection prophylaxis is usually instituted with antibiotics, antifungals, and antivirals.[48] There is no product that can be transfused to replace neutrophils, as these would be highly immunogenic and cause complications in the form of transfusion versus host disease. Neutropenia, then, is treated with colony-stimulating factors, commonly referred to as growth factors. The available growth factors in the United States are filgrastim (abbreviated G-CSF) and sargramostim (abbreviated GM-CSF). Filgrastim also is available in a 6 mg pegylated formulation that allows for one injection lasting up to 2 weeks versus daily injections for 10 to 14 days. The important difference between filgrastim and sargramostim is the major cell lines that are stimulated when they are given: filgrastim stimulates the granulocyte lineage only, meaning neutrophil production is the primary marker of efficacy with this agent,[50] while sargramostim has a broader cell lineage affected by its use, including the neutrophils, monocytes, and dendritic cells. Neither agent has any notable efficacy on platelets or red blood cells. In several head-to-head comparisons, neither sargramostim nor filgrastim have been shown to reduce infection rates after chemotherapy or readmission after chemotherapy administration significantly over the other.

SUMMARY

In conclusion, hematologic complications of critical illness can occur in any patient during any admission to the intensive care unit. Hematologic complications can be the primary reason for admittance to the ICU or can be an adverse event of the ICU stay. Hematologic complications can have drastic and sometimes fatal consequences and can prove to be very challenging to treat. Pharmacists working in the ICU setting must be cognizant of monitoring for hematologic adverse events of medication therapy and knowledgeable of the treatments for hematologic diseases that lead to admission to the ICU. Recognizing hematologic complications and disease presentations will help provide the patient with the best chance at a positive outcome.

KEY POINTS

- Hemorrhage from anticoagulation therapy is a major cause of morbidity and mortality in critical care.
- Prophylaxis against venous thromboembolism with mechanical devices or pharmaceuticals is necessary to reduce the risk of new thrombosis formation.
- Patients developing thromboembolism in the critical care setting can be difficult to manage with anticoagulation due to rapid changes in status.

- Important differences in anticoagulant medications exist, therefore a clear understanding is important to properly manage patients.
- Heparin-induced thrombocytopenia (HIT) is a rare but severe complication of anticoagulation therapy that requires careful monitoring for identification and treatment.
- Disseminated intravascular coagulopathy (DIC) is a common complication of critical illness, and sepsis in particular, that involves consumption of clotting factors with widespread systemic microemboli, causing organ ischemia and hypoperfusion.
- Liver disease is a complicated critical illness that can involve both severe hemorrhage requiring massive blood product replacement and thrombus formation.
- HELLP syndrome is an obstetric emergency involving the mother and fetus.
- Sickle cell anemia is a blood disorder that causes debilitating pain syndromes and thromboembolic disorders such as stroke and acute myocardial infarction.
- Patients with acute leukemias require complex medical care. Infection and tumor lysis syndrome are common scenarios requiring critical care admissions.

SELECTED SUGGESTED READINGS

- American College of Chest Physicians evidenced-based clinical practice guidelines (8th edition). *Chest* 2008;133.
- Raslan AM, Fields JD, Bhardwaj A. Prophylaxis for venous thrombo-embolism in neurocritical care: a critical appraisal. *Neurocrit Care.* 2010;12:297–309.
- Lehman CM, Frank EL. Laboratory monitoring of heparin therapy: partial thromboplastin time or anti-Xa assay? *Lab Medicine.* 2009;40(1):47–51.
- Lo GK, Juhl D, Warkentin TE, Sigouin CS, Eichler P, Greinacher A. Evaluation of pretest clinical score (4 T's) for the diagnosis of heparin-induced thrombocytopenia in two clinical settings. *J Thromb Haemost.* 2006;4:759–765.

REFERENCES

1. DeLoughery TG. Venous thromboembolism in the ICU and reversal of bleeding on anticoagulants. *Crit Care Clin.* 2005;21:497–512.
2. Schulman S, Beyth RJ, Kearon C, Levine MN. Hemorrhagic complications of anticoagulant and thrombolytic treatment: American College of Chest

Physicians evidenced-based clinical practice guidelines (8th edition). *Chest.* 2008;133:257–298.

3. Schulman S, Bijsterveld NR. Anticoagulants and their reversal. *Transfus Med Rev.* 2007;21(1):37–48.

4. Leissinger CA, Blatt PM, Hoots WK, Ewenstein B. Role of prothrombin complex concentrates in reversing warfarin anticoagulation: a review of the literature. *Am J Hematol.* 2008;83:137–143.

5. Geerts WH, Bergqvist D, Pineo GF, Heit JA, Samama CM, Lassen MR, Colwell CW. Prevention of venous thromboembolism: American College of Chest Physicians evidenced-based clinical practice guidelines (8th edition). *Chest.* 2008;133:381–453.

6. Raslan AM, Fields JD, Bhardwaj A. Prophylaxis for venous thrombo-embolism in neurocritical care: a critical appraisal. *Neurocrit Care.* 2010;12:297–309.

7. Broderick J, Connolly S, Feldmann E, Hanley D, Kase C, Krieger D, et al. Guidelines for the management of spontaneous intracerebral hemorrhage in adults: 2007 update: a guideline from the American Heart Association/ American Stroke Association stroke council, high blood pressure research council, and the quality of care and outcomes in research interdisciplinary working group. *Stroke.* 2007;38:2001–2023.

8. Vincent JL, Piagnerelli M. Transfusion in the intensive care unit. *Crit Care Med.* 2006;34(Suppl):S96–S101.

9. Corwin HL, Gettinger A, Pearl RG, Flink MP, Levy MM, Abraham E, et al. The CRIT study: anemia and blood transfusion in the critically ill—current clinical practice in the United States. *Crit Care Med.* 2004;32:39–52.

10. Asare K. Anemia of critical illness. *Pharmacotherapy.* 2008;28(10):1267–1282.

11. Mannucci PM. Desmopressin (DDAVP) in the treatment of bleeding disorders: the first 20 years. *Blood.* 1997;90(7):2515–2521.

12. Yank V, Tuohy CV, Logan AC, et al. Systematic review: benefits and harms of in-hospital use of recombinant factor VIIa for off-label indications. *Ann Intern Med.* 2011;154:529–540.

13. CRASH-2 trial collaborators. Effects of tranexamic acid on death, vascular occlusive events, and blood transfusion in trauma patients with significant haemorrhage (CRASH-2): a randomized, placebo-controlled trial. *Lancet.* 2010;376(9734):23–32.

14. Munoz JJ, Birkmeyer NJO, Birkmeyer JD, O'Connor GT, Dacey J. Is aminoca-proic acid as effective as aproptinin in reducing bleeding with cardiac surgery? *Circulation.* 1999;99:81–89.

15. Brown JR, Birkmeyer NJO, O'Connor GT. Meta-analysis comparing the ef-fectiveness and adverse-outcomes of antifibrinolytic agents in cardiac surgery. *Circulation.* 2007;115:2801–2803.

16. Lew W, Weaver F. Clinical use of topical thrombin as a surgical hemostat. *Biologics.* 2008;2(4):593–599.

17. Weaver F, Lew W, Granke K, et al. A comparison of recombinant thrombin to bovine thrombin as a hemostatic ancillary in patients undergoing peripheral arterial bypass and arteriovenous graft procedures. *J Vasc Surg.* 2008;47(6): 1266–1273.

18. Kearson C, Kahn SR, Agnelli G, Goldhaber S, Raskob GE, Comerota AJ. Antithrombotic therapy for venous thromboembolic disease: American College of Chest Physicians evidenced-based clinical practice guidelines (8th edition). *Chest*. 2008;133:454–545.

19. Hirsh J, Bauer KA, Donati MB, Gould M, Samama MM, Weitz JI. Parenteral anticoagulants: American College of Chest Physicians evidenced-based clinical practice guidelines (8th edition). *Chest*. 2008;133:141–159.

20. DeLoughery TG. Critical care clotting catastrophies. *Crit Care Clin*. 2005;21:531–562.

21. Lehman CM, Frank EL. Laboratory monitoring of heparin therapy: partial thromboplastin time or anti-Xa assay? *Lab Medicine*. 2009;40(1):47–51.

22. Douketis J, Cook D, Meade M, et al. Prophylaxis against deep vein thrombosis in critically ill patients with severe renal insufficiency with the low-molecular-weight heparin dalteparin an assessment of safety and pharmacodynamics: The DIRECT Study. *Arch Intern Med*. 2008;168(16):1805–1812.

23. Wood KE. Major pulmonary embolism. *Chest*. 2002;121:877–905.

24. Warkentin TE. Heparin-induced thrombocytopenia: pathogenesis and management. *British J Haematology*. 2003;121:535–555.

25. Warkentin TE, Cook RJ, Marder VJ, Sheppard JI, Moore JC, et al. Anti-platelet factor 4/heparin antibodies in orthopedic surgery patients receiving antithrombotic prophylaxis with fondaparinux or enoxaparin. *Blood*. 2005;106:3791–3796.

26. Warkentin TE, Greinacher A, Koster A, Lincoff AM. Treatment and prevention of heparin-induced thrombocytopenia: American College of Chest Physicians evidenced-based clinical practice guidelines (8th edition). *Chest*. 2008;133:340–380.

27. Kelton JG, Warkentin TE. Heparin-induced thrombocytopenia: a historical perspective. *Blood*. 2008;112(7):2607–2616.

28. Napolitano LM, Warkentin TE, AlMahameed A, Nasraway S. Heparin-induced thrombocytopenia in the critical care setting: diagnosis and management. *Crit Care Med*. 2006;34(12):2898–2911.

29. Lobo B, Finch C, Howard A, Minhas S. Fondaparinux for the treatment of patients with acute heparin-induced thrombocytopenia. *Thromb Haemost*. 2008;99:208–214.

30. Efird LE, Kockler DR. Fondaparinux for thromboembolic treatment and prophylaxis of heparin-induced thrombocytopenia. *Ann Pharmacother*. 2006;40:1383–1387.

31. Rota E, Bazzan M, Fantino G. Fondaparinux-related thrombocytopenia in a previous low-molecular-weight heparin (LMWH)-induced heparin-induced thrombocytopenia (HIT). *Thromb Haemost*. 2008;99:779–781.

32. Warkentin TE. Heparin-induced thrombocytopenia associated with fondaparinux. *N Engl J Med*. 2007;356(25):2653–2655.

33. Warkentin TE, Cook DJ. Heparin, low molecular weight heparin, and heparin-induced thrombocytopenia in the ICU. *Crit Care Clin*. 2005;21:513–529.

34. Lo GK, Juhl D, Warkentin TE, Sigouin CS, Eichler P, Greinacher A. Evaluation of pretest clinical score (4 T's) for the diagnosis of heparin-induced thrombocytopenia in two clinical settings. *J Thromb Haemost*. 2006;4:759–765.

35. Drews RE, Weinberger SE. Thrombocytopenic disorders in critically ill patients. *Am J Respir Crit Care Med.* 2000;162:347–351.

36. Aird WC. Sepsis and coagulation. *Crit Care Clin.* 2005;21:417–431.

37. Vincent JL, De Backer D. Does disseminated intravascular coagulation lead to multiple organ failure? *Crit Care Clin.* 2005;21:469–477.

38. Levy M. Disseminated intravascular coagulation: what's new? *Crit Care Clin.* 2005;21:449–467.

39. Kujovich JL. Hemostatic defects in end stage liver disease. *Crit Care Clin.* 2005;21:563–587.

40. Kelly DA, Tuddenham EG. Haemostatic problems in liver disease. *Gut.* 1986;27:339–349.

41. Martin JN, Rose CH, Briery CM. Understanding and managing HELLP syndrome: the integral role of aggressive glucocorticoids for mother and child. *Am J Obstet Gynecol.* 2006;195:914–934.

42. Montalembert M. Management of sickle cell disease. *BMJ.* 2008;337:626–630.

43. Verduzco LA, Nathan DG. Sickle cell disease and stroke. *Blood.* 2009;114(25):5117–5125.

44. Platt OS, Brambilla DJ, Rosse WF, Milner PF, Castro O, Steinberg MH, Klug PP. Mortality in sickle cell disease. *N Engl J Med.* 1994;331(15):1022–1023.

45. Platt OS. Hydroxyurea for the treatment of sickle cell anemia. *N Engl J Med.* 2008;358(13):1362–1369.

46. Ware RE. How I use hydroxyurea to treat young patients with sickle cell anemia. *Blood.* 2010;115(26):5300–5311.

47. Geller AK, O'Connor MK. The sickle cell crisis: a dilemma in pain relief. *Mayo Clin Proc.* 2008;83(3):320–323.

48. NCCN 1.2011. Guidelines for the treatment of AML. Cited with permission from the NCCN 1.2011 acute myeloid leukemia clinical practice guidelines in oncology. Copyright national comprehensive cancer network, 2010. Accessed December 29, 2010. http://www.nccn.org.

49. Cairo M, Coiffier B, Reiter A, Younes A. Recommendations for the evaluation of risk and prophylaxis of tumour lysis syndrome (TLS) in adults and children with malignant diseases: an expert TLS panel consensus. *British J Haematology.* 2010;149:578–586.

50. Stull DM, Bilmes R, Kim H, Fichtl R. Comparison of sargramostim and filgrastim in the treatment of chemotherapy-induced neutropenia. *Am J Health-Syst Pharm.* 2005;62:83–87.

Chapter 15

Pharmacotherapy of Neurotrauma and Neurologic Disease

Ron Neyens

LEARNING OBJECTIVES

1. Review general principles of cerebral physiology, oxygen delivery and consumption, and cerebral autoregulation.
2. Describe the common neurologic disease states encountered in the critically ill.
3. Explain pharmacologic principles and goals of managing intracranial hypertension.
4. Apply pharmacologic management principles for traumatic brain injury, ischemic stroke, hemorrhagic stroke, aneurysmal subarachnoid hemorrhage, status epilepticus, and spinal cord injury.
5. Be able to design basic care plans for critically ill patients with neurologic disease.

INTRODUCTION

Neurological injury may occur as a result of a traumatic, cerebrovascular, infectious, metabolic, or inflammatory insult. This chapter will focus on basic acute care pharmacological goals and principles for managing traumatic brain injury, ischemic stroke, hemorrhagic stroke, aneurysmal subarachnoid hemorrhage, status epilepticus, and spinal cord injury.

Following an acute neurological injury, a complex cascade of physiological events, known as secondary injury, may ensue.[1] Although the disease pathology varies between diagnoses, the primary initiating trigger of secondary injury is often ischemia. The brain is particularly susceptible due to its high resting energy expenditure and limited capacity to store oxygen and energy. An insult creating a supply and demand imbalance in oxygen and energy results in loss of ionic homeostasis, neuronal excitation, free radical generation, and lipid peroxidation.[1] Sustained ischemia leads to destruction of cellular integrity, progressing to cerebral edema, intracranial hypertension, and cellular death.

Pharmacotherapy is based on physiologic concepts and designed to prevent primary disease progression, ensure adequate oxygen delivery, control intracranial hypertension, curb secondary injury progression, and prevent associated medical complications.

Cerebral Anatomy and Physiology

The brain is encased within a closed, rigid compartment (the skull) containing brain tissue, cerebrospinal fluid, and blood volume. The Monroe–Kellie doctrine states that these structures reside in a state of equilibrium and that an increase in any one component must be compensated for by a decrease in another to ensure that the intracranial volume remains constant.[2] If homeostasis is lost and brain compliance decreases, the intracranial pressure (ICP) rises and cerebral blood flow (CBF) is compromised, risking cerebral ischemia and cellular death.

The brain has very little capacity to store oxygen, with its survivability dependent upon an adequate CBF and cerebral oxygen delivery (CDO_2). In normal physiologic conditions, homeostatic cerebral autoregulation is in place to ensure that *supply* (i.e., CBF and CDO_2), is coupled to meet *demand* (i.e., cerebral metabolic rate for oxygen consumption ($CMRO_2$)), despite variations in cerebral perfusion pressure (CPP). This occurs via a tight regulation of cerebral vascular resistance (CVR), stimulated by various interrelated processes involving pressure, chemical, and electrical gradients.[3] See Figure 15-1 detailing cerebrovascular autoregulation.

After brain injury, cerebrovascular autoregulation may be absent or impaired. The ability to detect the status of autoregulation creates clinical challenges since a definitive diagnostic tool does not currently exist. Hemodynamic management to ensure adequate CBF and CDO_2, without increasing cerebral blood volume (CBV) to the extent of increasing ICP, remains a cornerstone in the treatment of acute neurological injury. Table 15-1 details physiologic variables and their specific target parameters.[3,4]

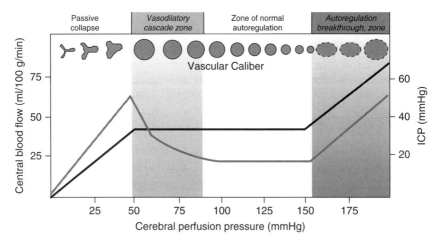

Figure 15-1 Cerebrovascular Autoregulation

Cerebral blood flow (CBF) is held constant by neuromyogenic modification of the diameter of precapillary arterioles. This occurs with cerebral perfusion pressures (CPP) between 50–150 mmHg, but may be shifted to the right in chronic hypertension. Beyond the upper and lower limits of autoregulation, CBF passively follows changes in CPP in a linear fashion, affecting intracranial pressures (ICP). In acute neurological injury, cerebral autoregulation may be impaired in zones of injury so that CBF becomes entirely pressure passive.

With kind permission from Springer Science+Business Media: Brigham and Women's Hospital Neurosurgery Group. Principles of cerebral oxygenation and blood flow in the neurological critical care unit. *Neurocrit Care.* 2006;4:77–82.

Table 15-1 Cerebral Physiologic Parameters[3, 4]

Definitions	Therapeutic Targets
Intracranial Pressure (ICP)	≤20 mmHg
Cerebral Perfusion Pressure (CPP)	50–70 mmHg
Jugular Venous Oxygen Saturation ($S_{jv}O_2$)	55–71%
Cerebral Oxygen Tension ($PbtO_2$)	>20%
Arterial Oxygen Percent Saturation (SaO_2)	92–100%
Cerebral Blood Flow (CBF)	Normal: 50–60 mL/100 g brain/min
	Ischemic: <20 mL/100 g brain/min
Arteriovenous Difference of Oxygen ($AVDO_2$)	6.3 ± 2.4 mL O_2/dL blood
Cerebral Metabolic Rate of Oxygen Consumption ($CMRO_2$)	150–160 µmol/100 g brain/min
Cerebral Oxygen Extraction (CEO_2)	25–45%

Neurological monitors and imaging can be used to direct appropriate therapy based on oxygen supply, demand, and utilization. ICP = measured variable with intracranial pressure monitor; CPP = mean arterial pressure (MAP) - ICP; $S_{jv}O_2$ = measured variable with intrajugular monitor; SaO_2 = measured variable from arterial blood gas (ABG); CBF = CPP/cerebral vascular resistance (CVR). Measured variable with intracranial blood flow monitor or functional imaging; $AVDO_2 = (SaO_2 - S_{jv}O_2) \times 1.39 \times$ hemoglobin; $CMRO_2 = CBF \times AVDO_2$; $CEO_2 = SaO_2 - S_{jv}O_2$.

TRAUMATIC BRAIN INJURY

Airway, Breathing, and Circulation

Hypoxemia and hypotension are predictors of poor outcomes following traumatic brain injury (TBI), and it stands to reason that the same is true for all patients with acute neurologic injury.[5] A patient airway with adequate oxygenation is the first priority for all acute neurological injuries; this is closely followed by resuscitation and restoration of hemodynamics with intravenous fluids, blood products, or vasopressors and/or inotropes to ensure adequate tissue perfusion and oxygen delivery.

The optimal resuscitation fluid remains unknown; however, it is best to avoid hypotonic solutions to prevent cerebral edema exacerbation.[1] The crystalloids versus colloids debate remains, though post-hoc analysis of the Saline versus Albumin Fluid Evaluation (SAFE) trial suggests a higher mortality with albumin resuscitation in TBI.[6] Isotonic or hypertonic crystalloids are most commonly utilized, with the latter gaining favor as they tend to augment intravascular volume and cardiovascular performance while improving intracranial compliance.[7] See Table 15–2 detailing characteristics of intravenous crystalloids.

Intracranial Hypertension

There are numerous pharmacologic and non-pharmacologic methods for managing intracranial hypertension. Non-pharmacologic methods may involve surgical decompression, cerebral spinal fluid diversion,

Table 15–2 Crystalloid Characteristics

Sodium Chloride Solution	Solution Sodium (mmol/L)	Tonicity (mOsm/L)
Lactated Ringers (LR)	130	273
0.9 %	154	308
2%	342	684
3%	513	1026
5%	855	1711
7.5%	1283	2566
10%	1711	3422
23.4%	4004	8008

hyperventilation, or hypothermia.[8] Figure 15–2 details a general approach for managing intracranial hypertension.

The cornerstone for pharmacologically treating acute ICP crisis (e.g., sustained ICP >20 mmHg) is osmotherapy with mannitol or hypertonic saline solutions, or hypnotics such as pentobarbital or propofol.[1,7–9] The goal is rapid restoration of normal ICP, allowing the clinician time to identify the etiology and devise a treatment plan. The medical literature has not clearly defined a therapeutic advantage between the two different osmotic strategies.[7–9] Although some controversy exists regarding comparative onset and duration of effect, potential pleotropic effects (e.g., free radical

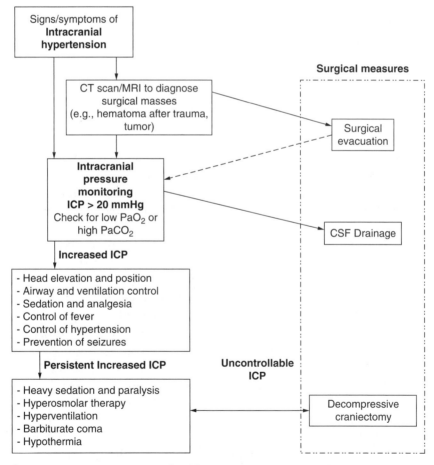

Figure 15–2 ICP Management Algorithm

From: Rangel-Castillo L, Gopinath S, Robertson CS. Management of intracranial hypertension. *Neurol Clin.* 2008;26:521–541

scavenging, inhibition of excitatory neurotransmitters), and associated adverse effects, it is well accepted that both therapies produce a rapid reduction in ICP. Expert opinion suggests that a more rapid effect may be observed with hypertonic saline solutions versus mannitol, which is attractive in a crisis situation.[9] The response tends to be biphasic, with the initial, rapid ICP reduction appearing to be related to blood viscosity reduction, optimization of CBF, and a resultant reflexive vasoconstriction and reduction in CBV and ICP. This phase is dependent upon the status of pressure autoregulation, with an impairment producing less pronounced clinical effects. The later phase, which is delayed 15 to 45 minutes after drug administration, is due to the maintenance of an osmotic gradient, cellular dehydration, and reduction in cerebral edema.

Mannitol can be given rapidly via peripheral access and is often available for rapid access from automated dispensing cabinets (ADCs). However, it can potentiate a profound diuresis, requiring aggressive volume management to ensure adequate systemic and cerebral perfusion. It is renally eliminated and best avoided if significant renal impairment exists, as it may lead to accumulation and rebound cerebral edema. If a multiple dose strategy is implemented, serum osmolarity should be maintained at <320 to 340 mOsm/L or the osmolar gap <10 to 15 from baseline to limit the risk of hyperosmolarity and its potential association with acute kidney injury (AKI).[10]

A hypertonic saline intermittent bolus dose strategy with concentrations between 3 and 23.4% follows similar principles as mannitol.[1,7-9] Administration of hypertonic solutions typically requires central access and concentrations greater than 3% may not be available for rapid access from ADCs. Continuous infusion of hypertonic solutions with concentrations of 1.5 to 3% is gaining acceptance. The goal is to maintain the serum sodium between 145 and 155 mEq/L (serum osmolarity approximately 300 to 320 mOsm/L), creating a continuous osmotic gradient with subsequent reduction in intracellular edema and ICP. The literature is abundant with small studies, with some suggesting fewer ICP crises with this therapeutic strategy.[7,8]

This strategy is not void of concerns, which include the development of homeostatic adaptation and generation of intracellular idioosmoles with rebound edema, particularly upon therapy discontinuation, as well as cardiopulmonary edema-associated decompensation and hyperosmolarity-associated AKI. One additional concern is the potential for central pontine myelinolysis associated with a rapid rise in serum sodium. However, this has only been reported in the setting of chronic hyponatremia rather than during induced hypernatremia for the management of cerebral edema and elevated ICPs.[11] If a continuous hypertonic saline strategy is implemented, it should be titrated to an established goal with frequent sodium checks—at least every 4 to 6 hours—and withdrawn carefully to ensure the potential for rebound edema is limited. Compounding a 75:25 or 50:50 (ratio by weight) sodium chloride:sodium acetate solution may help prevent hyperchloremic metabolic acidosis.

The mechanism of ICP reduction with the rapid acting barbiturate hypnotics remains unclear, but likely involves a coupled reduction in $CMRO_2$ and CBF.[1,8,9] Barbiturates commonly depress the myocardium and dilate the peripheral vasculature, creating hemodynamic instability requiring vasopressors. In refractory cases, an adequate response to a hypnotic may serve as a response predictor for a barbiturate-induced coma.[9]

In addition to managing acute ICP crisis, pharmacologic agents play an important role in maintaining homeostasis and curbing subsequent crises. It may include sedation and pain management optimization, fever control, CPP optimization, hyperosmolar therapy, chemical paralysis, and/or barbiturate coma.[1,8,9] The goal of sedation and pain management is a coupled reduction in $CMRO_2$ and CBF or CBV, while serving to prevent sympathetic-induced ICP crisis. Controversy exists regarding specific agents and their individual effects on cerebral physiology, with current data being limited by methodological quality and design.[12] It is generally accepted that benzodiazepines and propofol achieve a desired coupled reduction in $CMRO_2$ and CBF with variable effects on ICP. Opioids have minimal effects on $CMRO_2$, CBF or CBV, and ICP as long as a normotensive and normocarbic condition is preserved; therefore, agent selection is based on pharmacokinetic principles and the ability to provide adequate sedation, while facilitating frequent neurological exams. It is best to consider short acting combinations, such as propofol and intermittent fentanyl, particularly within the first 48 to 72 hours or until frequent (every 1 to 2 hours) neurological exams are no longer required.[1,13] Neurologically injured patients are at high risk for propofol infusion syndrome (PIS), so appropriate serological monitoring of CK, lactate, and triglycerides is warranted, particularly if high doses are utilized for long durations.[14]

Fever is associated with significant cerebrovascular vasodilation, increasing ICP via an increase in $CMRO_2$, CBF, and CBV.[8,15] In addition, fever may play a role in progressing secondary injury via excitotoxic neurotransmitter release and other inflammatory cascades. Normothermia should be targeted in all forms of acute neurological injury. Acetaminophen is the antipyretic of choice, inhibiting prostaglandin E_2 (PGE_2) production and its effects upon the hypothalamic thermostat. Ibuprofen may be used cautiously; however, an increased risk of intracranial bleeding may exist when used in patients with underlying intracranial hemorrhagic pathology or in those with an invasive intracranial monitor. In many cases, pharmacologic antipyretic therapy fails or additional reduction in core temperature is desired via therapeutic hypothermia. In this situation, alternative measures, including external surface or intravascular cooling devices, are employed.

Shivering is a common complication of therapeutic hypothermia, particularly during the initial cooling and rewarming phases. It is important to suppress this response, often with pharmacological measures, as it is known to increase oxygen consumption and ICP.[16] The best supporting data are for sedation optimization, monotherapy or combination therapy with buspirone and meperidine, dexmedetomidine, or magnesium infusions. Neuromuscular blocking agents may be considered if other pharmacotherapeutic alternatives fail.

A patient's optimal CPP goal can vary based on pathophysiology and the status of autoregulation. The Brain Trauma Foundation (BTF) recommends maintaining a CPP between 50 and 70 mmHg, with a target of around 60 mmHg to avoid excursions below the critical ischemia threshold.[17] A pharmacologically induced CPP >70 mmHg is associated with acute respiratory distress syndrome (ARDS).[18] If the CPP is <50 mmHg or signs of cerebral ischemia are detected at a higher CPP either clinically or via CBF monitors or other means of invasive ischemia monitors (e.g., Licox, intrajugular bulb, or cerebral microdialysis), a vasopressor or inotrope can be initiated to increase MAP or cardiac output (CO) with a resultant increase in CPP.[1,8,17] The optimal vasopressor in neurological injury remains unknown. Differences in their ability to alter cerebral physiology may exist; however, it is generally accepted that the patient's medical comorbidities and current hemodynamic status will dictate the best agent.[19]

Hypertension may be just as important to treat in specific cases. If a passive rise in ICP is observed as the systemic blood pressure and CPP increase, autoregulation may be impaired.[17,20] In this scenario, controlled reductions in blood pressure, hydrostatic pressure, and CPP with a short-acting intravenous antihypertensive may effectively reduce ICP by decreasing CBF, CBV, and cerebral edema. These manipulations should be accomplished with simultaneous cerebral oxygenation and ischemia monitoring. An antihypertensive with a reliable dose–response relationship and favorable safety profile is desirable. The optimal agent in neurological injury remains unknown, for similar concerns as described with vasopressors.[21] Conflicting data exist regarding sodium nitroprusside and its effects on increasing ICP via potent cerebral vasodilation. However, secondary to toxicity concerns of high dose or prolonged infusion of sodium nitroprusside, it is best to consider nicardipine, clevidipine, or labetalol as safer alternatives. The agent of choice depends on the patient's medical comorbidities, as well as the current clinical status.

Intractable ICP or crisis triggered by ventilator dyssynchrony that cannot be effectively managed with sedation and analgesia optimization may require chemical paralysis.[1,8] Paralysis may decrease motor activity trigger-induced ICP crisis and decrease intrathoracic pressure via diaphragmatic relaxation, which increases cerebral venous return and decreases CBV and ICP. Appropriate patient selection is essential as it compromises the ability to detect acute changes via a neurological exam. Paralytic agent selection is best directed by pharmacokinetic parameters, adverse effects, patient comorbidities, and end organ function.

Barbiturate-induced coma is often used as salvage therapy because of its many associated complications.[1,8,9] In a dose-dependent manner, it causes a coupled reduction in $CMRO_2$, CBF, and ICP. While the strategy is commonly used in practice and effective at reducing ICPs, it has not been shown to improve morbidity and mortality outcomes. If initiated, the incidence of hypotension and compromised CPP should be anticipated, often requiring vasopressor and/or inotropic support. Other associated complications include infections, hypothermia, cardiac depression, gastrointestinal ileus, and hypokalemia, with the possibility of severe rebound hyperkalemia upon discontinuation. Several different barbiturates have been investigated, with little comparable data, but pentobarbital is the most frequently utilized agent. Following initiation, the dose should be titrated to electroencephalogram (EEG) burst suppression. Goal pentobarbital levels are reported as 30 to 40 mg/L, but this is not correlated to clinical efficacy.[8,9] Levels are most useful following therapy discontinuation when trying to differentiate drug-induced versus lesion-induced effects on the neurological exam.

Glucocorticoids have a long-standing history in the treatment of cerebral edema.[9,22,23] They appear to be most effective in treating vasogenic edema versus other forms of cerebral edema, such as cytotoxic, hydrocephalic, and osmotic. They have been shown to increase mortality in TBI, and thus have no role in the management of cerebral edema in this patient population. It is generally considered that they only have a therapeutic role in the treatment of cerebral edema secondary to primary or metastatic brain tumors, brain abscesses, progressive neuroinflammatory processes, or severe pneumococcal meningitis.[9,22] They are believed to rapidly decrease cerebral edema by inhibiting the arachadonic acid cascade and decreasing the expression of vascular endothelial growth factor (VEGF), which is a very potent vascular permeability factor.[23] Dexamethasone is the most frequently used agent, given its long half-life and minimal mineralocorticoid activity. Dose ranges are 0.5 to 20 mg every 4 to 8 hours, titrated to clinical and radiological assessments. Table 15–3 provides an overview of pharmacological agents used for managing intracranial hypertension.[8,9]

Table 15-3 Pharmacological Agents Used for Intracranial Pressure (ICP) Control[8,9]

Agent	Dosing	Concerns	Comments
Mannitol	0.5–2 g/kg over 5–15 minutes—can be redosed every 4–6 hours	Rebound ICP Acute kidney injury Dehydration Hypotension	Dose response curve unknown Requires in-line filter—precipitates May be given via peripheral access Monitor serum osmolarity and osmolar gap
Hypertonic Saline	Crisis: 3%: 250–300 mL over 20 min 7.5%: 1.5–2.5 mL/kg over 20 min 10%: 75–100 mL over 20 min 23.4%: 30 mL over 20 min Maintenance: 2–3% continuous at 0.5–2 mL/kg/hr	Rebound ICP Myelinolysis Pulmonary edema Heart failure Acute Kidney Injury Coagulopathy	Central access if >2% Rapid availability may be limited Monitor serum sodium every 4–6 hours
Propofol	1–2 mg/kg	Hypotension Myocardial depression	Must ensure adequate CPP maintained
Pentobarbital	10 mg/kg over 30 min, then 5 mg/kg/ hr x 3 hrs, Maintenance: 1–4 mg/kg/hr	Hypotension Myocardial depression Immunosuppression Paralytic ileus	Must ensure adequate CPP maintained Monitor for propylene glycol toxicity Titrate to ICP control and/or EEG burst
Dexamethasone	10 mg IV x 1, then 4 mg IV q6h	Hyperglycemia Immunosuppression Psychosis	Only if edema caused by brain tumor, brain abscess, or progressive neuroinflammatory process (e.g., acute disseminated encephalomyelitis) Wean slowly to prevent rebound cerebral edema

CPP: cerebral perfusion pressure; EEG: electroencephalogram

Seizure Prophylaxis

A seizure can be particularly detrimental to a brain-injured patient as it can significantly increase $CMRO_2$ and ICP, potentiating cerebral ischemia.[24] It can also negatively impact long-term cognitive and psychosocial well-being.[25] Prophylactic antiepileptic drugs (AEDs) have been in use for several years, with many controversies evolving around agent selection, dosing, monitoring, and therapy duration. It is now well accepted that they appear to only be effective in preventing early seizures occurring within 7 days following injury.[24] Phenytoin, carbamazepine, valproic acid, and levetiracetam have all been studied with various methodologies for prophylactic use, with phenytoin dosed at 20 mg/kg, followed by 5 to 7 mg/kg/day divided every 8 to 12 hours for 7 days, having the most accepted and time-tested data.[24,26] Alterations in phenytoin pharmacokinetics during the acute phase of TBI are likely, including increased metabolism and the potential requirement for high doses.[27,28] Levetiracetam at a dose of 20 mg/kg, followed by 1,000 mg every 12 hours, is being used more frequently secondary to concerns with phenytoin-associated adverse effects and possibly worsened long-term cognitive outcomes in specific subtypes of acute stroke patients.[25,26]

ISCHEMIC STROKE

Approximately 85% of strokes are ischemic, with the remaining being of hemorrhagic origin.[29] The goals of therapy in ischemic stroke are medical stabilization, recanalization, and treatment of cerebral edema and intracranial hypertension, as well as the prevention of associated medical complications.

Hemodynamic Management

Medical stabilization is the first priority and may include intubation for airway management, volume replacement, and correction of any unstable cardiac arrhythmia, which is not uncommon in all types of stroke. Hypertension is common following an ischemic stroke and may serve as a physiologic compensatory response to provide adequate cerebral perfusion.[29-31] Blood pressure often declines spontaneously within the first few hours, but may require treatment in specific situations. Theoretical reasons to treat in the early phase include reducing new-onset end-organ damage, including cerebral edema, and preventing hemorrhagic transformation. The latter is particularly important in patients receiving thrombolysis with recombinant tissue plasminogen activator (rt-PA). Treating hypertension must be carefully balanced with potential neurological decline from treatment-induced hypoperfusion to ischemic brain penumbra surrounding the infarct core. The American Heart Association/American Stroke Association (AHA/ASA) guidelines recommend withholding antihypertensive therapy unless the systolic blood pressure (SBP) is >220 mmHg or the diastolic blood pressure (DBP) is >120 mmHg, unless end organ dysfunction is present.[29]

Antihypertensive treatment initiation should target a 15 to 25% reduction within the first 24 hours. If administration of rt-PA is considered, the targeted goal is a SBP <185 mmHg and a DBP <110 mmHg prior to administration and maintaining a SBP <180 mmHg and a DBP <105 mmHg after administration of rt-PA.[29] A safe lower limit for blood pressure during the acute phase remains undefined, yet is reported to be a SBP of 100 mmHg or a DBP of 70 mmHg; however, this is likely dependent upon the status of autoregulation.[29]

Some patients, particularly those with severe large vessel stenosis and vertebrobasilar disease, show an improved neurological exam when vasopressors are utilized to induce hypertension for CBF optimization. Large trials are lacking, but the goal is to typically titrate to a pressure 20 to 30% above baseline and wean based on the neurological exam and functional imaging.[19,29,31] The lack of neurological improvement within 30 to 60 minutes indicates a non-responder and induced hypertension should be aborted.

Revascularization

The most important therapy in ischemic stroke is restoration of blood flow to the ischemic penumbra, with the time of symptom onset directing candidacy for both intravenous and intra-arterial thrombolytic therapy.[29,30] rt-PA preferentially binds to clot-bound fibrin and catalyzes cleavage of entrapped plasminogen to plasmin. This process creates a local fibrinolysis with limited systemic proteolysis. In the National Institute of Neurologic Disorders and Stroke (NINDS) landmark study, neurological improvement did not differ within 24 hours, but an improvement in clinical outcomes was observed at 3 months.[32] The most significant associated harm is intracranial hemorrhage, which occurs at a rate of approximately 6%, as well as rare cases of anaphylaxis and angioedema. Based on this study, the number needed to treat (NNT) is 3, while the number needed to harm (NNH) is 30.[29,32]

Treatment with rt-PA should be considered at a dose of 0.9 mg/kg (maximum 90 mg), with 10% administered as a bolus and the remainder infused over 1 hour; this should be done in all acute ischemic stroke patients who meet criteria within 4.5 hours of symptom onset (the traditional time window had been 3 hours, but has now been extended to 4.5 hours per results of the European Cooperative Acute Stroke Study (ECASS-III)).[33] This extension in time does not create a situation that allows for further diagnostic work-up, as some estimate that 2 million neurons are lost every minute that treatment is delayed, with best outcomes in those receiving treatment within 90 minutes.[29,30] It is important that specific inclusion and exclusion criteria are considered to limit associated hemorrhagic complications. Table 15–4 lists inclusion and exclusion considerations.

Intra-arterial thrombolysis through a microcatheter provides an option to deliver high drug concentrations into the thrombus.[29,30] In comparison to the NINDS study, recanalization rates with intra-arterial thrombolysis appear to be higher; however, clinical outcomes are similar with a potential for a slightly higher rate of ICH.[29,34] Use of intra-arterial thrombolysis is growing in those with severe neurological deficits, presentation between 3 and 4.5 or even 6 hours after symptom onset, recent major surgery with contraindication to intravenous rt-PA, or occlusion of a major cervical or intracranial vessel that is unlikely to recanalize with intravenous rt-PA.

Table 15–4 rt-PA Inclusion and Exclusion Criteria

Inclusion	Relative Contraindications	Absolute Contraindications
Ischemic stroke onset within 3–4.5 hours*	Minor or rapidly improving symptoms	Multilobar infarct—hypodensity greater than one-third MCA
NIHSS >4 or potentially disabling	Seizure at onset of stroke	History of ICH or ruptured aneurysm
Age ≥18 years	Myocardial infarction in past 6 weeks	Another stroke or head trauma in past 3 months
	Hemorrhagic eye disorder	Major surgery or serious trauma in past 14 days
		Sustained SBP >185 mmHg or DBP >110 mmHg
		Gastrointestinal or urinary tract hemorrhage in past 21 days
		Arterial puncture at non-compressible site in past 7 days
		Heparin in past 48 hours with elevated aPTT
		Recent warfarin with INR >1.7
		Platelets <100 K/μL
		Glucose <50 or >400 explaining symptoms
		Recent lumbar puncture

*Excluding criteria in ECASS-III for intravenous rt-PA administered between 3–4.5 hours: age >80, NIHSS >25, oral anticoagulant regardless of INR, prior stroke plus diabetes mellitus

The decision analysis to proceed to intra-arterial therapy is often driven by perfusion mismatch and evidence of salvageable penumbra on radiological imaging. The intra-arterial dosing strategy is slightly different based on the type of catheter utilized, but a typical approach is one to two rt-PA boluses with 2 mg, followed by an infusion at 9 to 10 mg/hr until recanalization or a maximum of 22 mg has been administered.

To improve the efficiency and hopefully the efficacy of acute stroke recanalization in a way similar to the treatment of acute coronary syndromes (ACS), multimodal combination therapies are being investigated.[29,35,36] Ongoing studies are investigating the benefit of combined recanalization with lower dose intravenous rt-PA plus intra-arterial thrombolysis or mechanical thrombectomy, as well as the role of intracranial stenting. Other thrombolytic agents—tenecteplase, reteplase, and desmoteplase—and defibrinogenating agents such as ancrod, are being or have been tested; however, none have been established as effective or as a replacement for rt-PA.[29]

Anticoagulation and Antiplatelet Therapies

The role of emergency therapeutic anticoagulation with unfractionated heparin or low molecular-weight heparin in acute stroke remains controversial.[29,30] Early therapeutic anticoagulation is generally not considered beneficial as the majority of studies, with varying methodology, show an increased risk of symptomatic hemorrhagic transformation, particularly in those with moderate to severe strokes. However, adequate data do not exist for all subtypes of stroke and early therapeutic anticoagulation may be considered in specific scenarios, with careful consideration of risk versus benefit. These scenarios may involve strokes secondary to intracardiac or intra-arterial thrombi, vertebrobasilar disease, arterial dissection, large vessel atherosclerosis, or significant intracranial stenosis.[29] The AHA/ASA guidelines state that early therapeutic anticoagulation is generally not recommended, yet recognizes study limitations in regards to specific stroke subtypes. Deep vein thrombosis is a significant risk for stroke patients, and standard pharmacologic prophylaxis regimens are recommended.

Aspirin is the only oral antiplatelet agent evaluated for the treatment of acute ischemic stroke and is recommended at a daily dose of 325 mg. It may have a small reduction in recurrent stroke, NNT = 100, when initiated within 48 hours.[29] If rt-PA is administered, aspirin is withheld for 24 hours post-administration and initiated if the neurological exam is stable, repeat imaging confirms the absence of hemorrhagic transformation, and an emergent decompressive hemicraniectomy is not anticipated. It is generally considered that maintenance combination antiplatelet therapy may be harmful in patients with an ischemic stroke, as some data suggest an increased risk of intracranial hemorrhage with combination aspirin and clopidogrel. It is reasonable to consider combination therapy if a cardiac stent or an extra-cranial or intracranial stent was recently implanted, or for the management of atrial fibrillation if anticoagulation is contraindicated.[37] Patients should be stabilized on single antiplatelet therapy as soon as medically feasible. The intravenous glycoprotein IIb/IIIa inhibitors, abciximab, eptifibatide, and tirofiban are not recommended at this time as they have been shown to increase the risk of intracranial hemorrhage.[29]

The remainder of acute ischemic stroke therapy is largely supportive and directed towards management of cerebral edema and intracranial hypertension, which tends to be more common in large hemisphere strokes. The same medical ICP management principles apply as previously discussed. Treatment of residual effects and secondary prevention are beyond the scope of this text.

HEMORRHAGIC STROKE

Hemorrhagic stroke is associated with a high mortality.[38,39] Although a specific targeted therapy is lacking, studies suggest that many patients with small hemorrhages are readily survivable with aggressive medical care.[38,39] A small subset of patients may benefit from surgical management and clot evacuation, but the majority of care revolves around supportive medical measures. The goal of therapy is to reverse any existing coagulopathy, stabilize hematoma growth, and control hydrocephalus and intracranial hypertension.

Coagulopathy Management

Hematoma size and degree of progression are major risk predictors for poor outcome. Approximately 28 to 38% of patients experience hematoma growth within the first 24 hours, with the most rapid growth phase occurring within the first 1 to 3 hours.[38] The management for coagulopathic versus non-coagulopathic ICH differs, with the former having a greater risk of hematoma expansion that can occur over a longer period of time. Rapid reversal with blood products and pharmacologic agents targeted towards the specific anticoagulant or antiplatelet is advocated.[38-40] Intravenous vitamin K remains the antidote for reversing warfarin, but its ability to correct the coagulopathy is delayed for at least 6 to 24 hours; therefore, it serves as an adjunct to more rapid-acting agents. Reversal with blood products (e.g., fresh frozen plasma) can take several hours and potentially require large amounts of replacement volume, creating challenges in preventing pulmonary or cardiovascular decompensation in patients with renal or cardiopulmonary disease.

The use of recombinant activated factor VII (rFVIIa) or prothrombin complex concentrates (PCC) provides an opportunity for small volume, rapid reversal and is recommended per expert consensus.[38–40] However, currently, no study adequately compares rFVIIa with PCC. Recombinant FVIIa has been utilized at various dosages between 5 and 90 mcg/kg, with the most common dose being 20 or 40 mcg/kg. It may generate a thrombin burst, but does not replenish all of the vitamin K-dependent clotting factors and creates some concern that its effect may represent only a laboratory reversal of the internationalized ratio (INR) and not an actual coagulopathy reversal.

The use of PCC repletes additional vitamin K-dependent clotting factors, potentially offering an advantage over rFVIIa. There are several different PCC products, with each containing different quantities of clotting factors.[40,41] In general, they are classified as either four-factor products (factors II, VII, IX, and X) or three-factor products (II, IX, and X, but minimal to no factor VII). The majority of studies have used various dosing strategies of four-factor products, with less literature supporting three-factor product administration. There are some concerns that three-factor products may not adequately reverse the coagulopathy without concomitant administration of fresh frozen plasma (FFP) to supplement low quantities of factor VII.[42] Currently, only three-factor products are available in the United States. The majority of studies use between 25 to 50 units/kg, based on the presenting INR. If a three-factor PCC is utilized, 2 units of supplemental FFP or a 1 mg supplemental dose of rFVIIa should be considered.[41,42]

Dabigatran, an oral direct thrombin inhibitor, is now approved for anticoagulation in non-valvular atrial fibrillation.[43] Currently, there is no specific reversal antidote. Potential options may include rFVIIa or Factor Eight Inhibitor Bypass Agent (FEIBA). The most optimal pharmacologic reversal strategy remains undefined; however, it is imperative to ensure renal perfusion and adequate circulating platelets and fibrinogen.[44]

In addition to anticoagulants, many patients presenting with an ICH are taking antiplatelet agents. The utility of antiplatelet assays to assess platelet function and the benefits of platelet transfusion remain controversial.[38,40] It is reasonable to consider transfusing platelets in these patients, but the risk-to-benefit ratio must be assessed.

The management of non-coagulopathic ICH remains supportive. Recombinant FVIIa effectively reduced hematoma expansion in this population, but did not improve clinical outcomes, and so it is not currently recommended.[38,45] The primary study did have some methodological concerns and is being redesigned to better balance known risk factors (e.g., intraventricular hemorrhage) and to target patients with evidence of ongoing hematoma expansion on imaging.

Chapter 14 has further discussion on agent selection and coagulopathy reversal.

Hemodynamic and Seizure Management

Debate about the control of blood pressure in acute ICH revolves around two principles: hematoma growth and salvage of hypoperfused tissue surrounding the hematoma.[38,39] The current understanding suggests that an ischemic penumbra surrounding the hematoma likely does not exist and that intensive blood pressure control may prevent hematoma expansion and reduce cerebral edema. The AHA/ASA guidelines currently recommend a targeted SBP <160 mmHg or MAP <110 mmHg, or a CPP target of 50 to 70 mmHg if evidence of intracranial hypertension exists.[38]

The management of intracranial hypertension and cerebral edema follows the principles previously discussed. Investigative pharmacotherapy involves clot burden reduction with catheter directed rt-PA, intraventricular administration of rt-PA, and secondary oxidative stress reduction with the iron chelator, deferoxamine.[38,39]

The utility of prophylactic AEDs remains uncertain and they have not been shown to reduce the incidence of clinical seizures.[38] In fact, data have found an increased incidence of death or disability in patients with ICH receiving prophylactic AEDs, primarily phenytoin. It is best to not provide AED prophylaxis in ICH and only treat clinical or electrographic seizures if they occur.[38]

ANEURYSMAL SUBARACHNOID HEMORRHAGE

Pre-operative Phase

The primary concern immediately following presentation for an aneurysmal subarachnoid hemorrhage (aSAH) is resuscitation to ensure adequate cerebral perfusion, controlling hydrocephalus and intracranial hypertension, and preventing re-bleeding while waiting for a definitive aneurysm treatment plan.[46,47] Management of hydrocephalus is via CSF diversion through placement of a ventriculostomy or lumbar drain. Intracranial hypertension and ICP crisis management follow the same principles as previously discussed.

A few pharmacological modalities are typically implemented to prevent re-bleed. The most well-accepted therapy is emergent blood pressure control with short-acting intravenous antihypertensives. The optimal target range remains unknown, with literature suggesting a target SBP <140 to 160 mmHg with prevention of high systolic excursions.[46] The antihypertensive of choice follows the same principles as previously discussed, with a continuous infusion strategy limiting rebound excursions. The presence of intracranial hypertension may require a modified goal to target a CPP of 50 to 70 mmHg to ensure adequate cerebral perfusion.

Anti-fibrinolytics were effective and widely used as a prolonged infusion for the prevention of re-bleed before the 1980s.[46] However, the beneficial effects were offset by an increase in cerebral ischemic deficits and the therapy was largely abandoned. Today, the focus is on early treatment of the aneurysm and anti-fibrinolytics have reemerged. Tranexamic acid or aminocaproic acid initiated at presentation and continued until aneurysm repair or a maximum of 72 hours was associated with significant reduction in re-bleed without cerebral ischemic deficits.[46-48] Anti-fibrinolytic therapy may be reasonable to consider if no apparent high risk thromboembolic or ischemic factors are present and a predicted high rate of re-bleed exists.

The benefit of prophylactic AEDs during the perioperative period remains undefined. A short-course is reasonable in those requiring a craniotomy for aneurysm repair or those with an associated parenchymal hematoma or middle cerebral artery aneurysm.[46,47] It is common to use prophylactic AEDs until the aneurysm is repaired and then discontinue unless the patient remains comatose. Agent selection follows the same principles as discussed in TBI.

Neurogenic pulmonary edema and stunned myocardium with compromised left ventricular function can be observed during the acute phase of aSAH.[47] The condition is usually reversible, but may require supportive therapy to optimize brain perfusion and oxygenation. The therapeutic regimen targets the physiologic abnormality, but can include intravenous vasopressor (norephinephrine), inotropic (dobutamine or milrinone), or diuretic (furosemide or bumetanide) therapy.

Post-operative Phase

Post-operative goals following aneurysm repair are to prevent arterial vasospasm and delayed ischemic neurological deficits (DIND) and to treat medical complications.[46] Numerous pharmacological agents have been studied for the prevention or prophylaxis of vasospasm, with most failing to improve outcomes. Nimodipine (L-type calcium channel blocker) and pravastatin or simvastatin (HMG-CoA reductase inhibitors) have shown the most promise for either preventing vasospasm, DIND, and/or improving functional outcomes.[46,49] The only agent routinely accepted as standard of care is nimodipine 60 mg orally every 4 hours, initiated within 96 hours of ictus and continued for 21 days.[46,49] The most well-accepted data reveal an improvement in functional outcome by decreasing DIND, with no significant effect on angiographic vasospasm. The mechanism remains unclear, but is postulated to be neuroprotective through modulation of intracellular calcium and inhibition of thromboxane release and platelet aggregation.[50] The utility of other calcium channel blockers remains uncertain, with nimodipine being utilized largely for its comparative lipophilicity and possible higher cerebral distribution. A short, 14-day course of pravastatin or simvastatin is routinely utilized based on a risk-to-benefit assessment. They may provide clinical benefit by inhibiting superoxide production and enhancing endothelial nitric oxide production, thus decreasing the inflammatory response and increasing vasodilation, respectively.[46,51] The future utility of statin therapy is pending results of an on-going multi-center phase III trial utilizing simvastatin.[52]

Following aneurysm treatment, the systemic blood pressure control is typically relaxed and allowed to rise to a maximum SBP of 180 to 220 mmHg to ensure adequate cerebral perfusion.[46,47] Targeted blood pressure goals may change based on medical comorbidities (e.g., acute myocardial infarction, heart failure, intracranial hypertension). Prophylactic hypervolemia has shown no benefit and possibly more complications; however, it is imperative to ensure euvolemia in these patients.

The presence of blood in the subarachnoid space is thought to initiate a cascade of events that may result in vasospasm, or narrowing of the cerebral arteries, which may be accompanied by decreased CBF and ischemic sequelae.[46,53] It usually develops 3 to 5 days after aneurysm rupture, peaks at 5 to 14 days with symptom onset, and slowly resolves over 2 to 4 weeks. Treatment measures include Triple H (Hypertensive, Hypervolemic, and Hemodilution) and/or endovascular therapy to improve distal CBF and prevent DIND.[46,53,54] The term Triple H is still utilized, yet the typical target involves only hemodynamic augmentation, either targeting a goal MAP or cardiac index (CI) to ensure adequate cerebral perfusion. It has gained widespread acceptance, yet the efficacy and precise role remain uncertain. The morbidity and mortality of vasospasm can be high, thus the benefit of Triple H therapy is often counterbalanced by potential complications, such as pulmonary edema, decompensated heart failure, cerebral edema, ICP crisis, and re-bleed of any remaining unsecured or unruptured aneurysms. Vasopressors (phenylephrine or norepinephrine) or inotropes (dobutamine or milrinone) are utilized to target a MAP >120 mmHg (or >20% of baseline) or cardiac index >3.5 to 6 L/min/m^2.[46,47] Hemodynamic goals are adjusted based on clinical exam, patient tolerance, and functional imaging.

Endovascular therapy involves the administration of intra-arterial vasodilators directly at or near the site of vasospasm or utilizing balloon angioplasty if the spasm involves large proximal arteries.[54,55] It is generally accepted to initiate aggressive, early therapy, within 2-hours of clinical vasospasm onset.[46] Intra-arterial vasodilator therapy is usually reserved for small-vessel distal vasospasm where a balloon angioplasty catheter is not accessible.[55] Most studies show an increase in CBF with angiographic improvement, yet the duration of effect appears to be transient (1 to 24 hours) with only small improvements in neurological outcome. However, it is a reasonable therapy when considering the expected increase in morbidity and mortality with an aSAH patient who progresses towards vasospasm.

The pharmacologic agents most frequently utilized for endovascular therapy are papaverine (opium alkaloid with phosphodiesterase inhibition), nicardipine (L-type calcium channel blocker with vascular specificity), and verapamil (L-type calcium channel blocker lacking vascular specificity).[55] Nimodipine is not utilized in the United States for this indication because an intravenous formulation is not available. Papaverine is typically given at a dose of 150 to 300 mg (3 mg/mL solution), infused at 3 to 21 mg/min (1 to 7 mL/min). It results in a profound vasodilatory effect, risking an increase in CBV and ICP. It has also been associated with seizures, crystallization and microemboli, and possibly mitochondrial and neurotoxicity at higher doses. Nicardipine is typically given at a dose of 5 to 40 mg/procedure (0.83 to 1 mg/mL solution), infusing 0.5 to 1 mL over 60 seconds. Verapamil is typically given at a dose of 1 to 40 mg/procedure, infusing 1 to 5 mg boluses every 30 minutes. Each of them may contribute to systemic hypotension and ICP crisis, with the latter being more commonly described with the use of papaverine. General opinion is that verapamil and nicardipine may be safer alternatives in comparison to papaverine. Multiple daily treatments may be required to carry the patient through the period of most severe vasospasm.

STATUS EPILEPTICUS

Status epilepticus (SE) is associated with numerous triggering etiologies, most commonly from medication withdrawal or non-compliance in a known epilepsy patient or from acute neurologic or systemic insult and can be classified as convulsive or non-convulsive.[56-58] Definitions are conflicting, however any seizure persisting >5 minutes or two seizures without full recovery in between should be considered SE in order to facilitate the initiation of timely and appropriate treatment. The goals of therapy are rapid initiation of AEDs, treating any underlying triggering etiologies, and providing supportive medical care. See Table 15–5 detailing a pharmacological algorithm for SE.

Table 15–5 Treatment of Status Epilepticus in Adults

First 5 minutes	Diagnostic work-up
	ABCs (airway, breathing, and circulation)
	Obtain intravenous (IV) access
6–10 minutes	Thiamine 100 mg IV; D_{50} 50 mL IV unless adequate glucose known
	AND
	Lorazepam 0.1 mg/kg (or 4 mg) IV over 2 minutes; if still seizing, repeat once in 5 minutes
	OR
	If no IV access, give diazepam 20 mg PR or midazolam 10 mg IM or bucally
10–20 minutes	If seizures persist, begin fosphenytoin 20 mg PE/kg IV at 150 mg/min
	OR
	Valproate 30–40 mg/kg IV at 5 mg/kg/min
If seizures persist, give one of the following four options (intubation necessary, except for valproate)	Midazolam
	Load: 0.2 mg/kg, repeat 0.2–0.4 mg/kg IV boluses every 5 minutes until seizures stop, up to a maximum total loading dose of 2 mg/kg.
	Initial continuous infusion (cIV): 0.1 mg/kg/hr, titrate to response, range 0.05–2.9 mg/kg/hr. If still seizing, add or switch to propofol or pentobarbital.
	Propofol
	Load: 1 mg/kg, repeat 1–2 mg/kg IV boluses every 5 minutes until seizures stop, up to a maximum total loading dose of 10 mg/kg.
	Initial continuous infusion (cIV): 2 mg/kg/hr, titrate to response, range 1–10 mg/kg/hr. If still seizing, add or switch to midazolam or pentobarbital.
	Valproate
	Load: 30–40 mg/kg. If still seizing, additional 20 mg/kg. If still seizing, add or switch to midazolam or propofol.
	Phenobarbital
	Load: 20 mg/kg. If still seizing, add or switch to midazolam, propofol, or pentobarbital.
>60 minutes	Pentobarbital
	Load: 5–10 mg/kg, repeat 5 mg/kg IV boluses until seizures stop.
	Initial continuous infusion (cIV): 1 mg/kg/hr, titrate to response, range 0.5–5 mg/kg/hr; titrated to burst suppression on EEG.

Early initiation of pharmacological therapy may be more important than the particular agent selected. If AEDs are administered within the first 30 minutes of onset, an 80% response rate to first-line drugs has been observed, whereas a decline to 40% response rate occurred if therapy was delayed >2 hours.[56,57] The majority of supporting data for AED selection arises from the Veteran's Administration Cooperative study, which compared 4 intravenous regimens: phenobarbital (15 mg/kg), phenytoin (18 mg/kg), diazepam (0.15 mg/kg) plus phenytoin (18 mg/kg), and lorazepam (0.1 mg/kg). A trend towards improved efficacy was observed with lorazepam, while phenytoin monotherapy was shown to be less effective than lorazepam.[56,57] The remaining agents were shown to be equally effective as first-line agents, with very poor response rates to the second (7%) or third (2.3%) agent initiated. The first-line AED should be selected in consideration of each agent's pharmacokinetic/pharmacodynamic (PK/PD) profile, the patient's prior medical history, concomitant medications, allergies, hemodynamic status, and end organ function.

The benzodiazepines bind to high-affinity sites on the gamma aminobutyric acid (GABA) receptor, resulting in hyperpolarization of the neuronal cell membrane and decreased neuronal firing.[56-58] Diazepam is more lipophillic, potentially offering a faster cerebral distribution and therapeutic onset, whereas lorazepam is more hydrophilic, potentially offering a longer duration of antiseizure effect of 12 to 24 hours. If intravenous access is not available, diazepam 20 mg per rectum or midazolam 10 mg via the intranasal, bucal, or intramuscular route may be administered.

Phenytoin or fosphenytoin are the most frequently recommended agents following an initial benzodiazepine, but intravenous valproate is likely as effective and may offer some advantages.[56,57] The antiseizure activity of phenytoin is complex, however; its major action appears to block the voltage sensitive, use-dependent sodium channels. Hypotension and cardiac arrhythmias can occur with both of the hydantoins, but phenytoin has a slightly higher risk, which can be minimized by slowing the rate of administration. The maximum rate of administration for phenytoin is 50 mg/min, whereas fosphenytoin is 150 mg/min. Phenytoin is alkaline and can cause severe tissue necrosis, limiting it to intravenous administration via well-established access, whereas fosphenytoin is pH neutral and can be given via the intravenous or intramuscular route. Fosphenytoin requires dephosphorylation, which occurs over 10 to 15 minutes, to active phenytoin; however, this has not been shown to compromise clinical efficacy.[56,57] The dephosphorylation time is likely compensated by the ability to administer more rapidly in comparison to phenytoin. Pharmacokinetic variability can occur, particularly in patients with hypoalbuminemia, uremia, and interacting medications. The latter is common, particularly in refractory SE requiring multiple AED combinations. Free phenytoin levels targeting a goal of 1.5 to 2.5 mcg/mL should be monitored when readily available, particularly since excessively high levels potentially exacerbate seizures.

Valproate is a broad-spectrum AED with activity against all types of seizures. It is being more frequently used at an intravenous bolus dose of 30 to 40 mg/kg administered rapidly at a rate of 3 to 6 mg/kg/min, with a maintenance dose titrated to clinical response or a serum level of 50 to 100 mcg/mL.[56,57] One advantage over other first-generation AEDs is that it causes limited sedation and is not associated with hypotension at therapeutic doses. It is associated with auto protein displacement, particularly as levels exceeding 50 mcg/mL with normal albumin stores, and likely earlier in states of hypoalbuminemia. In these conditions, targeted total serum levels do not represent a linear relationship to free levels and toxicity may be observed despite "normal" total serum levels. Overall, it is very well tolerated, but some adverse effects are important to recognize, specifically hyperammonemia, hepatic failure, and thrombocytopenia. Hyperammonemia is common in many patients, but most remain asymptomatic and do not experience encephalopathy. Fatal hepatic failure is reported, but more common in patients <2 years of age or on multiple cytochrome CYP-450 enzyme inducers, as a metabolic shunting of the toxic metabolite occurs. It is important to monitor liver enzymes and liver synthetic function if patients are on valproic acid and multiple enzyme inducers. Thrombocytopenia is usually dose related and benign; however, some patients can experience platelet dysfunction and bleeding.

An alternative agent is intravenous phenobarbital 15 to 20 mg/kg administered at 50 to 100 mg/min.[56,57] It is an effective AED mediated through direct inhibitory GABA agonist activity, but can cause respiratory depression, myocardial depression, hypotension, and profound sedation. Sedation can potentially mask the neurological exam and limit the ability of the clinician to direct future treatment requirements.

If first-line therapeutic approaches fail, emergent intubation with rapid initiation of continuous benzodiazepines, propofol, or pentobarbital is indicated.[56-59] This should be considered very early in therapy and possibly immediately after failing a benzodiazepine trial, rather than waiting until a second-line agent has failed. The continuous agent should be titrated to burst suppression on EEG, most commonly a 5 to 10 second burst. Agent selection is largely based on PK/PD properties and anecdotal experience. In comparison to benzodiazepines and pentobarbital, propofol offers the advantage of a short alpha distribution half-life with the ability to perform rapid neurological exams and a mechanism involving both inhibitory GABA agonist activity and excitatory NMDA antagonist activity. The latter is particularly attractive, as experimental models have shown the development of pharmacoresistance as SE progresses, which is proposed to be mediated through GABA receptor uptake and down regulation, creating a dominant excitatory NMDA mediated seizure process.[58] For SE treatment, propofol is given as a loading dose of 1 to 2 mg/kg, repeated every 5 minutes until the seizure is terminated, followed by an infusion of 1 to 10 mg/kg/hr (15 to 150 mcg/kg/min). The disadvantage of propofol is concern for propofol infusion syndrome (PIS), particularly at high doses. It is best to limit infusions of more than 5 mg/kg/hr (83 mcg/kg/min) to <24 to 48 hours and monitor very closely for PIS. It may be reasonable to consider a combination of propofol plus midazolam as a propofol dose-sparing strategy. The preferred continuous benzodiazepine is midazolam, as it is lipophilic at body temperature and pH, offering a rapid onset, and it does not contain propylene glycol (PG) as a solubilizer.[56-59] In comparison, both lorazepam and the barbiturate pentobarbital contain PG.

Tachyphylaxis and pharmacoresistance can rapidly develop to GABA active agents, requiring very large lorazepam and pentobarbital doses and creating concern for PG toxicity. The disadvantage of midazolam is the potential for drug accumulation, particularly at high doses and long durations of therapy or in patients with end organ dysfunction and the inability to metabolize active drug or eliminate active metabolites. Midazolam is given as a loading dose of 0.2 to 0.4 mg/kg, repeated every 5 minutes until the seizure is terminated, followed by an infusion of 0.1 to 2.9 mg/kg/hr. Pentobarbital may have lower treatment failure rates in comparison to midazolam and propofol, but numerous methodological concerns exist with the particular comparative study.[56,57] Its major disadvantage is a long half-life and inability to perform rapid neurological exams, as well as a myriad of adverse effects, including myocardial depression, hypotension, immunosupression, and gastrointenstinal ileus.

Despite the continuous agent(s) selected for refractory SE, it is typical to continue for 12 to 24 hours after seizure termination and then begin a gradual taper over an additional 12 to 24 hours.[56,57] If seizures recur, consider treating for a longer duration and tapering more slowly, while maintaining high therapeutic levels of concomitant maintenance oral and intravenous agents.

A good clinical outcome with prolonged, highly refractory status epilepticus (RSE) is not common, with a greater chance for recovery in those who have an etiology secondary to medication withdrawal or non-compliance versus a structural, acute brain process. Multiple other pharmacological agents have been used in RSE and are mostly supported by case reports and anecdotal experience, with little direction regarding dosing strategies.[57,59] They may include levetiracetam, lacosamide, topiramate, zonisamide, oxcarbazepine, high-dose phenobarbital and/or continuous valproic acid, ketamine, lidocaine, or isoflurane. The utilization of isoflurane requires anesthesia equipment. Lidocaine can actually potentiate seizures at high doses, thus it is recommended to maintain serum levels <3 to 5 mcg/mL.[59]

SPINAL CORD INJURY

Pharmacotherapy for acute spinal cord injury remains very limited and is largely directed towards neuroprotection, hemodynamic stabilization and spinal cord perfusion, and management of associated medical complications.

Neuroprotection

Several pharmaceuticals have been tested for neuroprotective effects, with most failing to improve outcomes in acute spinal cord injury (SCI). The only agent to show benefit is high-dose methylprednisolone (MP) administered within 8 hours of blunt SCI, which is believed to inhibit lipid peroxidation, retard neuronal degeneration, and curb the inflammatory induced secondary injury cascade.[60] However, the methodology, analysis, and results of the NASCIS (National Acute Spinal Cord Injury Study) trials are fraught with controversy.[60,61] The traditional dose is 30 mg/kg intravenous bolus over 15 minutes, followed by an infusion of 5.4 mg/kg/hr to complete a 24-hour infusion if presentation is within 3 hours of injury, or a 48-hour infusion if presentation is within 3 to 8 hours of injury. The relatively small and questionable treatment effect may not outweigh the risk of patient harm and potential complications, including infections, delayed wound-healing, pulmonary embolism, myopathies, and avascular necrosis. Some clinicians suggest that the potential benefit in select patients as a small improvement in function, such as the ability to feel urinary urgency or the recovery of diaphragmatic function, may have a huge impact on activities of daily living, which supports use of steroids. An expert consensus panel does not definitively recommend MP to improve functional recovery.[62]

Hemodynamics and Neurogenic Shock

Neurogenic shock is not uncommon, particularly in SCI patients at a level above T1 through T6, secondary to sympathetic denervation and interruption of cardiac sympathetic innervation with unopposed vagal activity.[62]

The result is hemodynamic instability manifested by arteriolar dilation, hypovolemia, hypotension, relative bradycardia, and often hypothermia. Recovery is slow; it can take up to 2 to 6 weeks for the renin-angiotensin-aldosterone system (RAAS) to provide compensation for the loss of autonomic control. The immediate therapeutic goal is to restore systemic perfusion, thereby limiting hypoxic injury to the spinal cord, and to prevent symptomatic bradycardia or asystole. Small, uncontrolled studies suggest using fluids and vasopressors to maintain a MAP >85 mmHg for 7 days to ensure adequate spinal cord perfusion.[62] An agent with some beta$_1$-receptor activity is favored over those with selective alpha-receptor activity, as the latter may potentiate a reflex increase in vagal tone, worsening bradyarrhythmias. Secondary to the slow recovery in vasomotor tone, patients may require oral vasoactive or RAAS-active medications to maintain adequate perfusion while weaning off intravenous vasopressors. The use of midodrine (alpha$_1$-agonist), ephedrine or pseudoephedrine (mixed alpha/beta agonist), or fludrocortisone (mineralocorticoid) is not uncommon.

If bradycardia is contributing to hypotension or conduction block is evident, treatment with atropine 0.5 to 1 mg IV every 5 minutes, with a total of 3 mg or 0.04 mg/kg, is the drug of choice.[62] Atropine antagonizes the muscarinic (M$_2$) receptors in the sinoatrial (SA) and atrioventricular (AV) nodes, targeting the unopposed vagal response. If atropine fails or anticholinergic toxicity is evident, low-dose aminophylline has been effective in a few case reports.[63] The mechanism is reported to occur via antagonism of the adenosine (A$_1$) receptor in the SA and AV nodes or via inhibition of phosphodiesterase (PDE III), with a subsequent increase in circulating catecholamines. There is no established therapeutic range; however, it appears that low serum levels, <3.8 mcg/mL, are effective with minimal toxicity. The dose should be titrated based on individual patient response, with extreme caution utilized in those with a concomitant TBI for risk of a lowered seizure threshold with theophylline.

The remaining therapy for SCI injury involves pain management, bowel and bladder management, aggressive skin care, and prevention and treatment of autonomic dysreflexia.[62] All of these may occur and are important during the acute phase, but largely become a focus during the rehabilitation phase of SCI, and are beyond the scope of this text.

SUMMARY

Acute neurological injury can be a devastating disease and have major consequences on one's long-term functional and cognitive quality of life. The majority of pharmaceuticals targeted towards neuroprotection have unfortunately failed to improve morbidity and mortality. The best outcomes are in those who receive urgent treatment with the goal of minimizing the progression of the primary injury and preventing adverse events that contribute to secondary injury.

KEY POINTS

- Cerebral oxygen delivery is regulated by a complex mechanism that can be interrupted easily by injury.
- Stroke is the result of either an occlusive or hemorrhagic event and treatment varies based upon the underlying pathology.
- Management of patients with neurologic injury is primarily directed at improving oxygen delivery to minimize secondary damage due to swelling and inflammation.
- Seizure treatment in the critically ill can be particularly challenging and medications should be selected based upon an individual care plan and carefully monitored.

SELECTED SUGGESTED READINGS

- The Saline versus Albumin Fluid Evaluation (SAFE) study investigators. Saline or albumin for fluid resuscitation in patients with traumatic brain injury. *N Engl J Med.* 2007;357:874–884.
- Brain Trauma Foundation, American Association of Neurological Surgeons, Congress of Neurological Surgeons, Joint Section on Neurotrauma and Critical Care. Guidelines for the management of severe traumatic brain injury. *J Neurotrauma.* 2007;24(Suppl 1).
- Papangelou A, Lewin JJ, Mirski MA, et al. Pharmacologic Management of brain edema. *Curr Treat Op Neurol.* 2009;11:64–73.
- Adams HP, del Zoppo G, Alberts MJ, et al. Guidelines for the early management of adults with ischemic stroke: a guideline from the American Heart Association/American Stroke Association. *Stroke.* 2007;38:1655–1711.
- Morgenstern LB, Hemphill JC 3rd, Anderson C, et al. Guidelines for the management of spontaneous intracerebral hemorrhage: a guideline for healthcare professionals from the American Heart Association/American Stroke Association. *Stroke.* 2010;41: 2108–2129.
- Consortium for Spinal Cord Medicine. Early acute management in adults with spinal cord injury: a clinical practice guideline for health-care professionals. *J Spinal Cord Med.* 2008;31(4):403–479.

REFERENCES

1. Vincent JL, Berre J. Primer on medical management of severe brain injury. *Crit Care Med.* 2005;33:1392–1399.
2. Schaller B, Graf R. Different compartments of intracranial pressure and its relationship to cerebral blood flow. *J Trauma.* 2005;59(6):1521–1531.
3. Brigham and Women's Hospital Neurosurgery Group. Principles of cerebral oxygenation and blood flow in the neurological critical care unit. *Neurocrit Care.* 2006;4:77–82.
4. Brigham and Women's Hospital Neurosurgery Group. Neuromonitoring in neurological critical care. *Neurocrit Care.* 2006;4:83–92.
5. Brain Trauma Foundation, American Association of Neurological Surgeons, Congress of Neurological Surgeons, Joint Section on Neurotrauma and Critical Care. Guidelines for the management of severe traumatic brain injury. I. Blood pressure and oxygenation. *J Neurotrauma.* 2007;24(Suppl 1):S7–S13.
6. The Saline versus Albumin Fluid Evaluation (SAFE) study investigators. Saline or albumin for fluid resuscitation in patients with traumatic brain injury. *N Engl J Med.* 2007;357:874–884.
7. Forsyth LL, Liu-DeRyke X, Parker D, et al. Role of hypertonic saline for the management of intracranial hypertension after stroke and traumatic brain injury. *Pharmacotherapy.* 2008;28(4):469–484.
8. Rangel-Castillo L, Gopinath S, Robertson CS. Management of intracranial hypertension. *Neurol Clin.* 2008;26:521–541.
9. Papangelou A, Lewin JJ, Mirski MA, et al. Pharmacologic management of brain edema. *Curr Treat Op Neurol.* 2009;11:64–73.
10. Garcia-Morales EJ, Rohit C, Parvin CA, et al. Osmole gap in neurologic-neurosurgical intensive care unit: its normal value, calculation, and relationship with mannitol serum concentrations. *Crit Care Med.* 2004;32(4):986–991.
11. Greenberg, MS. *Handbook of Neurosurgery. 6th ed.* New York, NY:Thieme Medical Publishers; 2005:12–13.
12. Rhoney DH, Parker D. Use of sedative and analgesic agents in neurotrauma. *Neurol Res.* 2001;23:237–259.
13. Mirski MA, Lewin JJ. Sedation and pain management in acute neurological disease. *Semin Neurol.* 2008;28(5):611–630.
14. Hutchens MP, Memtsoudis S, Sadovnikoff N. Propofol for sedation in neuro-intensive care. *Neurocrit. Care* 2006;4:54–62.
15. Axelrod YK, Diringer MN. Temperature management in acute neurologic disorders. *Neurol Clin.* 2008;26:585–603.
16. Weant KA, Martin JE, Humphries RL, et al. Pharmacologic options for reducing the shivering response to therapeutic hypothermia. *Pharmacotherapy.* 2010;30(8):830–841.
17. Brain Trauma Foundation, American Association of Neurological Surgeons, Congress of Neurological Surgeons, Joint Section on Neurotrauma and Critical Care. Guidelines for the management of severe traumatic brain injury. IX. Cerebral perfusion thresholds. *J Neurotrauma.* 2007;24(Suppl 1):S59–S64.

18. Robertson CS, Valadka AB, Hannay HJ, et al. Prevention of secondary ischemic insults after severe head injury. *Crit Care Med.* 1999;27:2086–2095.
19. Muzevich KM, Voils SA. Role of vasopressor administration in patients with acute neurologic injury. *Neurocrit Care.* 2009;11(1):112–119.
20. Diringer MN, Axelrod Y. Hemodynamic manipulation in the neuro-intensive care unit: cerebral perfusion pressure therapy in head injury and hemodynamic augmentation for cerebral vasospasm. *Curr Opin Crit Care.* 2007;13:156–162.
21. Rose JC, Mayer SA. Optimizing blood pressure in neurological emergencies. *Neurocrit Care.* 2004;1:287–299.
22. Gomes JA, Stevens RD, Lewin JJ, et al. Glucocorticoid therapy in neurologic critical care. *Crit Care Med.* 2005;33:1214–1224.
23. Kaal EC, Vecht CJ. The management of brain edema in brain tumors. *Curr Opin Oncol.* 2004;16:593–600.
24. Brain Trauma Foundation, American Association of Neurological Surgeons, Congress of Neurological Surgeons, Joint Section on Neurotrauma and Critical Care. Guidelines for the management of severe traumatic brain injury. XIII. Antiseizure prophylaxis. *J Neurotrauma.* 2007;24(Suppl 1):S83–S86.
25. Rosengart AJ, Huo D, Tolentino J, et al. Outcome in patients with subarachnoid hemorrhage treated with antiepileptic drugs. *J Neurosurg.* 2007;107:253–260.
26. Frend V, Hons BP, Chetty M. Dosing and therapeutic monitoring of phenytoin in young adults after neurotrauma: are current practices relevant? *Clin Neuropharmacol.* 2007;30(6):362–369.
27. Temkin NR, Dikmen SS, Wilensky AJ. A randomized, double-blind study of phenytoin for the prevention of post-traumatic seizures. *N Engl J Med.* 1990;323:497–502.
28. Szaflarski JP, Sangha KS, Lindsell CJ. Prospective, randomized, single-blinded comparative trial of intravenous levetiracetam versus phenytoin for seizure prophylaxis. *Neurocrit Care.* 2010;12(2):165–172.
29. Adams HP, del Zoppo G, Alberts MJ, et al. Guidelines for the early management of adults with ischemic stroke: a guideline from the American Heart Association/American Stroke Association. *Stroke.* 2007;38:1655–1711.
30. Caulfield AF, Wijman CA. Management of acute ischemic stroke. *Neurol Clin.* 2008;26:345–371.
31. Urrutia VC, Wityk RJ. Blood pressure management in acute stroke. *Neurol Clin.* 2008;26:565–583.
32. National Institute of Neurological Disorders and Stroke rt-PA Stroke Study Group. Tissue plasminogen activator for acute ischemic stroke. *N Engl J Med.* 1995;333:1581–1587.
33. Hacke W, Kaste M, Bluhmki E, et al. Thrombolysis with Alteplase 3 to 4.5 hours after acute ischemic stroke. *N Engl J Med.* 2008;359:1317–1329.
34. The IMS II Trial Investigators. The interventional management of stroke (IMS) II study. *Stroke.* 2007;38:2127–2135.
35. The Internet Stroke Center at Washington University in St. Louis. IMS-III: the interventional management of stroke (IMS) III trial. http://www.strokecenter.org/trials/TrialDetail.aspx?tid=747. Accessed June 15, 2011.

36. The Internet Stroke Center at Washington University in St. Louis. SAMMPRIS: stenting vs. aggressive medical management for preventing recurrent stroke in intracranial stenosis. http://www.strokecenter.org/trials /TrialDetail.aspx?tid=819. Accessed June 15, 2011.

37. The ACTIVE Investigators. Effect of clopidogrel added to aspirin in patients with atrial fibrilliation. *N Engl J Med.* 2009;360(20):2066–2078.

38. Morgenstern LB, Hemphill JC 3rd, Anderson C, et al. Guidelines for the management of spontaneous intracerebral hemorrhage: a guideline for healthcare professionals from the American Heart Association/American Stroke Association. *Stroke.* 2010;41:2108–2129.

39. Nyquist P. Management of acute intracranial and intraventricular hemorrhage. *Crit Care Med.* 2010;38(3):946–953.

40. Beshay JE, Morgan H, Madden C, et al. Emergency reversal of anticoagulation and antiplatelet therapies in neurosurgical patients. *J Neurosurg.* 2010;112(2):307–318.

41. Bershad EM, Suarez JI. Prothrombin complex concentrates for oral anticoagulant therapy-related intracranial hemorrhage: a review of the literature. *Neurocrit Care.* 2010;12(3):403–413.

42. Holland L, Warkentin TE, Refaai M, et al. Suboptimal effect of a three-factor prothrombin complex concentrate (Profilnine-SD) in correcting supratherapeutic international normalized ratio due to warfarin overdose. *Transfusion.* 2009;49(6):1171–1177.

43. Connolly SJ, Ezekowitz MD, Yusuf S, et al. Dabigatran versus warfarin in patients with atrial fibrillation. *N Engl J Med.* 2009;361(12):1139–1151.

44. van Ryn J, Stangier J, Haertter S, et al. Dabigatran etexilate-a novel, reversible, oral direct thrombin inhibitor: interpretation of coagulation assays and reversal of anticoagulant activity. *Thromb Haemost.* 2010;103:1116–1127.

45. Mayer SA, Brun NC, Begtrup K, et al. Efficacy and safety of recombinant activated factor VII for acute intracerebral hemorrhage. *N Engl J Med.* 2008;358(20):2127–2137.

46. Bederson JB, Connolly ES, Batjer HH, et al. Guidelines for the management of aneurysmal subarachnoid hemorrhage: a statement for healthcare professionals from a special writing group of the stroke council, American Heart Association. *Stroke.* 2009;40:994–1025.

47. Komotar RJ, Schmidt JM, Starke, RM, et al. Resuscitation and critical care of poor-grade subarachnoid hemorrhage. *Neurosurgery.* 2009;64:397–411.

48. Starke RM, Kim GH, Fernandez A, et al. Impact of a protocol for acute antifibrinolytic therapy on aneurysm rebleeding after subarachnoid hemorrhage. *Stroke.* 2008;39:2617–2621.

49. Lazaridis C, Naval N. Risk factors and medical management of vasospasm after subarchnoid hemorrhage. *Neurosurg Clin N Am.* 2010;21(2):353–364.

50. Barker FG, Ogilvy CS. Efficacy of prophylactic nimodipine for delayed ischemic deficit after subarachnoid hemorrhage: a metanalysis. *J Neurosurg.* 1996;84: 405–414.

51. Trimble JL, Kocker DR. Statin treatment of cerebral vasospasm after aneurysmal subarachnoid hemorrhage. *Ann Pharmacother.* 2007;41:2019–2023.

52. The Internet Stroke Center at Washington University in St. Louis. STASH: Simvastatin in aneurysmal subarachnoid hemorrhage a multicentre randomised controlled clinical trial. http://www.strokecenter.org/trials/TrialDetail.aspx?tid=930. Accessed June 15, 2011.

53. Lee KH, Lukovits T, Friedman JA. "Triple-H" therapy for cerebral vasospasm following subarachnoid hemorrhage. *Neurocrit Care.* 2006;4:68–76.

54. Zwienenberg-Lee M, Hartman J, Rudisill N, et al. Endovascular management of cerebral vasospasm. *Neurosurgery.* 2006;59(2):53–147.

55. Weant KA, Ramsey CN, Cook AM. Role of intraarterial therapy for cerebral vasospasm secondary to aneurysmal subarachnoid hemorrhage. *Pharmacotherapy.* 2010;30(4):405–417.

56. Abou Khaled KJ, Hirsch LJ. Updates in the management of seizures and status epilepticus in critically ill patients. *Neurol Clin.* 2008;26:385–408.

57. Hirsch LJ, Arif H. Status epilepticus. *Continuum Lifelong Learning Neurol.* 2007;13(4):121–151.

58. Chen JW, Wasterlain CG. Status epilepticus: pathophysiology and management in adults. *Lancet Neurol.* 2006;5:246–256.

59. Robakis TK, Hirsch LJ. Literature review, case report, and expert discussion of prolonged refractory status epilepticus. *Neurocrit Care.* 2006;4:35–46.

60. Bracken MB, Shepard MJ, Holford TR, et al. Administration of methylprednisolone for 24 or 48 hours or tirilazad mesylate for 48 hours in the treatment of acute spinal cord injury. Results of the third national acute spinal cord injury randomized controlled trial. National Acute Spinal Cord Injury Study. *JAMA.* 1997;277(20):1597–1604.

61. Sayer FT, Kronvall E, Nilsson OG. Methylprednisolone treatment in acute spinal cord injury: the myth challenged through a structured analysis of published literature. *Spine J.* 2006;6:335–343.

62. Consortium for Spinal Cord Medicine. Early acute management in adults with spinal cord injury: a clinical practice guideline for health-care professionals. *J Spinal Cord Med.* 2008;31(4):403–479.

63. Whitman CB, Schroeder WS, Ploch PJ, et al. Efficacy of aminophylline for treatment of recurrent symptomatic bradycardia after spinal cord injury. *Pharmacotherapy.* 2008;28(1):131–135.

Chapter 16

Neonatal and Pediatric Intensive Care Basics

Wendy Jensen Bender

1. Define the neonatal and pediatric critically ill patient populations.
2. Describe pharmacokinetic changes seen in neonates, infants, and children.
3. Utilize knowledge of the unique differences in monitoring and treatment approaches in the pediatric critically ill patient to develop appropriate patient care plans.
4. Review neonatal and pediatric illnesses common to the critically ill patient population and describe appropriate treatments.

INTRODUCTION

Significant literature and attention is focused on the treatment of the critically ill adult patient, but a large amount of critical care practice occurs in the neonatal and pediatric patient populations. Pediatric patients can often be treated similarly to adults, but they are not "little adults." There are some general concepts, differing equipment, and specific physiology to consider when caring for a critically ill pediatric patient.

One of the first elements to understand is the terminology associated with different age groups, as different stages of development will lead to changes in the overall patient care plan. Table 16–1 delineates common definitions related to age. The intent of this chapter is to introduce the reader

Table 16–1 Defining Patient Populations

Pediatric Patients	Patients Under 18 Years of Age
Preterm/premature	Less than 37 weeks gestational age at birth
Term	37 to 40 weeks gestational age at birth
Neonate	Any infant birth to 28 days of age
Infant	1 month to 1 year of age
Child	1 to 11 years of age
Adolescent	12 to 16 years of age (often defined as up to 18 years of age)

to differences in pediatric practice by reviewing some basic differences in the pharmacokinetics of critically ill neonatal and pediatric patients, as well as common disease states encountered in these patient populations. It is important for any pharmacist working in an acute care setting to have at least fundamental knowledge of the differences in the neonatal and pediatric patient populations as compared to adult patients.

PHARMACOKINETICS OVERVIEW

Absorption, distribution, metabolism, and elimination of medications differ in infants, children, and adolescents as compared to adults. Generally speaking, organ function is not mature at birth and these differences affect the pharmacokinetics of medications. It is important to note that not only is organ function in pediatric patients different in comparison to adults, but that function also varies when comparing one pediatric age group to another.

Absorption

Medications can be administered via numerous routes, including oral, intravenous (IV), intramuscular (IM), rectally, and percutaneously, and differences among age groups can affect the preferred route of administration.[1-3] Newborns are relatively hypochlorhydric, so acid-labile drugs, such as penicillin, will achieve higher serum concentrations when given orally. Conversely, oral phenobarbital doses may need to be increased due to decreased absorption as a result of the weakly acidic nature of the drug. The rate of gastric emptying also affects drug bioavailability for oral medications. The effects of slowed gastric emptying in neonates on drug absorption is not well studied, but the delay would be expected to increase serum levels of medication absorbed in the intestine and increase the time to reach peak serum levels after oral administration. Administration via the IM route is difficult in low birth weight neonates due to a lack of muscle mass, and intramuscular absorption is also unreliable in patients with poor circulation and decreased muscle movement.[1-3] Transdermal administration of drugs in neonates is not well studied. At birth, neonatal skin has increased hydration and decreased stratum corneum thickness in comparison with adults, which would be expected to affect absorption rates, but the extent of the differences is unknown. Also, children have an increased body surface area per kilogram body weight, so adult BSA medication dosing cannot be assumed to be appropriate in children.

Distribution

Distribution is affected by total body water, protein binding, and adipose tissue, all of which differ to varying degrees in children in comparison to adults.[1-3] Premature and term infants have 85% and 75% total body water, respectively, and therefore will have an increased volume of distribution for hydrophilic drugs. The adipose tissue of the neonatal population also contains more water than adult adipose tissue. Very premature infants can have as little as 1% fat, which will decrease the volume of distribution of lipid soluble medications such as diazepam. Lastly, newborns have lower total protein and albumin levels in comparison to more mature patients. Fetal albumin binds to drugs poorly, increasing free drug levels of protein-bound medications.

Metabolism

Hepatic metabolism is much lower in the infant in comparison to an older child or adult. Enzyme pathway maturation varies depending on the patient and pathway; for example, sulfation enzymes are present at birth, but activity is lower than in an older patient. The conjugation pathway will reach adult levels by about 2 months of age, but the glucuronidation pathway does not reach adult activity until 6 to 18 months of age.[1-3] Despite the initially slowed hepatic metabolism, by about 1 year of age hepatic metabolism greatly exceeds that of adult metabolism. Therefore, children and adolescents may need much higher doses of medications to compensate for the increased hepatic activity.

Elimination

As with hepatic metabolism, renal function is also not mature at birth. Renal elimination of medications is much slower at birth due to immature glomerular filtration rates (GFR) and immature tubular secretion and reabsorption processes. In addition, GFR is slower in premature infants in comparison to term infants.[1-3] Generally, GFR reaches adult capacity by 8 to 12 months of age, even in premature infants. Renal elimination of medications in children and adolescents can be much faster than in adults, so pediatric patients must be monitored closely for drug efficacy.

UNIQUE ASPECTS OF NEONATAL AND PEDIATRIC CRITICAL CARE

There are some unique aspects of caring for critically ill neonates, infants, children, and adolescents. Understanding the unique equipment and intravenous access devices is one component necessary to provide optimal patient care. Further, many different disease processes may be seen in critically ill neonatal and pediatric patients. The more common problems will be addressed in this chapter; however, it is not possible to completely address all possible issues in one chapter, so the focus will be on problems and diseases where pharmacologic intervention is important.

Equipment

Premature neonates require special beds, warmers, and isolettes to assist in thermoregulation. Some isolettes can also be humidified to decrease insensible water loss through the premature skin barrier. Transcutaneous monitoring of partial pressure of oxygen and carbon dioxide is also possible due to the prematurity of the neonate's skin.[4]

Intravenous Access

Most forms of IV access have been discussed in Chapter 3, but in addition to IV access, the intraosseus (IO) catheter can be extremely useful in pediatric patients. In IO access, a needle is inserted into the intraosseus space, most often in the tibia, and can provide rapid access for fluid resuscitation or medication administration. Neonatal Intensive Care Unit (NICU) patients frequently have unique vascular access through an umbilical arterial catheter (UAC) and umbilical venous catheter (UVC). In addition to providing central intravenous access, umbilical catheters provide the opportunity for advanced monitoring, including arterial blood gas analysis and continuous monitoring of central venous pressure (CVP), blood pressure (BP), and mean arterial pressure (MAP). The UAC is threaded through one of the umbilical arteries in the umbilical stump and the tip resides in the aorta. The UVC is threaded through the umbilical vein and the tip will be in the inferior vena cava.[4,5]

Fluid Management

Prevention of overhydration, underhydration, and electrolyte imbalances in infants and children requires close attention. Infants and children normally exchange more extracellular fluid in a day in comparison to adults, so their body fluid reserve (i.e., the fluid that would not be excreted and replaced each day) is smaller. Fever and tachypnea both increase insensible water loss in pediatric patients. Assessment of hydration status includes skin color, mucous membrane moistness, tear production, heart rate, capillary refill, urine output, and weight, especially if an accurate baseline weight is available. Maintenance IV fluids should be isotonic and provide both dextrose for energy and electrolytes to prevent electrolyte imbalances.[6,7]

Respiratory Distress and Respiratory Failure in Infants, Children, and Adolescents

Infants and children have a higher oxygen requirement per kilogram in comparison with adults because of a higher metabolic rate.[8,9] As such, infants can require as much as twice the amount of oxygen an adult needs to oxygenate body tissues adequately. Infants and children experiencing respiratory distress can advance to respiratory failure, characterized by hypoxemia, hypercapnia, and ultimately cardiac arrest. Most pediatric cardiac arrest is preceded by respiratory distress and respiratory failure and can generally be avoided by rapid support of the patient in respiratory distress. Signs of hypoxemia include tachypnea, retractions, tachycardia, anxiety, and nasal flaring. Bradycardia and cyanosis are later signs of hypoxemia.

Elective intubation to prevent cardiac arrest in pediatric patients is common. Rapid sequence intubation (RSI) facilitates intubation in pediatric patients; this is because their smaller and more flexible airway makes it more difficult to place an endotracheal tube (ETT) and, in elective intubation, the patient is still somewhat alert and may not cooperate with intubation.[8,10-12] Rapid sequence intubation involves preoxygenation, which can be followed by administration of atropine to prevent bradycardia associated with ETT placement, as well as to decrease secretions; an induction agent for anesthesia (optional); a sedative agent; and a neuromuscular blocker to facilitate ETT placement and mechanical ventilation. Anesthetic agents that have evidence for use in RSI are etomidate and lidocaine.[10,12] Ketamine, thiopental, and midazolam have all been used as sedative agents in RSI as they act quickly and have relatively low rates of serious side effects.[11,12] Fentanyl is also frequently given with a sedative agent to facilitate intubation.[11,12] Choice of neuromuscular blocker is a matter of clinician choice, and agents with a rapid onset of activity that may be used include succinylcholine, pancuronium, vecuronium, or rocuronium.[10–12]

Pediatric Extubation

Because pediatric patients have smaller airways, they are more likely to experience problems related to airway swelling after extubation. Post-extubation larygnospasm, stridor, and reintubation prolong the intensive care stay and, therefore, practitioners should attempt to prevent those sequelae. Neonatal and pediatric patients commonly are given nebulized racemic epinephrine immediately after extubation to decrease airway swelling.[13] Additionally, corticosteroids given prior to extubation help prevent reintubation due to swelling and stridor. A short course of dexamethasone, 0.25 to 0.5 mg/kg every 8 hours for 3 doses, is commonly used for pediatric extubation. The course of dexamethasone is always started prior to extubation and some practitioners prefer to finish all three doses before extubation.

Shock in Infants, Children, and Adolescents

Shock in children can rapidly progress to cardiac arrest, therefore, early recognition and support are essential.[8] Shock results when oxygen delivery to tissues cannot meet the metabolic demands; untreated shock will lead to metabolic acidosis, end organ dysfunction, and death. In compensated shock, the child is able to maintain a normal blood pressure but is not able to meet the metabolic demands of the tissues. These patients will be tachycardic, pale, diaphoretic, have delayed capillary refill, and have weak peripheral pulses. It is important to treat compensated shock to prevent deterioration to hypotensive shock. Hypotensive shock in children is an ominous problem, as hypotension is a late sign of shock in a child and may quickly lead to cardiac arrest. Patients in hypotensive shock typically exhibit mental status changes caused by lack of oxygen reaching the brain.

The first steps in the treatment of shock are the basic ABCs of all critically ill patients: airway, breathing, and circulation. Inadequate oxygen delivery must be avoided in pediatric patients to improve outcomes.[14] As in adults, fluid boluses are important in the treatment of pediatric shock.[8,14] Once IV access is obtained, an isotonic IV fluid, frequently normal saline, is given at a dose of 20 ml/kg over 5 to 20 minutes. Fluids containing dextrose are not used for fluid resuscitation because they will increase serum osmolality and cause osmotic diuresis, which will worsen the patient's condition.

Practitioners may give a half bolus of 10 ml/kg of saline to children with a history of cardiac disease. Multiple boluses may be required in the pediatric patient and frequent assessment is important. Pharmacologic agents that are used in pediatric shock include inotropes such as dobutamine to increase heart rate and contractility, IV phosphodiesterase inhibitors like milrinone to increase contractility and decrease afterload, and vasopressor agents such as epinephrine to increase systemic vascular resistance.

Trauma and Preventable Injury

Trauma and preventable injuries are a significant cause of morbidity and mortality in the pediatric population.[15] Motor vehicle accidents claim more pediatric patients' lives than any other illness or traumatic event. Management of pediatric trauma is similar to adults, but the mechanisms of injury are often different and need to be considered to optimize care. Trauma surgeons often will specialize in pediatric trauma simply because of all the differences in care that have been previously discussed. Efforts to improve injury prevention are important in the care of pediatric patients. While pharmacists may not be able to decrease the rate of car accidents, pharmacists can decrease preventable injury due to poisoning by dispensing medications in child-proof bottles and educating the public regarding the safe use and storage of medications.

INFECTION

Viral infections are common in infants and children and, in some cases, can be life-threatening. Treatment is generally supportive and this section will focus on organisms that can be treated pharmacologically.

Sepsis

Sepsis is a potentially life-threatening disease in infants and children. Children may present with fever, tachycardia or bradycardia, tachypnea, petechiae, hypoxemia, and poor perfusion. Neonates may exhibit temperature instability rather than fever. Volume expansion is an important first step in the treatment of shock in pediatric patients. Septic patients frequently require vasopressor support for blood pressure and perfusion.

Sepsis in the NICU

Sepsis in the NICU can be particularly challenging to diagnose and treat. Premature infant adrenal glands may not respond sufficiently to the stress of serious illness and hydrocortisone may be used for blood pressure support if fluid boluses and vasopressors do not adequately increase blood pressure.[16] Neonates with sepsis are typically divided into early-onset or late-onset, which is differentiated based upon time after delivery. Late-onset sepsis definitions vary from more than 3 days to more than 7 days after delivery. Clinician judgment is important when selecting antibiotics for patients within the 3 to 7 day window to choose the most appropriate empiric regimen. In the NICU population, Group B *Streptococcus* (GBS) can be the cause of both early- and late-onset sepsis. *Escherichia coli, Haemophilus influenzae, Klebsiella,* and *Listeria monocytogenes* are also possible early-onset organisms.[17,18] *Escherichia coli, H. influenzae, L. monocytogenes, Staphylococcus aureus, Staphylococcus epidermidis, Pseudomonas, Enterococcus,* and *Candida sp.* may also be pathogens in late-onset sepsis in the neonatal period.[18,19]

Empiric therapy of early-onset sepsis in the NICU is usually ampicillin plus gentamicin. Empiric therapy of late-onset sepsis usually includes vancomycin to cover drug resistant *S. epidermidis.* Tobramycin or ceftazadime is normally chosen to cover the possibility of nosocomial *Pseudomonas* infection. Neonates with late-onset sepsis who did not receive 7 days of ampicillin should have it added to their regimen to cover for the possibility of *Listeria.* Very premature infants are at increased risk of *Candida* infections in late-onset sepsis and may be treated empirically with amphotericin or fluconazole. Acyclovir is used when there is a maternal history of herpes simplex virus (HSV) and suspected or confirmed lesions at delivery. A full course of antibiotic therapy for bacterial sepsis is generally 7 to 10 days. Treatment length for GBS meningitis is 14 to 21 days, dependent on whether or not the patient exhibited meningitis symptoms. Treatment length for HSV is 14 to 21 days, dependent on whether the disease is systemic sepsis or meningitis.

Pediatric Sepsis Outside the NICU

Neonates outside the NICU are at risk of infection from similar pathogens as their NICU counterparts.[17,18] However, nosocomial infection with *Pseudomonas, S. epidermidis,* and *Candida sp.* are not a significant worry. Empiric antibiotic therapy should consist of vancomycin to cover for drug resistant Gram positive species, ampicillin to cover *Listeria,* and Gram negative coverage, which may be provided by an aminoglycoside or a third generation cephalosporin. If HSV is a possibility, acyclovir should be added. As cultures are reported back, antibiotic coverage should be adjusted as necessary. In infants and children, *Neisseria meningitidis, Streptococcus pneumoniae, S. aureus, E. coli,* and *Klebsiella* are all possible organisms.[20] Group A *Streptococcus* and *S. aureus* especially should be considered if cellulitis is present. If the patient has had a significant amount of diarrhea, *Salmonella* should be considered as a cause. Patients with immunosuppression or chronic illness such as cystic fibrosis are at particular risk of *Pseudomonas* infection. Selection of empiric antibiotic coverage should take into consideration possible organisms and local sensitivity patterns. Commonly, empiric therapy can be started with vancomycin, if resistance patterns require it, plus a third generation cephalosporin.

Respiratory Distress Syndrome in Neonates

Respiratory distress syndrome (RDS) is most common in premature neonates and occurs with higher frequency at lower gestational ages.[21] As compared to acute respiratory distress syndrome (ARDS) in adults, RDS is mainly due to lack of surfactant production in the premature lung, which leads to atelectasis and decreases lung compliance. Surfactant production is normally developed at 34 to 36 weeks gestation. The high ventilatory pressures and high oxygen requirements needed to oxygenate the patient with poor lung compliance can lead to pulmonary damage and chronic lung disease (CLD) or bronchopulmonary dysplasia (BPD). RDS is a significant cause of morbidity and mortality in premature neonates, but symptoms can occur in term infants as well. In term neonates, meconium aspiration syndrome (MAS) and persistent pulmonary hypertension of the newborn (PPHN) are associated with symptoms of RDS. Clinically, RDS can present with grunting, retractions, nasal flaring, tachypnea, hypoxemia, hypercapnia, cyanosis, and acidosis. Breath sounds are described as "velcro-like" and chest X-ray will show a "ground glass appearance" over the lung fields. Patients can develop hypotension and respiratory failure either rapidly or slowly with RDS and frequently require vasopressors and mechanical ventilation. While much of the treatment of RDS is related to mechanical ventilation strategies, there are some pharmacologic measures for both prevention and treatment of RDS.

Lung maturity can be improved by administration of corticosteroids to a woman experiencing preterm labor before 34 weeks gestation and who may deliver within the next 7 days.[22] Corticosteroids appear to stimulate synthesis and secretion of endogenous surfactant in the neonate. The most commonly administered corticosteroid for fetal lung maturity is betamethasone, 12 mg IM every 24 hours for 2 doses. This regimen should be completed 24 hours prior to delivery for optimal results; dexamethasone, 6 mg IM every 12 hours for 4 doses, is an alternate therapy. There is no clear benefit for a neonate whose mother received multiple courses of corticosteroids and there may be adverse long-term sequelae to the infant. Therefore, multiple courses of steroids for lung maturity should be avoided.

After delivery, exogenous surfactant can be administered to the neonate to increase lung compliance and decrease the pressure needed to inflate the alveoli, which results in enhanced gas exchange with less damaging ventilator settings and less oxygen. Multiple exogenous surfactant products are available, but none match human surfactant exactly. Human surfactant is composed of phospholipids, neutral phospholipids, and protein.[23] Most of the phospholipid is dipalmitoylphosphatidylcholine (DPPC), which works to reduce surface tension. However, DPPC does not spread or adsorb well. The surface proteins important in enhancing spreading and adsorption of surfactant are SP-B and SP-C; the role of two other proteins, SP-A and SP-D, are less clear. Surfactant products available in the United States are natural surfactant products. Beractant (Survanta) is a bovine lung and synthetic product, calfactant (Infasurf) is derived from bovine calf lung lavage, and poractant (Curosurf) is derived from porcine lung. These products all contain surfactant phospholipids, SP-B, and SP-C and are administered via the endotracheal tube. It is important that the first dose be administered shortly after birth to minimize lung damage due to surfactant deficiency. Side effects that may be seen with any of the products are oxygen desaturation, apnea, bradycardia, blood pressure alterations, and endotracheal tube obstruction.

Bronchopulmonary Dysplasia

Bronchpulmonary dysplasia, the most common cause of CLD in infants, may develop due to pulmonary damage from ventilator support and supplemental oxygen.[21,23,24] BPD has become a less severe disease with the administration of antenatal corticosteroids, exogenous surfactant, and improvements in mechanical ventilation; however, the problem still exists. The pulmonary changes associated with this injury may persist until 10 years of age. Cardiac abnormalities and heart failure can also occur, but are not as common with less severe BPD. Patients with BPD exhibit hypoxia, hypercapnia, tachypnea, have pulmonary edema and increased mucous production, require supplemental oxygen, and grow poorly. Treatment of BPD includes nutritional support, supplemental oxygen, and fluid restriction. Pharmacotherapy of BPD may include diuretics and bronchodilators if respiratory hyperreactivity develops.

Furosemide is useful in treating pulmonary edema and decreasing pulmonary vascular resistance, leading to improved overall lung function. Side effects are common in infants and laboratory monitoring includes serum sodium, serum potassium, and serum chloride levels. Hypochloremic alkalosis can occur in infants, as can hypercalcuria, osteopenia, ototoxicity, and nephrocalcinosis. Infants receiving a potent loop diuretic frequently require sodium chloride and potassium chloride supplementation to replace electrolytes lost by the immature kidney. Thiazide diuretics have fewer side effects, but will not work as well or as reliably as furosemide. If a thiazide diuretic is used, spironolactone may also be added.

Albuterol is useful in treating bronchospasm in infants with bronchial hyperreactivity and BPD. Tachycardia may be seen with albuterol administration, but the drug is generally well tolerated in this age group.

Corticosteroids are no longer used in all, or even most, patients to prevent BPD. Besides the immediate side effects associated with corticosteroid use, there are significant long-term adverse sequelae. Patients given dexamethasone for BPD may develop cardiomyopathy or experience poor weight gain, poor head growth, and neurodevelopmental delays. As dexamethasone has not been shown to decrease mortality in BPD and is associated with significant side effects, it is no longer routinely used. However, there may be select patients who benefit from corticosteroid administration, such as those with the most severe disease.

Persistent Pulmonary Hypertension of the Newborn

Fetal circulation has high pulmonary vascular resistance, as fetal lungs are not responsible for oxygenation and blood shunts freely across the foramen ovale and ductus arteriosus.[25,26] At birth, the pulmonary vascular resistance should decrease and normal circulation commences. However, some infants have continued increased pulmonary vascular resistance, which results in the continued shunting of blood and fetal circulation; blood bypasses the lungs, which results in a lack of oxygenation. PPHN can result from MAS, RDS, or be a primary problem. It is mostly a disease of term and near term infants, but some premature infants can also be affected. Infants exhibit cyanosis, tachypnea, retractions, grunting, and hypoxemia without also having significant respiratory disease or a cyanotic heart defect.

Treatment of PPHN includes oxygen, continuous positive airway pressure devices, mechanical ventilation for severely hypoxic neonates, vasopressor support to improve cardiac function, inhaled nitric oxide (iNO), phosphodiesterase inhibitors, and extracorporeal membrane oxygenation (ECMO) for the most severely affected patients.[25,27] Inhaled nitric oxide is delivered at a maximum dose of 20 ppm and acts directly to cause vasodilation in the pulmonary vasculature. Patients on mechanical ventilation, continuous positive airway pressure, and oxygen can receive iNO. Monitoring includes frequent blood gases, methemoglobin levels, and oxygenation index (OI). Side effects of iNO are methemoglobinemia, hypotension, and withdrawal syndrome. Withdrawal syndrome, which is a worsening of the patient's condition, can generally be avoided by weaning the iNO to lower doses prior to discontinuing the inhalation. Patients who require longer term therapy or who no longer require respiratory interventions can be given sildenafil, an oral phosphodiesterase inhibitor, to treat PPHN.[28] Sildenafil appears to be well tolerated in this patient group.

ANALGESIA AND SEDATION DIFFERENCES IN PEDIATRICS

Appropriate analgesia and sedation in critically ill pediatric patients is important to improve patient comfort and, in mechanically ventilated patients, oxygenation.[29,30] Unfortunately, no clinical guidelines exist at this time to help guide the practitioner regarding pharmacotherapy for analgesia and sedation in pediatric patients. It is important to note that as pediatric patients tend to have better organ function in comparison to adults, higher doses of medications are frequently required to produce the desired sedative and analgesic effects. Titrating medications to effect and conscientious use of pain and sedation tools for patient assessment are very important in this patient population. Older agents such as midazolam, morphine, and fentanyl are popular medications in the pediatric patients. Newer agents, such as dexmedetomidine and propofol, are used as well. Caution should be exercised with propofol in pediatric patients since they are at increased risk of lactic acidosis and propofol infusion syndrome.[31] Only pediatric practitioners familiar with the use and side effects of propofol, along with having access to continuous monitoring and rapid laboratory results, should use propofol infusions for sedation in pediatrics.

SUMMARY

Pediatric patients are not merely "little adults," especially regarding medication administration, distribution, metabolism, and excretion (ADME). Differences in ADME should be considered when medicating critically ill infants and children. It is also helpful to remember some of the basic differences in disease states and disease progression when caring for this population.

KEY POINTS

- Neonatal and pediatric patients have unique pharmacokinetic profiles that must be considered when designing patient care plans.
- Most pediatric cardiac arrests are precipitated by respiratory compromise.
- Early recognition of shock in pediatric patients is important in prevention of cardiac arrest.
- Infections in infants and children can be rapidly life-threatening and empiric, broad-spectrum antibiotic coverage is important.
- Due to the early stages of development, neonates are at risk for unique disease processes that require special pharmacotherapy interventions.
- While sedation and analgesia are important in critically ill infants and children, no set guidelines for administration exist at this time.

SELECTED SUGGESTED READINGS

- Carcillo JA, Fields AI. Clinical practice parameters for hemodynamic support of pediatric and neonatal patients in septic shock. *Crit Care Med.* 2002;30:1365–1378.
- Wynn JL, Wong HR. Pathophysiology and treatment of septic shock in neonates. *Clin Perinatol.* 2010;37:439–479.

REFERENCES

1. Rodgers GC, Mayuynas NJ. Pharmacologic principles of drug therapy. In: McMillan JA, Feigin RD, DeAngelis C, Jones MD, eds. *Oski's Pediatrics Principles and Practice. 4th ed.* Philadelphia: Lippincott Williams & Wilkins; 2006: 44–49.
2. Nahata MC, Taketomo C. Pediatrics. In: DiPiro JT, Talbert RL, Yee GC, et al, eds. *Pharmacotherapy: A Pathophysiologic Approach. 7th ed.* New York: McGraw-Hill; 2008: 47--56.
3. Kearns GL, Adbel-Rahman SM, Alander SW, et al. Developmental pharmacology—drug disposition, action, and therapy in infants and children. *N Engl J Med.* 2003;349:1157–1167.
4. Bradshaw WT, Turner BS, Pierce JR. Physiologic monitoring. In: Merentein GB, Garnder SL, eds. *Handbook of Neonatal Intensive Care. 6th ed.* St. Louis: Mosby; 2006: 139–156.
5. Ehrenkranz RA. The newborn intensive care unit. In: McMillan JA, Feigin RD, DeAngelis C, Jones MD, eds. *Oski's Pediatrics Principles and Practice. 4th ed.* Philadelphia: Lippincott Williams & Wilkins; 2006: 201–220.
6. Neville KA, Verge CF, Rosenberg AR, et al. Isotonic is better than hypotonic saline for intravenous rehydration of children with gastroenteritis: a prospective randomized study. *Arch Dis Child.* 2006;91:226–232.
7. Taylor D, Durward A. Pouring salt on troubled waters. *Arch Dis Child.* 2004;89:411–414.
8. American Heart Association. *Pediatric Advanced Life Support.* Provider Manual. 2006.
9. Schweich PJ. Selected topics in emergency medicine. In: McMillan JA, Feigin RD, DeAngelis C, Jones MD, eds. *Oski's Pediatrics Principles and Practice. 4th ed.* Philadelphia: Lippincott Williams & Wilkins; 2006: 687–714.
10. McAllister JD, Gnauck KA. Rapid sequence intubation of the pediatric patient, fundamentals of practice. *Pediatr Clin N Am.* 1999;46:1249–1284.
11. Barone MA. Pediatric procedures. In: McMillan JA, Feigin RD, DeAngelis C, Jones MD, eds. *Oski's Pediatrics Principles and Practice. 4th ed.* Philadelphia: Lippincott Williams & Wilkins; 2006: 2671–2687.
12. Gerardi MJ, Sacchetti D, Cantor RM, et al. Rapid-sequence intubation of the pediatric patient. *Ann Emerg Med.* 1996;28:55–74.
13. Stein F, Karam JM. Extubation. In: McMillan JA, Feigin RD, DeAngelis C, Jones MD, eds. *Oski's Pediatrics Principles and Practice. 4th ed.* Philadelphia: Lippincott Williams & Wilkins; 2006: 2573–2574.

14. Carcillo JA, Fields AI. Clinical practice parameters for hemodynamic support of pediatric and neonatal patients in septic shock. *Crit Care Med.* 2002;30: 1365–1378.

15. Wilson MH, Levin-Goodman R. Injury prevention and control. In: McMillan JA, Feigin RD, DeAngelis C, Jones MD, eds. *Oski's Pediatrics Principles and Practice.* 4th ed. Philadelphia: Lippincott Williams & Wilkins; 2006: 134–146.

16. Wynn JL, Wong HR. Pathophysiology and treatment of septic shock in neonates. *Clin Perinatol.* 2010;37:439–479.

17. Koenig JM, Keenan WJ. Group B Streptococcus and early-onset sepsis in the era of maternal prophylaxis. *Pediatr Clin N Am.* 2009;56:689–708.

18. Edwards MS, Baker CJ. Sepsis in the newborn. In: Gershon AA, Hotez PF, Katz SL, eds. *Krugman's Infectious Diseases of Children.* 11th ed. Philadelphia: Mosby; 2004: 545–561.

19. Peterec SM, Warshaw JB. The premature newborn. In: McMillan JA, Feigin RD, DeAngelis C, Jones MD, eds. *Oski's Pediatrics Principles and Practice.* 4th ed. Philadelphia: Lippincott Williams & Wilkins; 2006: 220–235.

20. Thomas NJ, Tamburro RF, Hall MW, et al. Bacterial sepsis and mechanisms of microbial pathogenesis. In: Helfaer MA, Nichols DG, eds. *Rogers' Handbook of Pediatric Intensive Care.* 4th ed. Philadelphia: Lippincott Williams & Wilkins; 2009: 477–488.

21. Dudell GG, Stoll BJ. Respiratory tract disorders. In: Kleigman RM, Behrman RE, Jenson HB, Stanton BF, eds. *Nelson Textbook of Pediatrics.* 18th ed. Philadelphia: Saunders Elsevier; 2007: 728–754.

22. Walbrandt Pigarelli DL, Kraus CK, Potter BE. Pregnancy and lactation: therapeutic considerations. In: DiPiro JT, Talbert RL, Yee GC, et al, eds. *Pharmacotherapy: A Pathophysiologic Approach.* 7th ed. New York: McGraw-Hill; 2008:1297–1311.

23. Ghodrat M. Lung surfactants. *Am J Health-System Pharm.* 2006;63:1504–1521.

24. Amblavanan N, Carlo WA. Bronchopulmonary dysplasia: new insights. *Clin Perinatol.* 2004;31:613–628.

25. Bhandari A, Bhandari V. Pitfalls, problems, and progress in bronchopulmonary dysplasia. *Pediatrics.* 2009;123:1562–1573.

26. Konduri GG, Kim UO. Advances in the diagnosis and management of persistent pulmonary hypertension of the newborn. *Pediatr Clin N Am.* 2009;56:579–600.

27. Krishnan U. Management of pulmonary arterial hypertension in the neonatal unit. *Cardiol Rev.* 2010;18:73–75.

28. Leibovitch L, Matok I, Paret G. Therapeutic applications of sildenafil citrate in the management of paediatric pulmonary hypertension. *Drugs.* 2007;67:57–73.

29. Devlin JW, Roberts RJ. Pharmacology of commonly used analgesics and sedatives in the ICU: benzodiazepines, propofol, and opioids. *Crit Care Clin.* 2009;25:431–449.

30. Hartman ME, McCrory DC, Schulman SR. Efficacy and sedation regimens to facilitate mechanical ventilation in the pediatric intensive care unit: a systematic review. *Pediatr Crit Care Med.* 2009;10:246–266.

31. Zuppa AF, Barrett JS. Pharmacokinetics and pharmacodynamics in the critically ill child. *Pediatr Clin N Am.* 2008;55:735–755.

Abbreviations

Abbreviation	Name	Definition	Chapter
A/C	Assist/Control	Ventilator setting that provides full ventilatory support but allows patient-initiated breaths	4
AAA	Abdominal Aortic Aneurysm	Aneurysm of the descending aorta	9
ABCs	Airway, Breathing, and Circulation		16
ABG	Arterial Blood Gas	Measurement of pH, oxygen levels, and carbon dioxide levels within arterial blood	3
ACLS	Advanced Cardiac Life Support		9
ACS	Abdominal Compartment Syndrome	Blood pressure elevation within the abdominal cavity causing conditions such as acute renal failure	3
ACS	Acute Coronary Syndrome	Include unstable angina and non-ST segment elevation myocardial infarction	9

ACT	Activated Clotting Time		14
ADME	Administration, Distribution, Metabolism, and Excretion		16
ADQI	Acute Dialysis Quality Initiative		11
AEDs	Antiepileptic Drugs		15
AIN	Acute Interstitial Nephritis	Possible cause of acute kidney injury often associated with medications	11
AKI	Acute Kidney Injury		9
AKIN	Acute Kidney Injury Network		11
AMI	Acute Myocardial Infarction		3
APACHE	Acute Physiology and Chronic Health Evaluation	Commonly used scoring system to assess severity of illness in critically-ill patients	2
APRV	Airway Pressure Release Ventilation	Ventilator setting that maintains a relatively high airway pressure for the majority of the ventilatory cycle, with a release of pressure to allow for air exchange	4
APS	Acute Physiology Score	Component of the APACHE score that provides a measure of the acute process	2

ARDS	Acute Respiratory Distress Syndrome	Syndrome of lung dysfunction defined by acute onset, typically bilateral presentation, and significant inflammation	4
ARF	Acute Renal Failure		11
aSAH	Aneurysmal Subarachnoid Hemorrhage		15
ATC	Automatic Tube Compensation	Ventilator setting that provides air pressure to overcome the resistance of the endotracheal tube	4
ATN	Acute Tubular Necrosis	One of the primary causes of acute kidney injury	11
AUC/MIC	Area Under the Drug Concentration-Time Curve to Minimum Inhibitory Concentration Ratio	Marker of probable effectiveness for certain antibiotics, including vancomycin and levofloxacin	13
BD	Base Deficit	Amount of base that needs to be added to bring an acidemic patient to normal pH	6

BE	Base Excess	Amount of base that would need to be removed to bring an alkalemic patient to normal pH	6
BEE	Basal Energy Expenditure	Amount of energy needed by the body for basic needs	12
BiPAP	Bilevel Positive Airway Pressure	Non-invasisve ventilator setting that uses a tight fitting mask to provide two levels of postive pressure support to assist breathing	4
BMI	Body Mass Index		12
BNP	B-Type Naturetic Peptide	Protein produced by the heart, typically during periods of heart failure	9
BPD	Bronchopulmonary Dysplasia		16
BPH	Benign Prostatic Hyperplasia		11
bpm	Breaths Per Minute		4
BSA	Body Surface Area		3
BTF	Brain Trauma Foundation		15
CABG	Coronary Artery Bypass Graft	Surgical bypass of blocked coronary arteries	9

CAM-ICU	Confusion Assessment Method for the Intensive Care Unit	Scale designed for nonverbal, mechanically-ventilated, or restrained patients in ICU settings	5
CA-MRSA	Community-Associated MRSA		13
CAP	Community-Acquired Pneumonia		13
CAVH	Continuous Arteriovenous Hemofiltration		11
CAVHD	Continuous Arteriovenous Hemodialysis		11
CBF	Cerebral Blood Flow		15
CBV	Cerebral Blood Volume		15
CCU	Cardiac Care Unit		1
CDAD	*Clostridium Difficile*-Associated Disease		13
CDO_2	Cerebral Oxygen Delivery		15
CHE	Chronic Health Evaluation	Component of the APACHE score that provides a measure of the chronic conditions present	2
CHF	Congestive Heart Failure		9
CI	Cardiac Index	Cardiac output indexed for patient size	3
CLD	Chronic Lung Disease		16
$CMRO_2$	Cerebral Metabolic Rate for Oxygen Consumption		15

CMV	Controlled Mechanical Ventilation	Ventilator setting that typically does all of the work of breathing for the patient	4
CO	Cardiac Output	Volume of blood pumped by the heart per minute. Represented by HR X SV.	3
CPAP	Continuous Positive Airway Pressure	Ventilator setting that provides a continuous pressure to the airways. May be used in both invasive and non-invasive ventilation.	4
CPK	Creatinine Phosphokinase		13
CPN	Central Parenteral Nutrition		12
CPP	Cerebral Perfusion Pressure	Measure of overall perfusion to the cranial cavity. Calculated as MAP – ICP	3
CSF	Cerebral Spinal Fluid	Fluid that circulates around the brain and spinal cord	3
CTICU	Cardiothoracic Intensive Care Unit		1

CVICU	Cardiovascular Intensive Care Unit		1
CVP	Central Venous Pressure	Pressure within the superior vena cava. Similar to RAP.	3
CVR	Cerebral Vascular Resistance		15
CVVH	Continuous Venovenous Hemofiltration		11
CVVHD	Continuous Venovenous Hemodialysis		11
CVVHDF	Continuous Venovenous Hemodiafiltration		11
DAA	Drotrecogin Alfa (Activated)	Also known as recombinant human activated Protein C	10
DBP	Diastolic Blood Pressure		8
DIC	Disseminated Intravascular Coagulopathy	Condition of systemic clotting ultimately leading to bleeding or high risk of bleeding	9,14
DIND	Delayed Ischemic Neurological Deficits		15
DO_2	Oxygen Delivery	Amount of oxygen delivered by the blood to the tissues	3
DPI	Dry Powdered Inhaler		4
DPPC	Dipalmitoylphosphatidylcholine		16
DSM-IV	*Diagnostic and Statistical Manual of Mental Disorders*, fourth edition		5

ECG	Electrocardiograph (or Electrocardiogram)	Electrical evaluation of the conduction pathways of the heart	3
ECMO	Extracorporeal Membrane Oxygenation	Process for oxygenating blood when patient in severe pulmonary failure	16
ED	Emergency Department		3
EEG	Electroencephalogram		15
EF	Ejection Fraction	Percentage of blood pumped from ventricles with each beat	3
EGDT	Early-Goal Directed Therapy		10
EN	Enteral Nutrition		12
Epi	Epinephrine		8
EPS	Extrapyramidal Symptoms		5
ESBLs	Extended Spectrum Beta-Lactamases		13
ETT	Endotracheal Tube	Tube that passes through the vocal cords and allows for invasive mechanical ventilation	4
FEIBA	Factor Eight Inhibitor Bypass Agent		15

FeNa	Fractional Excretion of Sodium	Diagnostic calculation that helps determine etiology of acute kidney injury	11
FFP	Fresh Frozen Plasma		15
FiO_2	Fraction of Inspired Oxygen	Percentage of oxygen in air breathed in and out	3,4
GABA	Gamma Amino Butyric Acid	Inhibitory neuroreceptor that causes central nervous system depression when stimulated	5
GALT	Gut-Associated Lymphoid Tissue		12
GBS	Group B Streptococcus		16
GCS	Glascow Coma Score (or Scale)	Measure of the alertness of a patient. Score ranges from 3 to 15 and is composed of verbal response, eye opening, and motor response.	2
GFR	Glomerular Filtration Rate	Measured or estimated filtration rate that represents kidney function	2,11

GI	Gastrointestinal	Generic term referring to the gastrointestinal tract and can include structures from the esophagus to the rectum	1
GRV	Gastric Residual Volume	Amount of fluid remaining in the stomach. Typically associated with tube feedings.	4
HAP	Hospital-Acquired Pneumonia		13
HCAP	Healthcare-Associated Pneumonia		13
HELLP	Hemolysis (H), Elevated Liver Enzymes (EL), and Low Platelets (LP).	Syndrome associated with eclampsia/pre-eclampsia	14
HIT	Heparin-Induced Thrombocytopenia		14
HPA	Hypthalamic-Pituitary-Axis		8
HR	Heart Rate	Beats per minute	3
HSV	Herpes Simplex Virus		16
IABP	Intra-Aortic Balloon Pump	Mechanical device that augments blood pressure and circulation in cardiac patients	3
IAH	Intra-Abdominal Hypertension	Elevated pressure within the abdominal compartment	3

IAP	Intra-Abdominal Pressure	Measurement of pressure within abdominal compartment	3
IC	Indirect Calorimetry	Tool for energy expenditure measurement using volume of carbon dioxide exhaled and oxygen used by the patient	4
ICP	Intra-Cranial Pressure	Pressure within the intra-cranial cavity	3
ICU	Intensive Care Unit		1
IHD	Intermittent Hemodialysis		11
IHI	Institute for Healthcare Improvement		10
IL-6	Interleukin-6	Pro-inflammatory mediator	10
IMV	Intermittent Mandatory Ventilation	Ventilator setting that allows for fully supported breaths and patient-initiated breaths	4
iNOS	Inducible Nitric Oxide Synthase		11
IO	Intraosseus		16
ISS	Injury Severity Score	Scoring system used primarily for trauma patients	2
IV	Intravascular or Intravenous		3
IVFE	Intravenous Fat Emulsions		12
LMWH	Low Molecular-Weight Heparin		9

LVAD	Left Ventricular Assist Device	Mechanical pump that is utilized to increase cardiac output and organ perfusion	9
MAAS	Motor Activity Assessment Scale		5
MALT	Mucosal-Associated Lymphoid Tissue		12
MAP	Mean Arterial Pressure	Calculation that represents the average pressure within the arterial system. Calculated as [SBP + 2(DBP)]/3	3
MAS	Meconium Aspiration Syndrome		16
MDI	Metered Dose Inhaler		4
MDR	Multi-Drug Resistant		13
MI	Myocardial Infarction		3
MIC	Minimum Inhibitory Concentration		13
MICU	Medical Intensive Care Unit		1
MODS	Multiple Organ Dysfunction Score	Scoring system for outcomes measurement in critically-ill patients	2
MODS	Multiple Organ Dysfunction Syndromes		11
MRSA	Methicillin-Resistant *Staphylococcus aureus*		13
MSSA	Methicillin-Susceptible *Staphyloccus aureus*		13

MTM	Medication Therapy Management	Medication review and management for patients with multiple medications	1
MV	Minute Ventilation	Amount of air breathed in and out during one minute. Equal to respiratory rate x Vt.	4
NE	Norepinephrine		8
NICU	Neonatal Intensive Care Unit		1
NIF	Negative Inspiratory Force	Amount of force able to be generated by the patient on inspiration	4
NMB	Neuromuscular Blockers	Medications used to chemically induce paralysis	4
NNH	Number Needed to Harm	Statistical representation that describes adverse events in terms of how many patients will be treated for one patient to experience an adverse event	15

NNT	Number Needed to Treat	Statistical representation that describes positive events in terms of how many patients will be treated for one patient to experience that positive outcome	15
NPPV	Noninvasive Positive Pressure Ventilation	Ventilation support that does not require an endotracheal tube	4
NRS	Numeric Rating Scale	Pain scale	5
NSTEMI	Non ST Segment Elevation Myocardial Infarction		9
NTG	Nitroglycerin		8
O_2ER	Oxygen Extraction Ratio	Amount of oxygen pulled from hemoglobin to be used by the tissues	3
PA	Pulmonary Artery	Typically used in reference to an intravascular device	3
PAI-1	Plasminogen-Activator Inhibitor 1		10
PAOP	Pulmonary Artery Occlusion Pressure	Another name for PCWP or PAWP. Pressure measurement that represents left ventricular end diastolic pressure.	3

PAWP	Pulmonary Artery Wedge Pressure	Another name for PCWP or PAOP. Pressure measurement that represents left ventricular end diastolic pressure.	3
PBP	Penicillin Binding Protein		13
PCC	Prothrombin Complex Concentrate		14
PCI	Percutaneous Coronary Intervention	Intervention where a cardiologist uses a catheter to open blocked arteries	9
PCR	Polymerase Chain Reaction		13
PCWP	Pulmonary Capillary Wedge Pressure	Another name for PAWP or PAOP. Pressure measurement that represents left ventricular end diastolic pressure.	3
PD	Pharmacodynamic		13
PDE	Phosphodiesterase-3 Inhibitors		9
PEEP	Positive End Expiratory Pressure	Ventilator setting that provides pressure to the airways at the end of expiration	4

PEG	Percutaneous Endoscopic Gastrostomy	Tube inserted through the abdominal wall into the stomach	12
PEJ	Percutaneous Endoscopic Jejunostomy	Tube inserted through the abdominal wall that terminates in the jejunum	12
PGY1	Post Graduate Year 1	Designation given to the first year of residency training with broad educational goals and objectives	1
PGY2	Post Graduate Year 2	Designation given to the second year of residency training that is typically specialty-focused residency	1
PICU	Pediatric Intensive Care Unit		1
PIP	Peak Inspiratory Pressure	Maximal airway pressure during the respiratory cycle	4
PK	Pharmacokinetic		13
PN	Parenteral Nutrition		12
PNA FISH	Peptide Nucleic Acid Fluorescent In Situ Hybridization		13

Ppeak	Peak Inspiratory Pressure	Maximal airway pressure during the respiratory cycle	4
PPHN	Persistent Pulmonary Hypertension of the Newborn		16
Pplat	Plateau Pressure	Measure of airway pressures at end inspiration, reflecting pressure in the alveoli	4
PPN	Peripheral Parenteral Nutrition		12
pRBCs	Packed Red Blood Cells		7
PS	Pressure Support	Ventilator setting that provides pressure at the beginning of a breath	4
PSVT	Paroxysmal Supraventricular Tachycardia	Ventricular arrhythmia initiated in the atria	9
PVC	Premature Ventricular Contraction	Arrhythmia where a premature beat occurs that is generated from the ventricles	3
PVR	Pulmonary Vascular Resistance	Afterload for the right side of the heart. The amount of resistance in the pulmonary circulation.	3

RAAS	Renin-Angiotensin-Aldosterone System		11
RAP	Right Atrial Pressure	Pressure within the right atrium of the heart. Similar to CVP.	3
RASS	Richmond Agitation Sedation Scale		5
RDS	Respiratory Distress Syndrome		16
REE	Resting Energy Expenditure	Amount of energy needed by the body for basic needs	4
rFVIIa	Recombinant Factor VII Activated	Factor VII made from a recombinant process	6
RIFLE	Risk, Injury, Failure, Loss, End-Stage Renal Disease	Scoring and classification system for acute kidney injury	2
RN	Registered Nurse		3
RRT	Renal Replacement Therapy		11
RSBI	Rapid Shallow Breathing Index	Resipiratory rate divided by tidal volume (in liters)	4
RSI	Rapid Sequence Intubation	A process to rapidly sedate, often paralyze, and intubate a patient	16
rt-PA	Recombinant Tissue Plasminogen Activator		15
SaO_2	Arterial Oxygen Saturation	The oxygen saturation of arterial hemoglobin	3

SAPS	Simplified Acute Physiology Score	Relatively simple scoring system to allow comparison of two groups of critically ill patients	2
SAS	Sedation–Agitation Scale	Also known as the Riker scale	5
SBP	Systolic Blood Pressure		8
SBT	Spontaneous Breathing Trial	Allowing the patient to breath spontaneously to assess ability to wean from ventilator	4
SCI	Spinal Cord Injury		15
SCUF	Slow Continuous Ultrafiltration		11
ScVO$_2$	Central Venous Oxygen Saturation	Central venous oxygen saturation of hemoglobin, typically measured in the superior vena cava and primarily represents the venous return from the head and upper body	3
SE	Status Epilepticus		15
SIADH	Syndrome of Inappropriate Antidiuretic Hormone	Condition often leading to hyponatremia	7
SICU	Surgical Intensive Care Unit		1

SIMV	Synchronized Intermittent Mandatory Ventilation	Ventilator setting that allows for fully supported breaths and patient-initiated breaths	4
SIRS	Systemic Inflammatory Response Syndrome	Syndrome defined by alteration in heart rate, respiratory rate, temperature, and white blood cell count	5
SjO_2	Jugular Oxygen Saturation	Oxygenation of jugular venous blood	3
SLED	Sustained Low Efficiency Dialysis		11
SOFA	Sequential Organ Failure Assessment	Scoring system most useful for tracking progression of patient condition	2
SSG	Surviving Sepsis Guidelines		10
SSTIs	Skin and Soft Tissue Infections		13
STEMI	ST-Elevation Myocardial Infarction		9
SV	Stroke Volume	Amount of blood pumped by the ventricles with a single beat	3
SVO_2	Venous Oxygen Saturation	Venous oxygen saturation of hemoglobin from all sources of venous return. Typically measured in right atrium.	3

SVR	Systemic Vascular Resistance	Often synonymous with afterload. The amount of resistance in the systemic circulation.	3
SVV	Stroke Volume Variation	The amount of variation in volume pumped by the heart per heartbeat	3
SWI	Stroke Work Index		3
TBI	Traumatic Brain Injury		15
TISS	Therapeutic Intervention Scoring System	Scoring system used primarily to measure acuity level based on nursing interventions	2
TLR-4	Toll-Like Receptor 4		10
TNA	Total Nutrient Admixture		12
TNF-α	Tumor Necrosis Factor-Alpha	Pro-inflammatory mediator	10
TPN	Total Parenteral Nutrition		12
UAC	Umbilical Arterial Catheter		16
UFH	Unfractionated Heparin		9
UVC	Umbilical Venous Catheter		16
V/Q	Ventilation/Perfusion	Representation of ventilation (air) compared to perfusion (blood) within the lungs	4

VAP	Ventilator-Associated Pneumonia	Pneumonia that occurs after a patient has been mechanically ventilated	4,13
VAS	Visual Analog Scale	Pain scale	5
Vd	Volumes of Distribution		11
V_{DS}	Physiologic Dead Space	The sum of anatomic (trachea, bronchus) and alveolar components that do not participate in CO_2 elimination	4
VEGF	Vascular Endothelial Growth Factor	A very potent vascular permeability factor	15
VF	Ventricular Fibrillation	Heart rhythm considered a medical emergency, as it is a non-perfusing rhythm	3
VICS	Vancouver Interaction and Calmness Scale		5
VO_2	Oxygen Demand	Amount of oxygen needed by the tissues	3
VRS	Verbal Rating Scale	Pain scale	5
Vt	Tidal Volume	Amount of air breathed in and out during a ventilatory cycle	4

| VTE | Venous Thromboembolism | Term that broadly includes events such as deep vein thrombosis and pulmonary embolism | 1,14 |
| WOC | Wound Ostomy Continence | Specific nursing practice focused on wound and ostomy care | 3 |

Index

Tables and figures are indicated by an italic *t* and italic *f* respectively.

A

abciximab, 174–175, 175*t*
abdominal aortic aneurysm, 181
acetaminophen, 86, 341
acetazolamide therapy, 120
acid-base management
  acetazolamide, 120
  acid therapy, 120
  bicarbonate therapy, 119–120
  medications in, 121
acid-base physiology, 112–113
acid-base status assessment
  acid, 113–114
  acidosis or alkalosis, 116
  alternate techniques, 116–117, 117*f*
  base, 115
  base deficit/excess, 115
  diuresis/dialysis, 121
  pH, 113
acidemia/acidosis, 112–113, 116
acid-fast stains, 276
acid therapy, 120
Acinetobacter species, 274, 290
acquired resistance, 289
activated clotting time (ACT), 315–316
activated factor VII (rFVIIa), 313, 324, 325, 327
activated partial thromboplastin time (aPTT), 315–316, 322
acute arrhythmia, 185–187
acute bacterial endocarditis, 298–299
acute cholecystitis, 275
acute coronary syndrome (ACS), 172–178
acute decompensated heart failure, 181–184
Acute Dialysis Quality Initiative (ADQI), 217
acute glomerulonephritis, 220
acute hemorrhagic events
  and anticoagulant therapy, 311
  blood products for, 309*t*

causes and treatments, 308
  HIT, 321–323
  reversal of, 310*t*
acute illness scoring systems
  APACHE, 15–17, 16*f*
  ISS, 18
  MODS, 18
  RIFLE, 18–19
  SAPS, 17
  SOFA, 17–18
  TISS, 18
  usefulness of, 13–15
acute interstitial nephritis (AIN), 220
acute intrinsic kidney injury, 219–221
acute kidney injury (AKI)
  classification of, 217
  etiologies, 217–221, 218*t*
  morbidity and treatments, 221–222
Acute Kidney Injury Network (AKIN), 217
acute leukemia, 328–330
acute myocardial infarction, 178–179
Acute Physiology Score (APS), 15
acute renal failure (ARF). *See* acute kidney injury (AKI)
acute tubular necrosis (ATN), 219–220
acyclovir, in obstructive AKI, 221
ADDRESS trial, 206
ADME (absorption, distribution, metabolism, elimination), in pediatric patients, 368–370, 378
ADQI (Acute Dialysis Quality Initiative), 217
advanced cardiac life support, 188–190, 189*t*
adverse consequences
  of amphotericin B, 292
  of anticoagulation therapy, 320
  of antimicrobial therapy, 275, 299–300
  of daptomycin, 287
  of linezolid, 286